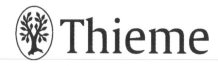

Invasive Skull Base Mucormycosis

New Perspectives

Editors-in Chief

Narayanan Janakiram, MS, DLO
Managing Director
Royal Pearl Group of Hospitals
Tiruchirappalli, Tamil Nadu and Hyderabad, Telangana, India

Sampath Chandra Prasad Rao, MS, DNB, FACS, FEB-ORLHNS, FEAONO
Consultant Skull Base, Hearing Implantology
Otolaryngology-Head and Neck Oncosurgeon
Manipal Hospital;
Managing Director
Bangalore Head and Neck Sciences and Bangalore Skull Base Institute
Bangalore, Karnataka, India

Associate Editors:

Shilpee Bhatia Sharma, MS (ENT)
Senior Consultant
Department of Otorhinolaryngology
Royal Pearl Hospital
Tiruchirappalli, Tamil Nadu, India

Lekshmy R. Kurup, MS, DNB (ENT)
Junior Consultant
Department of Otorhinolaryngology
Royal Pearl Hospital
Tiruchirappalli, Tamil Nadu, India

Sathyanarayanan Janakiram, MS (ENT)
Junior Consultant
Department of Otorhinolaryngology
Royal Pearl Hospital
Tiruchirappalli, Tamil Nadu, India

Harshita Singh, DNB (ENT)
Junior Consultant
Department of Otorhinolaryngology
Royal Pearl Hospital
Tiruchirappalli, Tamil Nadu, India

Thieme
Delhi • Stuttgart • New York • Rio de Janeiro

Publishing Director: Ritu Sharma
Senior Development Editor: Dr. Gurvinder Kaur
Director-Editorial Services: Rachna Sinha
Project Manager: Shipra Sehgal
Managing Director & CEO: Ajit Kohli

Thieme Medical and Scientific Publishers Private Limited.
A - 12, Second Floor, Sector - 2, Noida - 201 301,
Uttar Pradesh, India, +911204556600
Email: customerservice@thieme.in
www.thieme.in

Cover design: Thieme Publishing Group
Page make-up by RECTO Graphics, India

Printed in India by Nutech Print Services

5 4 3 2 1

ISBN: 978-93-95390-31-6
Also available as an e-book:
eISBN (PDF): 978-93-95390-34-7
eISBN (epub): 978-93-95390-35-4

I dedicate this book to my family. My father Mr. Narayanan, my mother Mrs. N. S. Kalyani, my son Dr. Sathyanarayanan, and my daughter Shreyani Ram, who wholeheartedly supported me during my tough COVID-19 times.

I also want to thank a special person, Late Mrs. Savitha, who was instrumental in helping me during the time when I was admitted with advanced COVID-19 disease.

I also dedicate this book to all my residents, who played a crucial role in getting this book in shape.

Narayanan Janakiram, MS, DLO

Contents

Video Contents

Foreword

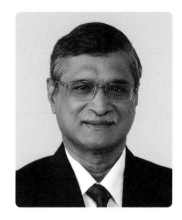

India has faced several waves of COVID-19 pandemic, which have had devastating effects on the population. To make matters worse, there was an outbreak of mucormycosis among the infected patients, with extensive involvement of the nose and paranasal sinuses and often involving the orbit, the soft tissues of the face, and invading the skull base. The problem was further compounded by lack of availability of appropriate antifungal drugs in the initial period. Treatment of these patients with mucormycosis involves extensive surgical debridement, antifungal agents, and correction of metabolic problems. Many ear, nose, and throat (ENT) and maxillofacial surgeons operated on these difficult cases during the pandemic, unmindful of the dangers they were exposing themselves to.

Dr. Narayanan Janakiram and his team, whose expertise in the field of endoscopic sinus surgery and skull base surgery is well known, did yeoman service during the pandemic, operating on several patients with extensive mucormycosis and saving their lives. This experience has been now translated into a book, which offers insight into the problems of diagnosis and medical and surgical management of this dreaded disease and its complications.

Dr. Janakiram has teamed up with Dr. Sampath Chandra Prasad Rao, a renowned skull base surgeon, and the duo has put together their experience in this book, which is amply illustrated with over 200 scans, 370 clinical images, and 20 videos which can be accessed using a QR code.

This book serves as an efficient guide to those clinicians who may face the challenge of treating patients with this dreaded invasive disease of mucormycosis.

M.V. Kirtane, MS, DORL, FNAMS, DSc
Professor Emeritus
Seth G S Medical College and KEM Hospital
Mumbai, Maharashtra, India

From Author's Desk

Invasive skull base mucormycosis (ISBM) has rampaged this subcontinent and caused extensive mutilation in patients who suffered from this disease, both cosmetically and functionally. It was particularly seen in large numbers in India, and hence gave every skull base surgeon an opportunity to study this disease in detail.

This book is a culmination of the unvarying routine faced by each resident and consultant who have worked day and night to treat this disease in our tertiary care center—Royal Pearl Hospital, India. As we saw varying stages of the disease, manifested by post-COVID-19 patients, we could study and classify mucormycosis into various stages which led us to propose an updated classification for ISBM. The earlier classifications were based on limited number of patients and hence were ambiguous. Our attempt was to study the patient population in a systematic and methodic manner wherein the spread, progress, and other clinical manifestations of the disease were analyzed in a comprehensive manner, which enabled us to arrive at a classification that could be used to prognosticate and form protocols in planning treatment strategies.

For the past two decades, skull base surgery has remained our area of focus. Our experience and expertise with all the essential instruments like the advanced IMAGE1 S Rubina camera by Karl Storz, endoscopic Doppler system, and the latest imaging studies to diagnose and treat patients enabled us to tackle this pandemic in an efficient and effective manner. Our experience is a testament to our view that mucormycosis is necessarily a disease that needs to be handled by a skull base surgeon.

ISBM has always been there in the past, but not so rampant as we saw in the post-COVID-19 era. In the past, the surgeries described for this disease were confined to only limited debridement. But we espied that it was clearly not enough to give complete surgical clearance. We also operated on a large number of revision cases, which made us comprehend the nuances involved in the treatment of ISBM. We used endoscopic approaches in majority of cases and did not hesitate to do open approaches whenever it was deemed necessary.

In this book, we have included several case scenarios, videos, and new signs like the "holy cross sign" as seen postoperatively in several cases. Hence, I am sure this attempt will help the readers to understand the disease, the treatment protocols, and the postoperative care in detail.

I want to thank all my residents, especially Dr. Shilpee Bhatia Sharma, who was involved in the "four-handed technique" in most of my cases. I would also like to thank Dr. Lekshmy R. Kurup, Dr. Harshita Singh, Dr. Sathyanarayanan, Dr. Manoj Gunde, Dr. Deepak Phulwani, Dr. Avinash Nalluri, and Dr. Chinta Sangeetha for their unstinted work which paved the way to summarizing our experience, leading to the culmination of this wonderful textbook.

I hope this book will open new vistas in the management of ISBM and will be a valuable guide to every doctor treating patients with this intriguing pathology.

Narayanan Janakiram, MS, DLO

About the Author

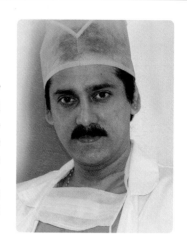

Narayanan Janakiram, MS, DLO, is the Managing Director of "Royal Pearl Group of Hospitals," Tiruchirappalli, Tamil Nadu and Hyderabad, Telangana, India. He is internationally acclaimed for his work in skull base surgery. He is also a pioneer in endoscopic management of juvenile nasopharyngeal angiofibroma. Dr. Janakiram has authored several books in skull base surgery: *The Atlas of Sellar, Suprasellar, and Parasellar Lesions; Step-By-Step Approach to Endoscopic Cadaveric Dissection; and Juvenile Nasopharyngeal Angiofibroma* to name a few. He has also written multiple chapters and articles pertaining to skull base surgery and is known for his passion for teaching. He was conferred with "The Heinz Stammberger Award for Excellence in Teaching" in the year 2022.

Contributors

Akshay Gopinathan Nair, DNB (Opthamology), FACS
Consultant
Ophthalmic Plastic Surgery and Ocular Oncology Services
Advanced Eye Hospital and Institute
Navi Mumbai, Maharashtra, India

Ananth Chintapalli, MS
Associate Consultant
Department of ENT-Skull Base Surgery
Bangalore Head and Neck Sciences and Bangalore Skull Base
    Institute
Bangalore, Karnataka, India

Ashritha M.C.V., MDS
Junior Consultant
Department of Conservative Dentistry and Endodontics
Royal Pearl Hospital
Tiruchirappalli, Tamil Nadu, India

Balamurugan Chinnasamy, DA
Senior Consultant
Department of Anaesthesia
Royal Pearl Hospital
Tiruchirappalli, Tamil Nadu, India

Chinta Sangeetha Mahalakshmi, MS (ENT)
Junior Consultant
Department of Otorhinolaryngology
Royal Pearl Hospital
Tiruchirappalli, Tamil Nadu, India

Ganga Kamath Kudva, MS (ENT), DNB (ENT)
Fellow in Training in Skull Base Surgery
Bangalore Head and Neck Sciences
Bangalore Skull Base Institute
Bangalore, Karnataka, India

Harshita Singh, DNB (ENT)
Junior Consultant
Department of Otorhinolaryngology
Royal Pearl Hospital
Tiruchirappalli, Tamil Nadu, India

Lekshmy R. Kurup, MS, DNB (ENT)
Junior Consultant
Department of Otorhinolaryngology
Royal Pearl Hospital
Tiruchirappalli, Tamil Nadu, India

Muralidhar Thondebhavi, MD, FRCA, FFPMRCA, MBA
Senior Consultant
Anesthesiology and Pain Management
Apollo Hospitals
Bangalore, Karnataka, India

Narayanan Janakiram, MS, DLO
Managing Director
Royal Pearl Group of Hospitals,
Tiruchirappalli, Tamil Nadu and Hyderabad, Telangana, India

**Neha Mishra, MD (Medicine), Post Doctoral Fellowship
    (Infectious Diseases)**
Consultant
Infectious Diseases and Control
Manipal Hospital
Bengaluru, Karnataka, India

P. Subramanian, MDS
Senior Consultant
Department of Oral and Maxillofacial Surgery
Royal Pearl Hospital
Tiruchirappalli, Tamil Nadu, India

**Pallavi Rao, DNB (Radiodiagnosis), European Diploma in
    Radiology**
Consultant Radiologist and Senior Scientific Officer
Image Core Lab;
Director
Aadhya Healthcare Private Ltd.
Bengaluru, Karnataka, India

**Raghuraj Hegde, MS (Opthamology), FAICO (Oculoplastic
    Surgery)**
Consultant
Orbit, Ophthalmic Plastic Surgery Service and Ophthalmic
    Oncology Service
Department of Ophthalmology
Manipal Hospitals
Bangalore, Karnataka, India

Rath P.K., MD
Professor
Department of Pathology
Dhanalakshmi Srinivasan Medical College
Perambalur, Tiruchirappalli, Tamil Nadu, India

Renuka Bradoo, MS (ENT)
Consultant ENT and Skull Base Surgeon
Fortis Hospital, Mulund;
Professor and Head
Department of ENT
L.T.M Medical College and General Hospital
Mumbai, Maharashtra, India

S.K. Priyadarshini, MDS
Assistant Professor
Department of Oral Medicine and Radiology
Dhanalakshmi Srinivasan Dental College
Perambalur, Tiruchirappalli, Tamil Nadu, India

Sampath Chandra Prasad Rao, MS, DNB, FACS, FEB-ORLHNS, FEAONO
Consultant Skull Base, Hearing Implantology
Otolaryngology-Head and Neck Oncosurgeon
Manipal Hospital;
Managing Director
Bangalore Head and Neck Sciences and Bangalore Skull Base Institute
Bangalore, Karnataka, India

Sathyanarayanan Janakiram, MS (ENT)
Junior Consultant
Department of Otorhinolaryngology
Royal Pearl Hospital
Tiruchirappalli, Tamil Nadu, India

Shilpee Bhatia Sharma, MS (ENT)
Senior Consultant
Department of Otorhinolaryngology
Royal Pearl Hospital
Tiruchirappalli, Tamil Nadu, India

Sunena Saju, MS
Associate Consultant
Department of ENT
Bangalore ENT Institute and Research Center
Bangalore, Karnataka India

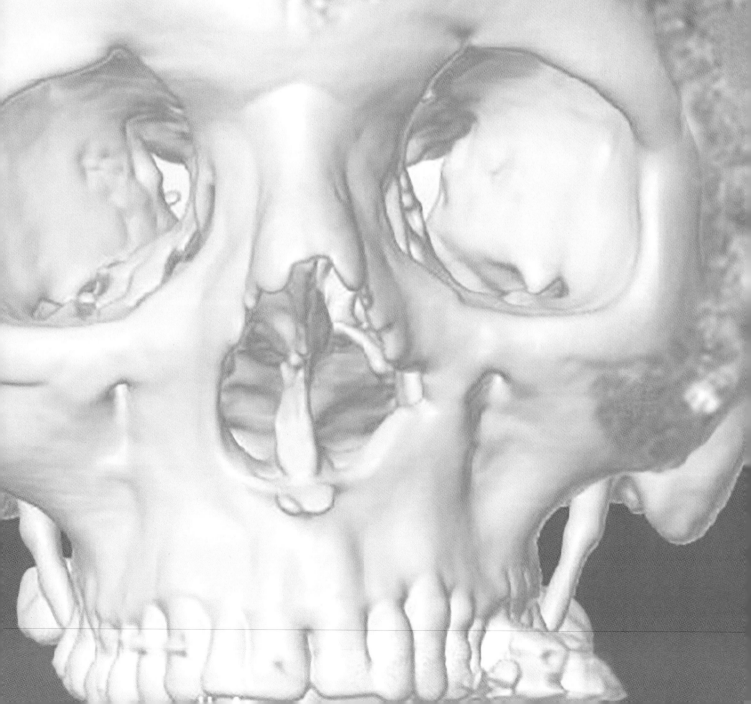

1

Mucormycosis in Pre-COVID-19 Era

Mucormycosis in Pre-COVID-19 Era

Sampath Chandra Prasad Rao, Ananth Chintapalli, and Sunena Saju

Introduction

Zygomycetes class of fungi comprises of the order Mucorales and Entomophthorales. The Entomophthorales are rare cause of subcutaneous and new cutaneous infection known as entomophthoramycosis. The order Mucorales comprise of 55 genera with 261 species.

Not all 261 species cause human infection. Just a subset of this order, about 38 species, have been proved to cause infection in human being (**Table 1.1**).

Table 1.1 Current nomenclature of medically important mucoralean species according to updated taxonomy[1]

Current species names	Previous names/synonyms
Lichtheimia corymbifera	*Absidia corymbifera, Mycocladus corymbifer*
Lichtheimia ornata	*Absidia ornata*
Lichtheimia ramosa	*Absidia ramosa, Mycocladus ramosus*
Mucor ardhlaengiktus	*Mucor ellipsoideus, Mucor circinelloides* f. *circinelloides*
Mucor circinelloides	*Rhizomucor regularior, Rhizomucor variabilis* var. *regularior*
Mucor griseocyanus	*Mucor circinelloides* f. *griseocyanus*
Mucor irregularis	*Rhizomucor variabilis*
Mucor janssenii	*Mucor circinelloides* f. *janssenii*
Mucor lusitanicus	*Mucor circinelloides* f. *lusitanicus*
Rhizopus arrhizus (incl. var. *delemar*)	*Rhizopus oryzae*
Rhizopus microsporus	*Rhizopus microsporus* var. *azygosporus*, var. *chinensis*, var. *oligosporus*, var. *rhizopodiformis*, var. *tuberosus*

In 1876, Furbinger from Germany described fungal hyphae and few sporangia within hemorrhagic infarct in the lungs of a patient who died of cancer.[2] This is considered the first ever documented case of mucormycosis. Arnold Paltauf in 1885 published the first case of disseminated mucormycosis coma which he named mycosis mucorina.[3] In 1943, a case series of three fatal cases of advanced rhinocerebral mucormycosis in patients with diabetic ketoacidosis (DKA) were reported where typical findings like proptosis and ophthalmoplegia were described.[4] It was only in 1955, after the development of amphotericin, the first cured case of mucormycosis was reported.[5]

Incidence of the disease went up from zero over the years and now is considered the third most common opportunistic fungal infection after candidiasis and aspergillosis.[6] Increase in incidence of mucormycosis was documented well in literature but determination of exact incidence was a dilemma because population-based studies would vary in time period, population definition, and diagnostic parameters. Rising trend of mucormycosis in India is well documented in literature by various studies like by Chakrabarti et al. In their study, data from three consecutive studies from a single center reflected an incidence of 12.9 cases per year in the first decade, 35.6 cases per year over a period of 5 years, and 50 cases per year for 18 months.[7–9] Similar rising trend was shown in a population-based study by Bitar et al in France between 1997 and 2006 and by Saegeman et al from Belgium in 2010.[10,11] An alarming shift in mucormycosis cases from community acquired to nosocomial infection in susceptible host is also noted.[12] Various studies like those by Mitchell et al and Verweij et al discuss the incidence of mucormycosis due to the use of contaminated wooden tongue depressor in preterm neonates and contaminated wooden applicator used to mix drugs in immunocompromised patients, respectively.[13,14] A clear understanding of pathogenesis is important and inevitable in preventing and treating mucormycosis.

Pathogenesis

Pathogenesis of mucormycosis begins with inhalation or ingestion of sporangiospores, or inoculation of conidia via puncture wounds or trauma.[15,16] The pathogenesis can be discussed under the following subheadings:
- Host defense mechanisms.
- Role of iron in pathogenesis.
- Fungal endothelial interactions.

Host Defense Mechanisms

Mucorales need to evade host defense mechanism, invade vascular system, and scavenge host immune system for growth and to cause disease.

In a normal healthy individual (host), primary defense mechanism against Mucorales includes:

- Specialized iron binding protein sequestering serum iron from organism.
- Endothelial cells which regulate vascular tone and permeability.
- Circulating mononuclear and polymorphonuclear (PMN) phagocytes which generate oxidative metabolites and cationic peptides (defensins).
- Neutrophils which on exposure to Mucorales upregulate expression of toll-like receptor 2 and rapidly induce NF-kB pathway related genes.[17]

Any condition resulting in imbalance of the above defense system can make an individual prone to mucormycosis like malignant hematological disease with or without stem cell transplantation, neutropenia, diabetes mellitus (DM) poorly controlled with or without DKA, iron overload, and major trauma.

Role of Iron in Pathogenesis

Iron plays a crucial role in the pathogenesis of mucormycosis. Mucorales have multiple pathways to acquire iron from the host. In the first mechanism, in patients with DKA or any state of systemic acidosis the available iron level in serum is high predisposing the individual to mucormycosis. This is because acidosis per se disrupts the capacity of transferrin to bind iron.

Second, an increased incidence of invasive mycosis is noted in patients with iron overload and patients on treatment with iron chelator deferoxamine. Fungi can obtain iron from the host with high affinity and permit low molecular weight iron chelator.[18,19]

Rhizopus species utilizes deferoxamine as a siderophore for acquiring iron from the host. A few species of *Rhizopus* can accumulate greater amounts of iron supplied by deferoxamine than *Aspergillus fumigatus* and *Candida albicans*.

There is a linear correlation between iron uptake by *Rhizopus* and its growth in serum.[20] The latest iron chelators like deferiprone and deferasirox do not have siderophore activity. Fungi has high affinity iron permease which contain redundant surface reductases that reduce ferric into the soluble ferrous form. The protein complex comprising of a multicopper oxidase and ferrous permease captures the reduced ferrous iron.[19]

Rhizopus is also known to secrete rhizoferrin, a siderophore which supplies iron through an energy-dependent receptor-mediated process.[21] Rhizoferrin lacks ability to take iron from serum, and the organism adapts to use of xenosiderophore like desferoxamine to obtain iron more efficiently. The third mechanism adopted by fungi to obtain iron is through the use of heme. The *Rhizopus oryzae* homologues of heme oxygenase enable it to obtain iron from lost hemoglobin which explains the angioinvasive nature of *R. oryzae*. High affinity iron permease gene (FTR1) in *R. oryzae* facilitates intracellular heme uptake by acting as cytoplasmic membrane permease, followed by heme oxygenase which degrade heme and release ferric iron. Sre A, a transcriptional regulator gene, and genes encoding for two ferritin orthologues for storage of iron, are other genes likely involved in the iron uptake mechanism of *R. oryzae*.[22]

Fungal Endothelial Interactions

R. oryzae strains adhere to type IV collagens and extracellular matrix laminin. Recently, GRP78 glucose regulated protein was identified to act as a receptor that mediates penetration through and damage of endothelial cells by Mucorales. GRP78 is also known as BiP/HSPAS member of HSP70 family in endoplasmic reticulum. It functions as a cellular chaperone protein, and recent studies report translocation of a fraction of GRP78 to cell surface.[23]

It is also interesting to find that along with elevated levels of glucose and iron, there is also enhanced expression of GRP78 surface protein which result in penetration through and damage of endothelial cells by Mucorales.

Other putative virulence factors are:

- Circulatory mononuclear and PMN lymphocytes are a major line of host defense which in presence of hyperglycemia and low pH is found to be dysfunctional.[24] They have impaired chemotaxis and defective intracellular killing by both oxidative and nonoxidative[24] mechanisms.
- In a study by Waldorf et al, they describe how critical it is for inhaled sporangiospores to germinate for establishing infection.[25] In immunocompetent mice, although the alveolar macrophages harvested revealed limited capacity to kill the organism, they did show inhibition to germination of spores. While in immunosuppressed mice, pulmonary alveolar macrophages are unable even to prevent germination of sporangiospores.[25]

Risk Factors

Major risk factors for development of mucormycosis are as listed in **Box 1.1**.

Box 1.1   Risk factors for mucormycosis[27]

- Diabetes mellitus (poorly controlled, ketoacidosis).
- Hematologic malignancy with neutropenia or graft versus host disease; organ transplantation (hematopoietic stem cell transplantation more common than solid organ transplantation).
- Autoimmune disorders.
- Immunosuppressive therapy.
- Human immunodeficiency virus.
- Iron overload.
- Burns.
- Trauma including surgery.
- Peritoneal dialysis.
- Malnutrition.
- Prior treatment with voriconazole.

A recent meta-analysis between 2000 and 2017 comparing 851 cases across 600 publications worldwide identifies the following risk factors for development of mucormycosis[26]: Diabetes mellitus (40%), trauma (33%), heme M (32%), diabetic ketoacidosis (20%), neutropenia (20%), no underlying disease (18%), solid organ transplant recipients (SOTR) (14%), burns (11%), and natural disasters (5%). In Asia, diabetes mellitus is the most common risk factor whereas organ transplant and heme M are more common in Europe and North America.[26]

Details of the clinical features, diagnostic, and treatment methods are discussed in the subsequent chapters of this book.

References

1. Walther G, Wagner L, Kurzai O. Updates on the taxonomy of Mucorales with an emphasis on clinically important taxa. J Fungi (Basel) 2019;5(4):106

2. Fürbringer P. Beobachtungen über Lungenmycose beim Menschen. Virchows Arch 1876;66:330–365

3. Paltauf A. Mycosis mucorina: Ein Beitrag zur Kenntnis der menschilchen Fadenpiltzer-krankungen. Virchows Arch Pathol Anat 1885;102:543–564

4. Gregory JE, Golden A, Haymaker W. Mucormycosis of the central nervous system: a report of three cases. Bull Johns Hopkins Hosp 1943;73:405–419

5. Harris JS. Mucormycosis; report of a case. Pediatrics 1955; 16(6):857–867

6. Slavin M, van Hal S, Sorrell TC, et al; Australia and New Zealand Mycoses Interest Group. Invasive infections due to filamentous fungi other than Aspergillus: epidemiology and determinants of mortality. Clin Microbiol Infect 2015;21(5):490.e1–490.e10

7. Chakrabarti A, Das A, Sharma A, et al. Ten years' experience in zygomycosis at a tertiary care centre in India. J Infect 2001;42(4):261–266

8. Chakrabarti A, Das A, Mandal J, et al. The rising trend of invasive zygomycosis in patients with uncontrolled diabetes mellitus. Med Mycol 2006;44(4):335–342

9. Chakrabarti A, Chatterjee SS, Das A, et al. Invasive zygomycosis in India: experience in a tertiary care hospital. Postgrad Med J 2009;85(1009):573–581

10. Bitar D, Van Cauteren D, Lanternier F, et al. Increasing incidence of zygomycosis (mucormycosis), France, 1997–2006. Emerg Infect Dis 2009;15(9):1395–1401

11. Saegeman V, Maertens J, Meersseman W, Spriet I, Verbeken E, Lagrou K. Increasing incidence of mucormycosis in University Hospital, Belgium. Emerg Infect Dis 2010;16(9):1456–1458

12. Ibrahim AS, Spellberg B, Walsh TJ, Kontoyiannis DP. Pathogenesis of mucormycosis. Clin Infect Dis 2012; 54(Suppl 1):S16–S22

13. Mitchell SJ, Gray J, Morgan ME, Hocking MD, Durbin GM. Nosocomial infection with Rhizopus microsporus in preterm infants: association with wooden tongue depressors. Lancet 1996;348(9025):441-443

14. Verweij PE, Voss A, Donnelly JP, de Pauw BE, Meis JF. Wooden sticks as the source of a pseudoepidemic of infection with Rhizopus microsporus var. rhizopodiformis among immunocompromised patients. J Clin Microbiol 1997;35:2422-2423

15. Petrikkos G, Skiada A, Lortholary O, Roilides E, Walsh TJ, Kontoyiannis DP. Epidemiology and clinical manifestations of mucormycosis. Clin Infect Dis 2012;54(Suppl 1):S23–S34

16. Lelievre L, Garcia-Hermoso D, Abdoul H, et al; and the French Mycosis Study Group. Posttraumatic mucormycosis: a nationwide study in France and review of the literature. Medicine (Baltimore) 2014;93(24):395–404

17. Chamilos G, Lewis RE, Lamaris G, Walsh TJ, Kontoyiannis DP. Zygomycetes hyphae trigger an early, robust proinflammatory response in human polymorphonuclear neutrophils through toll-like receptor 2 induction but display relative resistance to oxidative damage. Antimicrob Agents Chemother 2008; 52(2):722–724

18. Howard DH. Acquisition, transport, and storage of iron by pathogenic fungi. Clin Microbiol Rev 1999;12(3):394–404

19. Stearman R, Yuan DS, Yamaguchi-Iwai Y, Klausner RD, Dancis A. A permease-oxidase complex involved in high-affinity iron uptake in yeast. Science 1996;271(5255): 1552–1557

20. Boelaert JR, de Locht M, Van Cutsem J, et al. Mucormycosis during deferoxamine therapy is a siderophore-mediated infection. In vitro and in vivo animal studies. J Clin Invest 1993;91(5):1979–1986

21. Thieken A, Winkelmann G. Rhizoferrin: a complexone type siderophore of the Mucorales and entomophthorales (Zygomycetes). FEMS Microbiol Lett 1992;73(1-2):37–41

22. Schrettl M, Kim HS, Eisendle M, et al. SreA-mediated iron regulation in Aspergillus fumigatus. Mol Microbiol 2008;70(1):27–43

23. Wang M, Wey S, Zhang Y, Ye R, Lee AS. Role of the unfolded protein response regulator GRP78/BiP in development, cancer, and neurological disorders. Antioxid Redox Signal 2009;11(9):2307–2316

24. Chinn RY, Diamond RD. Generation of chemotactic factors by Rhizopus oryzae in the presence and absence of serum: relationship to hyphal damage mediated by human neutrophils and effects of hyperglycemia and ketoacidosis. Infect Immun 1982;38(3):1123–1129

25. Waldorf AR, Ruderman N, Diamond RD. Specific susceptibility to mucormycosis in murine diabetes and bronchoalveolar macrophage defense against Rhizopus. J Clin Invest 1984;74(1):150–160

26. Jeong W, Keighley C, Wolfe R, et al. The epidemiology and clinical manifestations of mucormycosis: a systematic review and meta-analysis of case reports. Clin Microbiol Infect 2019;25(1):26–34

27. Reid G, Lynch JP III, Fishbein MC, Clark NM. Mucormycosis. Semin Respir Crit Care Med 2020;41(1):99–114

2

COVID-19 and Its Aftermath— Mucormycosis

Chapter 2

COVID-19 and Its Aftermath—Mucormycosis

Sampath Chandra Prasad Rao and Ananth Chintapalli

Introduction

Sinonasal mucormycosis as an acute invasive infection is a rare, opportunistic, saprophytic, potentially fatal condition of the severely immunocompromised individuals. Poorly controlled diabetes mellitus is the forerunner of the etiological conditions rendering the individuals susceptible to the uncommon yet dreadful disease, solid organ transplant, bone marrow suppression, etc., being the other clinical conditions.

The prevalence of mucormycosis is reported to be 0.14 per 1,000 in India, 80 times higher when pitched against its prevalence in developed countries globally, which is 0.005 to 1.7 per million population.

Rhino-orbito-cerebral mucormycosis (ROCM) caused by the group of filamentous molds belonging to the order Mucorales accounts for 70% of all cases of mucormycosis and represents the complete spectrum ranging from sinonasal tissue invasion to rhino-orbital disease and rhino-orbito-cerebral disease. Despite aggressive surgical therapies which include extensive debridement and advanced antifungal therapy like liposomal amphotericin-B (LAMB), the management of mucormycosis remains challenging with fatality rates being as much as 50 to 80% of the cases, and an accompanying COVID-19 infection further increases the odds. This chapter is about the fundamental pathophysiology along with clinical aspects of the ROCM from SARS-CoV-2 outlook.

Pathophysiology of SARS-CoV-2 (COVID-19) and Associated Rhino-Orbito-Cerebral Mucormycosis

The atypical respiratory viral pandemic "COVID-19" is caused by the novel coronavirus that belongs to the family Coronaviridae and is named as severe acute respiratory syndrome coronavirus-2 (SARS-CoV-2). This section describes the pathophysiology of the infection from otolaryngology and upper airway perspective.

The virus transmitting via aerosols and respiratory microdroplets from one person to the other enters the host cells through endocytosis or membrane fusion after binding to the host cell receptor, mainly the angiotensin converting enzyme 2 (ACE-2) which is seen highly expressed in adult nasal epithelium. The corona viruses structurally have four proteins, namely, the spike (S), membrane (M), envelope (E), and a nucleocapsid (N) proteins, of which the S protein, protruding from the viral surface, is the most crucial for the virus attachment and penetration into the host. The S protein further comprises two subunits (S1 and S2), of which the S1 subunit helps the virus bind to the host cell receptor and S2 plays a role in the fusion of the viral and host cell membranes. The host immune response to the COVID-19 infection, as understood, is complex with several studies showing lymphopenia, particularly reduced T cells in the peripheral blood circulation. The plasma concentrations of proinflammatory cytokines (IL-6, IL-10, granulocyte colony stimulating factor, macrophage inflammatory protein 1alpha, and tumor necrosis factor alpha) increase the inflammation of the endothelium of the blood vessels and their subsequent damage, as occurs in severe COVID-19 infection, along with lymphopenia, and decrease in CD4+ and CD8+ T cell counts predisposes the individual to secondary opportunistic fungal infection.

These host changes bring about thrombosis and pulmonary embolism in severe diseases as observed in elevated D-dimer and fibrinogen levels. The elevated serum ferritin levels with increased availability of free iron, metabolic acidosis, hypoxemia, and hypercoagulability in addition to high doses of systemic steroid therapy used as a part of treatment to address the crisis renders the individual highly susceptible to contracting opportunistic bacterial and fungal infections. While long-term corticosteroid therapy is implicated in opportunistic fungal infections in poorly controlled diabetics is well documented, reports have suggested that even short-term usage of steroid therapy can as well be associated with developing mucormycosis in such individuals. The world in general, and India in particular, has seen a sharp rise in mucormycosis cases during the second wave of the pandemic.

Etiopathogenesis of Mucormycosis

The pathogenesis of the mucormycosis based on the anatomic localization is in six forms—ROCM, pulmonary, gastrointestinal, cutaneous, disseminated, and mucormycosis of uncommon sites. Of these, ROCM, which is particularly invasive and the most common, is the focus of this chapter.

The order Mucorales comprise numerous genera (*Rhizopus, Mucor, Lichtheimia, Rhizomucor, Cunninghamella, Apophysomyces, Saksenae,* and others). The most involved genus in mucormycosis is *Rhizopus,* followed by *Mucor* and *Lichtheimia.* The order Entomophthorales are significantly different from Mucorales and are involved in chronic subcutaneous infections in immunocompetent individuals, usually in the tropical and subtropical climate zones.

Exposure to contaminated bandages, medical equipment, and ventilation systems has of late been a major cause for nosocomial outbreaks. Individuals infected with COVID-19 disease, and specifically those with already pre-existing conditions such as uncontrolled diabetes mellitus and immune suppressed state, are more susceptible. The impaired metabolism, hypercoagulability, hypoxia, elevated free iron in the body, hyperglycemia (as seen in patients with pre-existing diabetes mellitus or secondary to high dose systemic steroid therapy in management of COVID-19 infection) coupled with oxygen inhalation with unhygienic humidifiers, and usage of antibiotics make the individual prone to opportunistic infections.

Host Defense and Mucormycosis

The clinical data reveals substantial evidence that individuals with incompetent immune system, who lack phagocytes or have impaired phagocytic function, are at a higher risk of mucormycosis as in the case of severely neutropenic patients. In diabetes mellitus, which is an independent risk factor for both COVID-19 and mucormycosis, hyperglycemia and low pH, coexisting as in diabetic ketoacidosis (DKA), render the phagocytes impaired by deranging their chemotaxis, making oxidative and nonoxidative mechanisms ineffective to neutralize the fungi. Hyperglycemia, regardless of whether due to pre-existing diabetes or de novo or DKA, is the single most important risk factor observed in majority of the cases of mucormycosis in patients affected with COVID-19 infection.

Role of Iron Uptake in Mucormycosis Pathogenesis

Iron being an essential element for the vital metabolic processes of cell growth and development, the fungi possess the ability to acquire iron from the host and thereby succeed as a pathogen. The levels of available, unbound iron in the serum play a crucial role in putting patients with DKA at a higher risk of mucormycosis. Hence, iron in mammals is bound to

carrier proteins such as transferrin, ferritin, and lactoferrin as a sequestration, thus avoiding its toxic effects on the host body, and not making it available for pathogens is indeed a major universal host defense mechanism. Acidic conditions decrease the iron-binding capacity of the carrier proteins, probably by proton-mediated displacement of the ferric iron. Fungi obtain iron from the host by either using high-affinity iron permeases as a part of oxidative reductive system that reduce ferric iron into more soluble ferrous form, or by using low molecular weight iron chelators (siderophores) such as rhizopherrin, a siderphore of polycarboxylate family secreted by *Rhizopus*. The other mechanism by which the fungi obtain iron from the host is through heme, which explains the angioinvasive nature resulting in vessel thrombosis and subsequent tissue necrosis, thereby impeding the reach of the lymphocytes to these areas. The angioinvasion likely contributes to the dissemination of the pathogen throughout the host body. Elevation of proinflammatory cytokines especially interleukin-6, and concomitant acidosis, increases free iron by increasing the ferritin levels due to enhanced synthesis and decreased iron transport. Acidosis also reduces the ability of transferrin to chelate iron thus making iron more available.

Mucormycosis Infection in COVID-19 Pandemic

Taking into consideration the various patient factors such as hyperglycemia and metabolic acidosis, neutropenia, raised serum ferritin levels, corticosteroid-induced immune suppression, misuse of antibiotics, and mutant strain of the COVID-19 virus reasons for rise in the mucormycosis cases, there are several other environmental factors that need to be taken into account when considering mucormycosis in COVID-19 infection.

Home Care Isolation

With many people developing COVID-19 infections not requiring hospitalization but only home isolation, individuals with uncontrolled diabetes mellitus or several other immune compromised state may get exposed to unhygienic indoor conditions such as indoor dampness, mold odor, and visible mold exposure especially in warm subtropical climate zone. Since the pathogenesis of ROCM is thought to be inhalation of the fungal spores by a susceptible host, the indoor sites particularly associated with fungi, where humid organic material is exposed to heat, such as soils of potted indoor plants, can become a potential source of fungal infection.

Steam Inhalation

Airborne fungal spores are almost ubiquitous and can be found on all human surfaces in contact with air, especially on the upper and lower airway mucosa. Despite inhaling these sporangiospores being a daily occurrence, the members of the family are seldom found to be affected on checking the nasal mucus, suggesting that spores in the mucus of airway mucosa are cleared by mucociliary transport as a competent first line of defense. However, unwarranted use of steam inhalation can cause scalding of the nasal mucosa and provide a point of entry for fungi.

Nosocomial Sources

Mucormycosis, a formerly community-acquired condition and often seen in the setting of DKA, is rapidly becoming a nosocomial infection in patients with malignancy or undergoing organ or hematopoietic cell transplantation. Possibility of cross contamination of infection is also high in hospitals. Investigations about increased airborne fungal load should be conducted especially during hospital renovation and construction activities in the vicinity of the care units. In emerging countries, some operating theaters are equipped with air conditioners but inefficient air filters, which may lead to a significantly increased fungal risk. Hospital water is also a potential reservoir for fungi.

Humidifiers

Respiratory care equipment such as oxygen humidifiers and nebulizers has been identified as a potential vehicle causing major nosocomial infections if colonized by fungi or bacteria. In a study, 75.71% samples from the humidifiers showed fungal growth, out of which 69.70% were from the intensive care unit (ICU), 80% were from the wards, and 85.71% were from the outpatient departments. Bacteria grew on 76.66% of swabs from the central line humidifiers, 78.26% swabs from the O_2 cylinder humidifiers, and 47.5% swabs from the nebulizers. Fungi grew on 86.79% of swabs from O_2 humidifiers and 41.17% swabs from Hudson's chambers.

A potential advantage of early detection and prompt initiation of treatment is reduction of the disease course with better outcomes. Mucorales responsible for the disease are not only known to produce false-negative results in microbiological analysis, but also enigmatic clinical presentation, delayed diagnosis, and increased mortality.

The prognosis and outcome of the mucormycosis significantly depend on the comorbidities of the patient. Considering the fact that host factors such as hyperglycemia and acidosis, neutropenia, raised serum ferritin levels,

corticosteroid-based immunosuppression, injudicious usage of antibiotics, and mutant strain of the COVID-19 did play a major role in the sharp rise of mucormycosis cases, the observation that there has not been any significant rise of more common fungi like candida and aspergillus is something which needs to be evaluated more fundamentally. It is apparent that despite similar management protocols being followed for the management of COVID-19 infection during the first wave, there has not been any surge in the mucormycosis cases during that period in contrast to what, India particularly, was witnessed during the second wave of COVID-19, forcing to be declared an epidemic. As in every epidemic where the host and source factors have their roles to play, the source factors in this scenario of mucormycosis epidemic in the COVID-19 pandemic need to be thoroughly evaluated and be considered along with the host factors. While giving importance to the host factors, the environmental factors need to be researched as mucormycosis is very rare and essentially a nosocomial infection in the West. India has a 70% higher baseline incidence of mucormycosis compared to the rest of the world suggesting there are significant source-related factors that need to be investigated.

References

1. Song G, Liang G, Liu W. Fungal co-infections associated with global COVID-19 pandemic: a clinical and diagnostic perspective from China. Mycopathologia 2020;185(4): 599–606

2. Baker RD. Mucormycosis; a new disease? J Am Med Assoc 1957;163(10):805–808

3. Sugar AM. Agents of mucormycosis and related species. In: Mandell GL, Bennett JE, Dolin R, eds. Mandell, Douglas, and Bennett's Principles and Practice of Infectious Diseases. 5th ed. New York, USA: Churchill Livingstone; 2000:2685–2695

4. Chander J, Kaur M, Singla N, et al. Mucormycosis: battle with the deadly enemy over a five-year period in India. J Fungi (Basel) 2018;4(2):46

5. Prakash H, Chakrabarti A. Global epidemiology of mucormycosis. J Fungi (Basel) 2019;5(1):26

6. Skiada A, Pagano L, Groll A, et al; European Confederation of Medical Mycology Working Group on Zygomycosis. Zygomycosis in Europe: analysis of 230 cases accrued by the registry of the European Confederation of Medical Mycology (ECMM) Working Group on Zygomycosis between 2005 and 2007. Clin Microbiol Infect 2011;17(12):1859–1867

7. Deutsch PG, Whittaker J, Prasad S. Invasive and non-invasive fungal rhinosinusitis—a review and update of the evidence. Medicina (Kaunas) 2019;55(7):319

8. Garg D, Muthu V, Sehgal IS, et al. Coronavirus disease (Covid-19) associated mucormycosis (CAM): case report and systematic review of literature. Mycopathologia 2021;186(2):289–298

9. Saldanha M, Reddy R, Vincent MJ. Title of the article: paranasal mucormycosis in COVID-19 patient. Indian J Otolaryngol Head Neck Surg 2021;1–4. doi: 10.1007/s12070-021-02574-0. Online ahead of print

10. Sen M, Lahane S, Lahane TP, Parekh R, Honavar SG. Mucor in a viral land: a tale of two pathogens. Indian J Ophthalmol 2021;69(2):244–252

11. Satish D, Joy D, Ross A, Balasubramanya. Mucormycosis coinfection associated with global COVID-19: a case series from India. Int J Otorhinolaryngol Head Neck Surg 2021;7(5):815–820

12. Moorthy A, Gaikwad R, Krishna S, et al. SARS-CoV-2, uncontrolled diabetes and corticosteroids—an unholy trinity in invasive fungal infections of the maxillofacial region? A retrospective, multi-centric analysis. J Maxillofac Oral Surg 2021;20(3):418–425

13. Hanley B, Naresh KN, Roufosse C, et al. Histopathological findings and viral tropism in UK patients with severe fatal COVID-19: a post-mortem study. Lancet Microbe 2020;1(6):e245–e253

14. Dallalzadeh LO, Ozzello DJ, Liu CY, Kikkawa DO, Korn BS. Secondary infection with rhino-orbital cerebral mucormycosis associated with COVID-19. Orbit 2022;41(5):616–619

15. Placik DA, Taylor WL, Wnuk NM. Bronchopleural fistula development in the setting of novel therapies for acute respiratory distress syndrome in SARS-CoV-2 pneumonia. Radiol Case Rep 2020;15(11):2378–2381

16. Johnson AK, Ghazarian Z, Cendrowski KD, Persichino JG. Pulmonary aspergillosis and mucormycosis in a patient with COVID-19. Med Mycol Case Rep 2021;32:64–67

3A

Imaging Spectrum of COVID-19-Associated Rhino-Orbito-Cerebral Mucormycosis

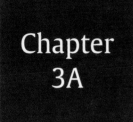

Chapter 3A

Imaging Spectrum of COVID-19-Associated Rhino-Orbito-Cerebral Mucormycosis

Pallavi Rao, Sampath Chandra Prasad Rao, and Ganga Kamath Kudva

Introduction

Rhino-orbito-cerebral mucormycosis (ROCM) is known to be the most common form of mucormycosis in patients with diabetes mellitus and immunocompromised status.[1] Recently, higher incidence is being reported in patients who have recovered from COVID-19 infection. The nonspecific clinical manifestations and elusive presentation of ROCM often lead to delay in diagnosis, with resultant poor prognostic outcome. In patients with limited involvement of paranasal sinus and early diagnosis, survival rate of 50 to 80% has been reported; however, in patients with intracranial extension, mortality rate increases to more than 80% despite aggressive treatment.[2] Hence, a high index of suspicion based on appropriate risk stratification and improved laboratory diagnosis is important for the timely diagnosis of ROCM. A definitive diagnosis is based on the histopathological demonstration of nonseptate and right-angled branching fungal hyphae typical for Mucormycetes in biopsies of affected tissues. Hence, radiological imaging plays a vital role in early diagnosis, assessment of extent of involvement, and in planning treatment outcomes.[3]

Clinico-Radiological Correlation

Radiological imaging aids in the early diagnosis and surgical management of ROCM by understanding the extent and pathway of spread. The hallmark of invasive ROCM is tissue necrosis resulting from angioinvasion and subsequent thrombosis. Radiological features of COVID-19-related ROCM have shown common initial infection in nasal cavity and paranasal sinuses spreading inferiorly to the palate, posteriorly to the sphenoid sinus, laterally into orbits and cavernous sinus, and intracranially to extra-axial spaces and brain parenchyma.[4] The route of spread to cranium is either through the orbital apex or cribriform plate of the ethmoid bone. Occasionally, cerebral vascular invasion can lead to hematogenous dissemination of the infection with or without development of mycotic aneurysms.[4] Clinical signs and symptoms that suggest ROCM in susceptible individuals include epistaxis, nasal discharge/obstruction, palatal perforation, multiple cranial nerve palsies, unilateral periorbital facial pain, orbital inflammation, eyelid edema, proptosis, ophthalmoplegia, headache, and acute vision loss.[3] A black necrotic eschar, which is typically even seen in radiological imaging, is the hallmark of mucormycosis. However, the absence of this finding should not exclude the possibility of mucormycosis.[5]

Radiological Features

Computed tomography (CT) and magnetic resonance imaging (MRI) help in assessing the extent of disease and are indispensable for surgical planning. Imaging spectrum also helps in identification of complications like internal carotid artery (ICA) thrombosis, and orbital and intracranial extensions.[6] CT is better to assess bony erosions; MRI is superior in evaluating soft tissue involvement, and perineural, intracranial, and intraorbital extension of the disease. Imaging techniques including MRI show only nonspecific features during the early stage of the disease like mucosal thickening which may delay diagnosis (**Fig. 3A.1**).

There is a higher incidence of bony erosions in COVID-19-associated ROCM than in the pre-COVID-19 era. Intraorbital spread can occur through intact orbital walls through angioinvasion and intracranial extension via erosion of cribriform plate. Sphenoid sinus involvement is most often associated with intracranial and intraorbital involvement[7] (**Fig. 3A.2**).

Computed Tomography

CT scan is the preferred modality for evaluating bone destruction and signs of invasion, although soft tissue necrosis precedes bone involvement. Findings include bone rarefaction, septal perforations, erosions, and permeative destruction involving sinus walls and contiguous bony structures (**Figs. 3A.3** and **3A.4**).

Noncontrast CT demonstrates hypoattenuating mucosal thickening or an area of soft tissue attenuation of the involved paranasal sinus and nasal cavity. Preoperative contrast-enhanced CT is useful in defining the extent of ROCM.[8]

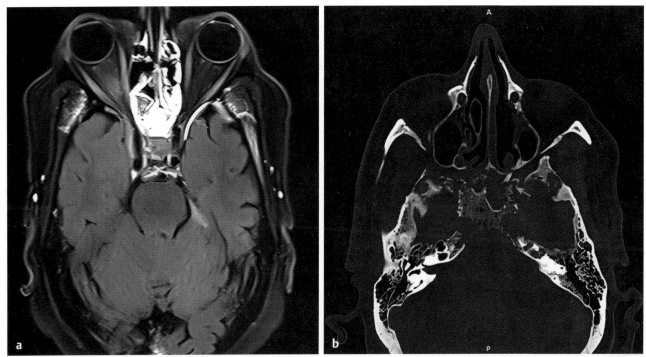

Fig. 3A.1 A 50-year-old male, post COVID-19, presented with severe headache. **(a)** T2 fluid-attenuated inversion recovery (FLAIR) magnetic resonance imaging (MRI) demonstrating mucosal thickening in bilateral ethmoid and sphenoid sinuses with dural thickening in the anterior left temporal region (*arrow*). The patient was medically managed for acute sinusitis. **(b)** High-resolution computed tomography (HRCT) of the same patient 1 month later showed extensive erosions of the floor and lateral walls of the sphenoid sinus (*arrow*), greater wing of sphenoid, and pterygoid plates.

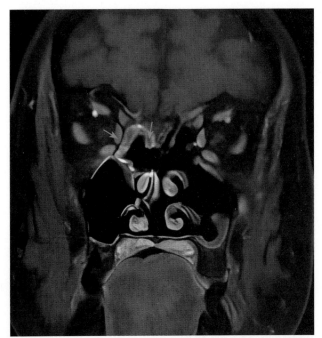

Fig. 3A.2 A 50-year-old male with diabetes presented with headache and blurring of vision in the right eye. Contrast enhanced T1-weighted (T1W) magnetic resonance imaging (MRI) demonstrating enhancement of medial wall of right orbit (*arrow, on the left*) and dura along the cribriform plate (*arrow, on the right*).

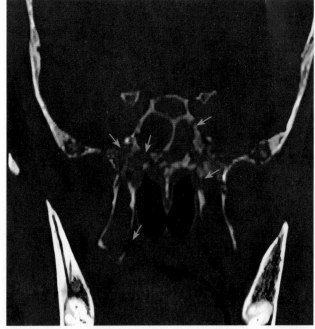

Fig. 3A.3 A 44-year-old male with diabetes presented with severe headache and postnasal drip. Noncontrast, coronal computed tomography of paranasal sinus (CTPNS) demonstrating extensive erosions of the floor and lateral walls of the sphenoid sinus, greater wing of sphenoid, and pterygoid plates (*arrows*).

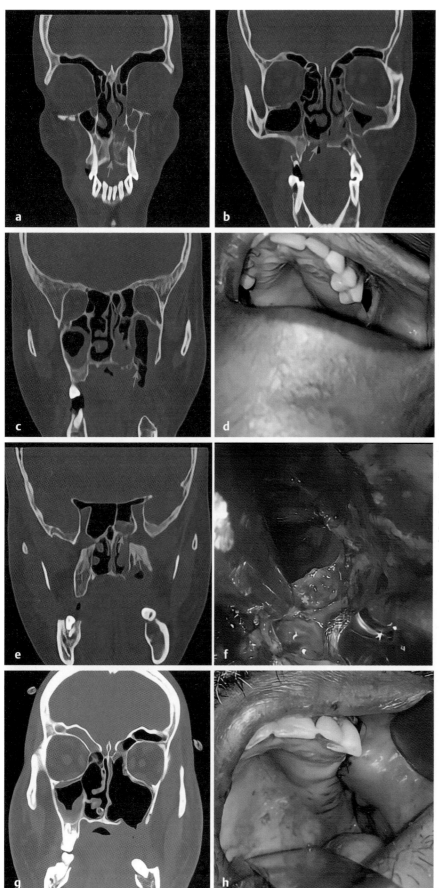

Fig. 3A.4 A post-COVID-19, 35-year-old male presented with left side cheek swelling and palatal defect post teeth extraction. Bone window, coronal, reformat computed tomography (CT) image, sequentially anterior to posterior, demonstrating **(a)** bony defect in the hard palate (*arrow*) with erosion of the floor and lateral wall of the left nasal cavity, **(b)** mucosal thickening in the left maxillary sinus with erosions of the walls of the sinus and floor of the left orbit, inferior turbinate (*arrow, above*), hard palate (*arrow, below*), and maxillary alveolus on the left, and **(c)** oroantral fistula (*arrow*) with erosions of the maxillary alveolus, hard palate, and lateral wall of the left nasal cavity. **(d)** Corresponding clinical examination image showing the oroantral fistula. **(e)** Erosions of the floor of the sphenoid sinus (*arrow, above*); lateral wall of left nasal cavity with sclerotic changes (*arrow, below*) in the left maxilla. **(f)** Intraoperative picture showing erosions of floor of sphenoid with unhealthy mucosa and necrotic tissue (*). **(g)** Corresponding postsurgical coronal CT image demonstrating disease clearance in the left maxillary sinus with the sinus merging with the nasal cavity; surgical reconstruction and repair of the oroantral fistula. **(h)** Postsurgical primary closure of the oroantral fistula preserving the hard palate mucosa.

The "seven variable" CT based model proposed by Middlebrooks et al was found to be effective as a screening tool to triage patients at risk for acute invasive fungal sinusitis.[7]

The presence of any one of the seven variables (extension of disease into the periantral fat, orbital invasion, pterygopalatine fossa involvement, septal perforation, involvement of nasolacrimal duct, lacrimal sac, and bone dehiscence) had a 95% sensitivity and 86% specificity for fungal etiology.

The presence of any two variables gave 88% sensitivity, 100% specificity, and 100% positive predictive value for the diagnosis of invasive fungal sinusitis.[9]

Due to the angioinvasive nature of the disease, disease progression results in skull base osteomyelitis and extensive bone involvement indicating advanced disease.[2] The involved bones show erosions, expansion, sclerosis, and irregular lytic destruction (**Fig. 3A.5**).

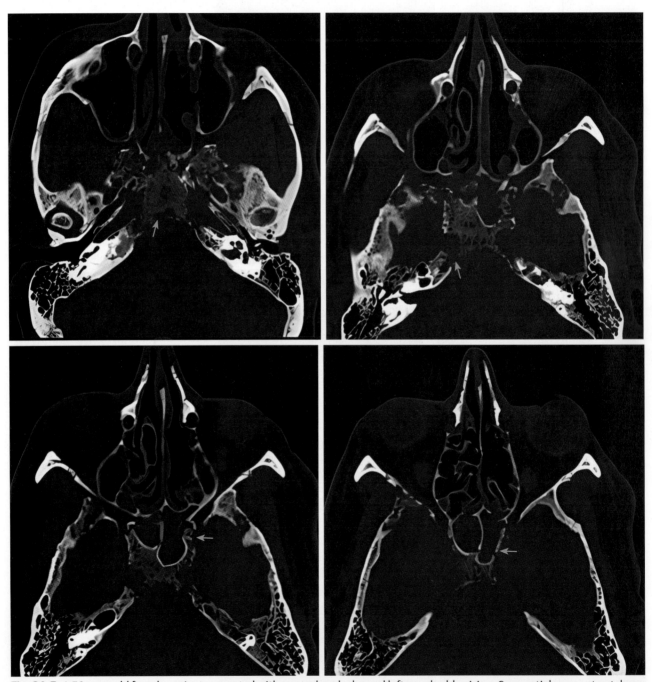

Fig. 3A.5 A 50-year-old female patient presented with severe headache and left eye double vision. Sequential noncontrast, bone window, axial computed tomography of paranasal sinus (CTPNS) demonstrating erosion of walls of the sphenoid sinus, clivus, and left inferior turbinate with opacification of the sphenoid sinuses (*arrows*).

Magnetic Resonance Imaging

MRI is useful in identifying the soft tissue extent of disease, orbital involvement, cavernous sinus thrombosis, ICA occlusion, and intradural and intracranial extent of ROCM. Multiplanar MRI is also a better choice than CT when there is potential nephrotoxicity that may result from the iodinated contrast use in CT because of the coincident therapy with nephrotoxic drugs.[10] Typical MRI findings described in progressive ROCM include a hyperintense sinus, T2 hyperintense lesion extending from paranasal sinuses along the orbital apex into intracranial compartment, and narrowing or slow flow in the ipsilateral ICA[11] (**Figs. 3A.6** and **3A.7**). MRI demonstrates variable T1 and T2 intensities with focal lack

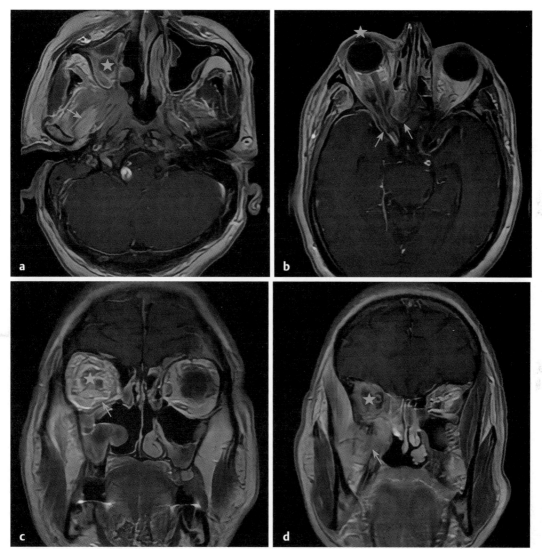

Fig. 3A.6 A 58-year-old male presented with complaints of headache, nasal discharge, numbness of right side of face, proptosis, and sudden onset of loss of vision suggestive of orbital apex syndrome. **(a)** Postcontrast, T1-weighted (T1W), axial magnetic resonance imaging (MRI) demonstrating peripherally enhancing mucosal thickening within the right maxillary sinus with nonenhancing central debris (*), enhancing soft tissue thickening in the infratemporal fossa involving the pterygoid muscles (*arrow*), and enhancing areas within the ramus of the mandible on the right side. **(b)** Postcontrast, axial, T1W MRI demonstrating right-sided proptosis (*), enhancing soft tissue cellulitis in the retroorbital fat (*arrows*), perineural enhancement surrounding the optic nerves, and peripherally enhancing abscess surrounding the optic nerve extending to the orbital apex. **(c)** Coronal, postcontrast, T1W MRI demonstrating extensive soft tissue enhancement involving the right retroorbital fat with enlargement (*), ill-defined margins and enhancement involving the extraocular muscles (*arrow*), and thickening and enhancement of the posterior scleral margins. Perineural enhancement around the optic nerve. **(d)** Postcontrast, coronal, T1W MRI demonstrating retrobulbar soft tissue enhancement with a peripherally enhancing abscess (*); extensive osseous hyperintensities involving the roof, floor, and medial and lateral walls of the right orbit; soft tissue involvement with enhancement in the region of the infratemporal fossa (*arrow*); and enhancing mucosal thickening involving the bilateral sphenoid sinuses.

of enhancement in areas of devitalized mucosa. Contrast-enhanced MRI can also demonstrate perineural, intraorbital, and intracranial spread of the disease.[12]

The most commonly reported signal characteristics on MRI of the sinuses (**Fig. 3A.7**) and brain include:

- T1: Isointense lesions relative to brain parenchyma and hypointense mucosal thickening in the paranasal sinuses.
- T2: Variable signal intensities with around 20% showing hyperintense lesions. Fungal elements most commonly tend to have low signal on T2 images.
- T1 contrast (gadolinium [Gd]): On contrast-enhanced MRI, the devitalized mucosa appears as contiguous foci of nonenhancing tissue leading to the black turbinate

sign (**Fig. 3A.8**). Fungal spores germinate to produce hyphae that cause infarction as they invade the nasal mucosa due to occlusion of small vessels. This results in a "black" area of nonenhancing mucosa which stands out against the normal enhancing mucosa.[13]

- Diffusion-weighted imaging (DWI) and apparent diffusion coefficient (ADC): Restricted diffusion may be seen as increased signal intensity on DWI and decreased intensity on ADC. Restricted diffusion is a documented finding in invasive fungal infections due to ischemia and necrosis related to the angioinvasive nature of the disease. Thus, DWI and ADC have potential to differentiate ROCM from other forms of invasive lesions like carcinomas.

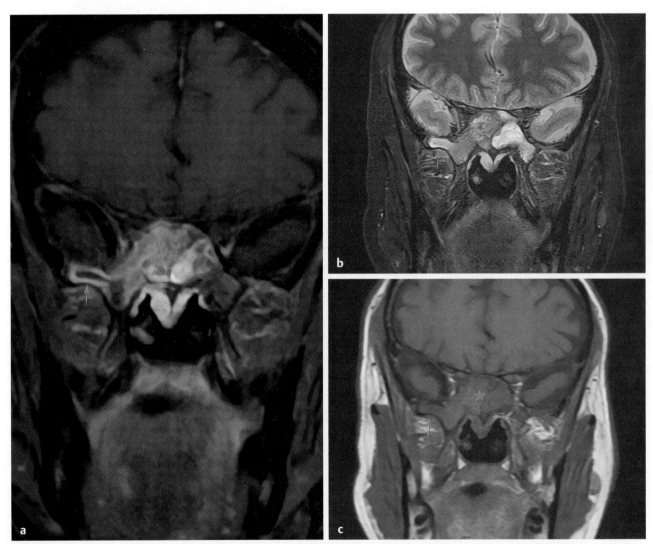

Fig. 3A.7 (a–c) Postcontrast, T1-weighted (T1W), T2-weighted (T2W), and noncontrast, T1W, coronal magnetic resonance (MR) images demonstrating extensive enhancing soft tissue lesions within the sphenoid sinuses (*) with peripherally enhancing necrotic lesion extending along the floor of the right middle cranial fossa (*arrow*).

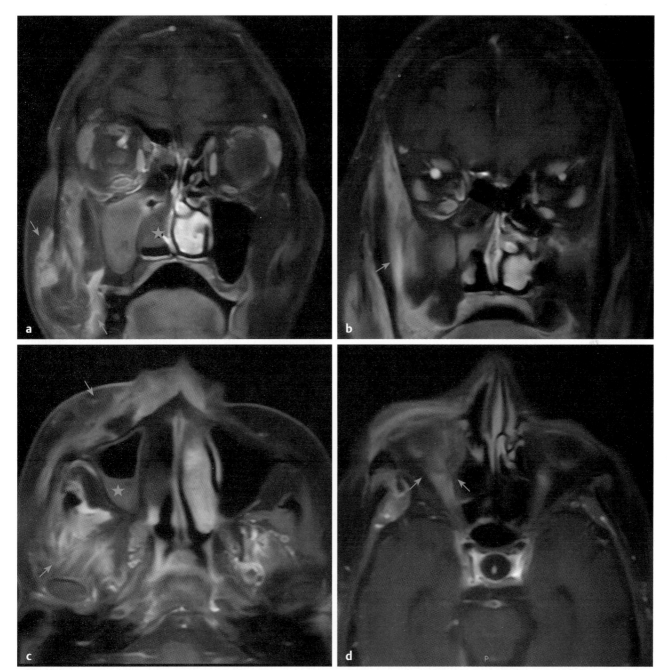

Fig. 3A.8 A 57-year-old male presented with mild proptosis, nasal obstruction, and headache post COVID-19. **(a)** Noncontrast, T2-weighted (T2W) and **(b)** coronal magnetic resonance imaging (MRI) images demonstrating hypointense right inferior turbinate (black turbinate sign shown with *asterisk*), right maxillary sinus mucosal thickening, and edema involving adjacent facial soft tissues (*arrows*). Right orbital extension has involved the inferior rectus muscle. **(c)** Axial, T2W MRI demonstrating fluid level in the right maxillary sinus (*), and soft tissue swelling with hyperintensities in the infratemporal and premaxillary regions on the right (*arrows*). **(d)** Axial, T2W images at the level of the orbits demonstrating right proptosis with retroorbital, periorbital, and optic nerve hyperintensities (*arrows*) suggesting cellulitis and left infratemporal inflammatory changes.

Sinonasal

Sinonasal imaging findings include unilateral or bilateral pansinus inflammatory changes such as polypoidal mucosal thickening with debris, fluid levels and may be nonspecific. The most commonly involved sinuses are maxillary and ethmoid.[12] Foci of hyperdense areas in the affected sinus on CT scans are highly suggestive of fungal etiology.[14] On MRI, sinus contents have a variety of signal, including T2 hyperintensity to marked hypointensity on all sequences, possibly due to presence of iron and manganese in the fungal elements.[2]

Soft Tissue Involvement

Infiltration of periantral fat is the earliest sign of soft tissue involvement. Extension of mucormycosis beyond the sinus without any bony destruction is possible due to its spread along vascular channels and nerves.[9] Spread of mucormycosis from nasal cavity to sphenopalatine foramen and ipsilateral pterygopalatine fossa occurs along either the posterior nasal nerves or the sphenopalatine artery.

This pattern of extension of disease beyond the margins of the sinuses is best observed on fat-suppressed, T2-weighted (T2W) and fat-suppressed, postcontrast T1-weighted (T1W) images, as edema and bony wall enhancement. Spread can be assessed with soft tissue infiltration and obliteration of the normal fat planes in the pterygopalatine fossa, infratemporal fossa, and pterygomaxillary fissure. On MRI, periantral fat involvement is seen as signal changes and enhancement within the premaxillary and retroantral fat. Further extension into the infratemporal fossa shows enhancement within the muscles of mastication. Extension of the pathology into the pterygopalatine fossa is seen as replacement of normal fat signal intensity surrounding the branches of the internal maxillary artery and presence of soft tissue enhancement.

Orbital

The most common sites of extrasinus involvement are orbit and facial soft tissues, followed by orbital apex, masticator space, pterygopalatine fossa, pterygoid plates, anterior and lateral skull base, cavernous sinus, brain, and ICA. Nonspecific findings on CT scan include mass effect, bony dehiscence and erosions, thickening of the extraocular muscles, and inflammatory changes of the orbit and orbital apex (**Fig. 3A.9**). T1W and T2W MRI images may demonstrate variable soft tissue intensity of retroorbital fat with thickening of extraocular muscles and proptosis indicating raised intraorbital pressure

(**Fig. 3A.8**). Postcontrast, T1W MRI show enhancing areas in retroorbital fat, thickening and enhancement of extraocular muscles, and periorbital soft tissue enhancement.[15] Involvement of lacrimal gland and lacrimal sac may cause asymmetric enlargement and enhancement as compared to contralateral structures. MRI shows thickening and lateral displacement of medial rectus muscle which is characteristic of orbital invasion of ROCM from ethmoid sinuses.[16] Vasculitis and thrombosis of the superior ophthalmic vein or ophthalmic artery and internal carotid arteries can be seen as lack of enhancement on contrast-enhanced CT scan.[17] Flow-sensitive gradient-echo MR sequences or MR angiography may also be used for this purpose.

Cavernous Sinus

Involvement of the cavernous sinus on contrast-enhanced CT scans may show lack of enhancement in venous phase, which is consistent with thrombosis from the invasive fungus. On postcontrast T1 MR images, enhancing soft tissue in orbital apex and cavernous sinus indicates cavernous sinus involvement. Changes in signal intensity, size and contour of cavernous sinus, and increased dural enhancement along the lateral border of cavernous sinus indicate cavernous sinus thrombophlebitis (**Figs. 3A.10** and **3A.11**). MR venogram and CT venogram may better demonstrate sinus thrombosis.

Internal Carotid Artery

ICA involvement may be seen as perivascular soft tissue enhancement initially. Advanced disease may cause complete thrombosis of ICA with resultant extensive cerebral infarctions that increase morbidity and mortality.[18] Invasion of branches of external carotid arteries may also cause thrombosis, most common being ophthalmic artery.

Intracranial Extension

Intracranial involvement occurs by invasion through superior orbital fissure, cribriform plate, angioinvasion, and perineural or hematogenous route. Spread of mucormycosis can cause vasculitis and inflammation of the meninges leading to meningitis. Dural abscesses with peripherally enhancing loculated dural collections may precede brain parenchymal involvement in some cases (**Fig. 3A.12**). Involvement of brain parenchyma is suggestive of cerebritis and may progress to abscess formation. DWI sequence is more specific for fungal abscess, which shows restricting wall and intracavitary projections while sparing the core of the lesion.[19,20]

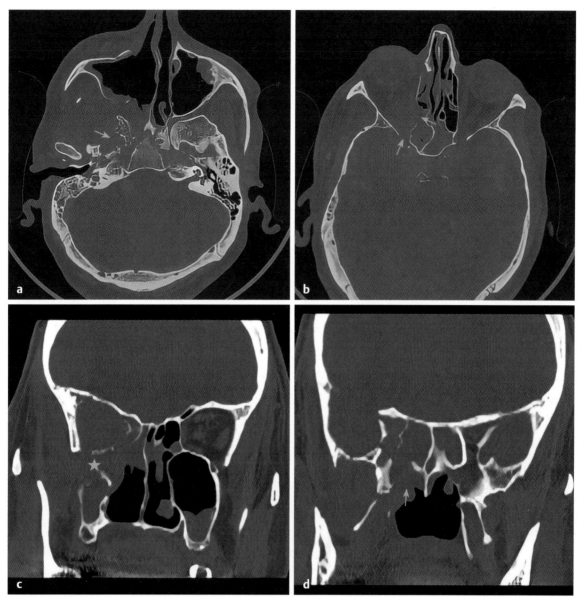

Fig. 3A.9 A case of right orbital cellulitis. **(a)** Axial, bone window computed tomography (CT) image demonstrating postsurgical changes in the posterior and medial wall of the right maxillary sinus, with excision of the turbinates. Erosions in the middle cranial fossa and greater wing of sphenoid extending to the clivus (*arrow*). Soft tissue density within the right middle ear and mastoid air cells. **(b)** Axial, bone window CT image demonstrating erosions of the medial wall of the right orbit, enlargement of the right orbital fissures, soft tissue density lesion in the posterior aspect of the right retroorbital region (*arrows*), and extensive soft tissue density within the bilateral sphenoid sinuses extending to the ethmoid sinuses and the nasal cavity. Right periorbital soft tissue swelling. **(c, d)** Coronal, bone window CT image demonstrating erosions of the floor of the right orbit with retroorbital fat replaced by soft tissue density, soft tissue thickening in the infraorbital region with erosions of the roof and medial wall of the right maxillary sinus (*), polypoidal mucosal thickening in bilateral maxillary sinuses, postsurgical changes in the right nasal cavity with defects in the lateral wall and roof, and soft tissue thickening extending to the roof of the nasal cavity (*arrow*). Bony defects are seen in the floor of the sphenoid sinus and pterygoid plates.

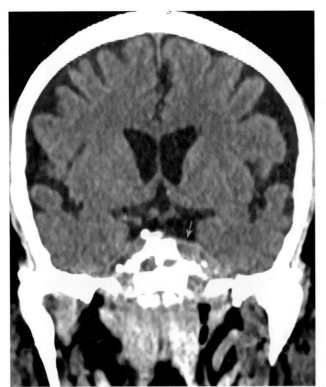

Fig. 3A.10 Noncontrast, coronal computed tomography (CT) of brain demonstrating hyperdensity in the region of left cavernous sinus in this known case of rhino-orbito-cerebral mucormycosis (ROCM) is suggestive of thrombosis.

Follow-Up Scan

Imaging plays a vital role in detecting immediate and long-term postsurgical complications as well as recurrent disease. Postsurgical CT scan can detect immediate complications like hemorrhage, mass effect on the brain, and infarcts due to vascular compromise or thrombus. During continued medical management with antifungal treatment in the post-operative period, imaging helps assess response or progression (**Fig. 3A.13**). Postsurgical complications may include subdural abscess, meningitis, encephalitis, intraparenchymal brain abscess, and arterial and venous thrombosis with secondary infarcts. Re-exploration may be planned based on imaging findings if disease progression necessitates debridement. Due to aggressive medical and surgical management, acute and fulminant forms of ROCM can be controlled, but the risk of mucormycosis-associated skull base osteomyelitis (SBO) needs to be considered in long-term follow-up. Indeed, ROCM with SBO can be recognized with high-resolution CT. The characteristic finding on MRI, especially nonenhanced T1W sequence, is loss of T1 hyperintensity of skull base marrow fat[19] (**Fig. 3A.14**).

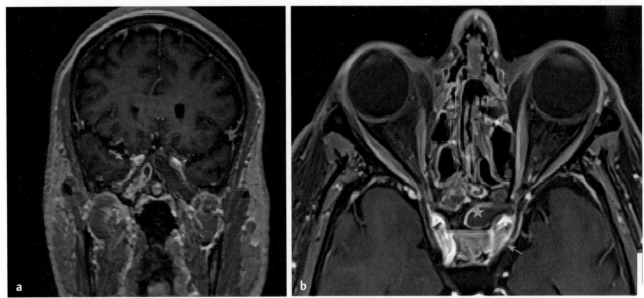

Fig. 3A.11 A case of known rhino-orbito-cerebral mucormycosis (ROCM) presented with severe headache, double vision, and nasal obstruction. (Magnetic resonance imaging [MRI] findings at presentation described in **Fig. 3A.7.**) Surgical debridement and 3 months of antifungal treatment was completed at follow-up MRI. **(a)** Postcontrast, coronal, T1-weighted (T1W) MRI demonstrating decreased enhancement in the region of the sphenoid sinus with resolution of abscess. **(b)** Postcontrast, axial, T1W MRI demonstrating reduced enhancement in the region of the bilateral cavernous sinus (*arrow*) and decreased enhancement within the sphenoid sinus with peripherally enhancing organized collection.

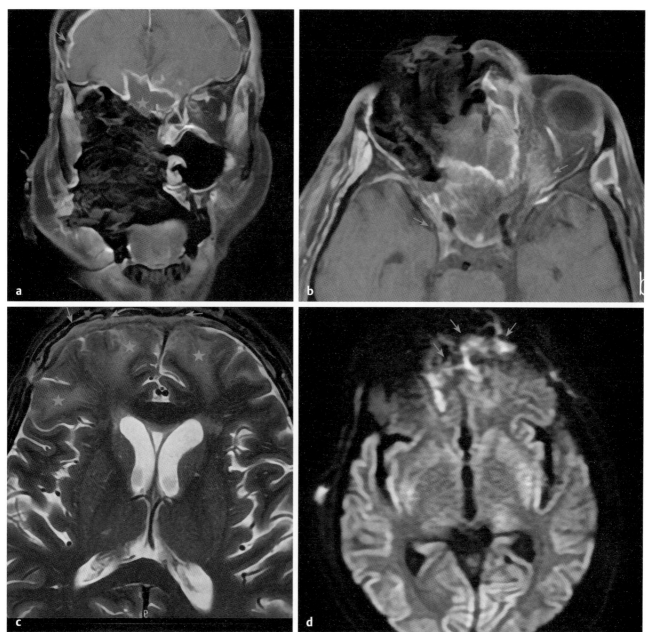

Fig. 3A.12 A known case of rhino-orbito-cerebral mucormycosis (ROCM), post orbital exenteration and maxillectomy, presented with seizures and altered sensorium. **(a)** Postcontrast, coronal, T1-weighted (T1W) magnetic resonance imaging (MRI) showing extensive postsurgical changes in the nasal cavity, orbit, and right maxilla. A peripherally enhancing extraaxial abscess is seen in the basifrontal region (*) with dural thickening and meningeal enhancement in the cerebral convexities suggesting meningitis (*arrow*). **(b)** Corresponding postcontrast, T1W, axial image demonstrating enhancement within the sphenoid and ethmoid sinuses, region of the cavernous sinuses bilaterally, left retroorbital fat (*arrows*), and in the left lateral temporal scalp region suggesting inflammation and soft tissue cellulitis. **(c)** Axial, T2W MRI demonstrating diffuse white matter T2 hyperintensities in the bilateral frontal lobes (*) with dural and meningeal thickening (*arrows*) in the frontal region suggesting meningoencephalitis. **(d)** Axial diffusion-weighted imaging (DWI) demonstrating restricted diffusion in the bilateral, extraaxial, basifrontal regions in the region of the abscess (*arrow*).

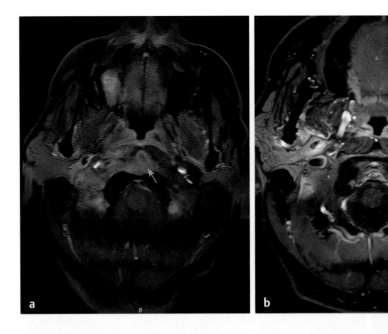

Fig. 3A.13 A known case of rhino-orbito-cerebral mucormycosis (ROCM). **(a)** Preoperative axial, postcontrast T1-weighted (T1W) magnetic resonance imaging (MRI) demonstrates peripherally enhancing abscess in the prevertebral/clival region. **(b)** Corresponding posttreatment (surgical and medical management) follow-up MRI image demonstrates complete resolution of the abscess.

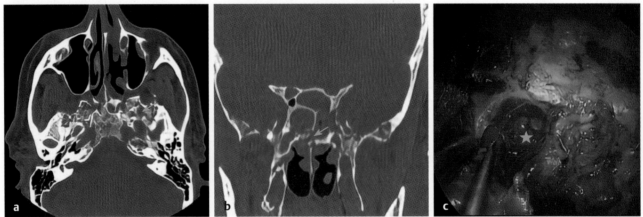

Fig. 3A.14 A 66-year-old male presented with complaints of severe headache, nasal discharge, and postnasal drip, few weeks post-COVID-19 infection. He underwent endoscopic, right, wide, middle meatal antrostomy with endoscopic, left medial maxillectomy and bilateral sphenoethmoidectomy with left infratemporal fossa clearance. Based on histopathological diagnosis of mucormycosis, he was on medical management for 5 months. Follow-up computed tomography (CT) and magnetic resonance imaging (MRI) scans showed osteomyelitic changes. In view of persistent disease in the clival area, the patient underwent endoscopic transnasal transphenoidal approach for sphenoclival debridement. Histopathology showed chronic inflammation. The patient was continued on medical management for two more months. **(a)** Axial, bone window CT image demonstrating extensive erosions involving the clivus, greater wing and lesser wing of sphenoid (*arrow*), walls of the sphenoid sinuses, and inter-sphenoid septum. There are erosions extending to the carotid canals bilaterally. **(b)** Coronal CT in bone window setting demonstrating erosions of the walls of the sphenoid and maxillary with extensive soft tissue density within the sinuses. There are erosions of the roof of the nasal cavity and the nasal septum in the posterosuperior aspect (*arrow*). Erosions of the pterygoid plates, greater wing of sphenoid bone, middle cranial fossa is noted bilaterally. **(c)** Intraoperative findings showing exposed left infratemporal fossa with necrotic tissue (*).

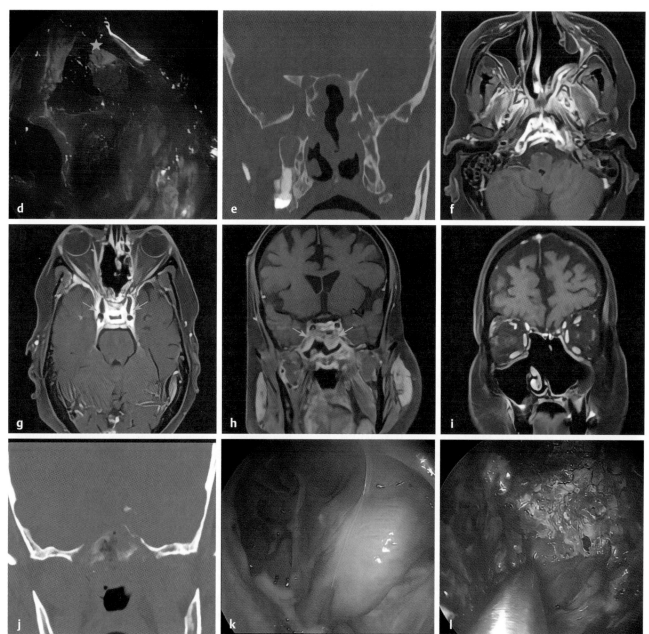

Fig. 3A.14 *(Continued)* **(d)** Sphenoid sinus with eroded inter-sphenoid septum and floor of sphenoid. Unhealthy mucosa with fungal debris noted superiorly (*). **(e–h)** Follow-up scan 2 months post-surgery. **(e)** Coronal, bone window CT image demonstrating interval development of sclerosis in the walls of the sphenoid sinus with postsurgical changes in the inter-sphenoidal septum. Interval development of sclerosis in the pterygoid plates and the greater wing of sphenoid is also noted. There is persistent soft tissue density within the sphenoid sinus. **(f)** Postcontrast, T1-weighted (T1W) MRI demonstrating enhancing soft tissue areas in the infratemporal fossa involving the pterygoid muscles with extension to involve the clivus. **(g)** Postcontrast, T1W, axial MRI demonstrating enhancing soft tissue areas in the region of bilateral cavernous sinus (*arrows*) and roof of the sphenoid sinus regions extending to the clivus. **(h)** Postcontrast, T1W, coronal MRI demonstrating peripherally enhancing area in the clivus (*arrows*), bilateral cavernous sinus, and parasellar regions suggesting persisting clival osteomyelitis. Post medical management with antifungal for 5 months. **(i)** Postcontrast, T1W, coronal MRI demonstrating postsurgical changes in the medial wall of bilateral maxillary sinuses and interval healing of polypoidal mucosal thickening. No residual disease seen in the region of the nasal cavity and the orbits. **(j)** Coronal, bone window CT image demonstrating postsurgical changes in the region of the clivus with soft tissue air loculi and bone debridement changes. Interval development of sclerosis is seen in the greater wing of sphenoid and middle cranial fossa bilaterally. **(k)** Complete mucosalization of the operated cavity with healthy Hadad flap in the region of infratemporal fossa. Polypoidal changes noted in the sphenoid sinus. **(l)** Bony sequestra and serous discharge noted with erosions of clivus and floor of sphenoid sinus suggestive of chronic osteomyelitis.

Conclusion

Multimodality imaging in ROCM is helpful in early diagnosis and for timely surgical intervention. It aids in planning treatment strategies and vigilant follow-up on the progression or regression of the disease. CT and MRI complement each other as CT scan demonstrates bony changes whereas multiplanar MRI provides better evaluation of soft tissue, skull base invasion, and intracranial, perineural, and vascular involvement.

References

1. Roden MM, Zaoutis TE, Buchanan WL, et al. Epidemiology and outcome of zygomycosis: a review of 929 reported cases. Clin Infect Dis 2005;41(5):634–653

2. Ribes JA, Vanover-Sams CL, Baker DJ. Zygomycetes in human disease. Clin Microbiol Rev 2000;13(2):236–301

3. Orguc S, Yücetürk AV, Demir MA, Goktan C. Rhinocerebral mucormycosis: perineural spread via the trigeminal nerve. J Clin Neurosci 2005;12(4):484–486

4. Petrikkos G, Skiada A, Lortholary O, Roilides E, Walsh TJ, Kontoyiannis DP. Epidemiology and clinical manifestations of mucormycosis. Clin Infect Dis 2012;54(Suppl 1):S23–S34

5. Mossa-Basha M, Ilica AT, Maluf F, Karakoç Ö, İzbudak I, Aygün N. The many faces of fungal disease of the paranasal sinuses: CT and MRI findings. Diagn Interv Radiol 2013;19(3):195–200

6. Franquet T, Giménez A, Hidalgo A. Imaging of opportunistic fungal infections in immunocompromised patient. Eur J Radiol 2004;51(2):130–138

7. Middlebrooks EH, Frost CJ, De Jesus RO, Massini TC, Schmalfuss IM, Mancuso AA. Acute invasive fungal rhinosinusitis: a comprehensive update of CT findings and design of an effective diagnostic imaging model. AJNR Am J Neuroradiol 2015;36(8):1529–1535

8. Chan LL, Singh S, Jones D, Diaz EM Jr, Ginsberg LE. Imaging of mucormycosis skull base osteomyelitis. AJNR Am J Neuroradiol 2000;21(5):828–831

9. Garces P, Mueller D, Trevenen C. Rhinocerebral mucormycosis in a child with leukemia: CT and MRI findings. Pediatr Radiol 1994;24(1):50–51

10. Safder S, Carpenter JS, Roberts TD, Bailey N. The "Black Turbinate" sign: an early MR imaging finding of nasal mucormycosis. AJNR Am J Neuroradiol 2010;31(4):771–774

11. Rao VM, el-Noueam KI. Sinonasal imaging. Anatomy and pathology. Radiol Clin North Am 1998;36(5):921–939, vi

12. Bawankar P, Lahane S, Pathak P, Gonde P, Singh A. Central retinal artery occlusion as the presenting manifestation of invasive rhino-orbital-cerebral mucormycosis. Taiwan J Ophthalmol 2020;10(1):62–65

13. Mathur M, Johnson CE, Sze G. Fungal infections of the central nervous system. Neuroimaging Clin N Am 2012;22(4):609–632

14. Awal SS, Biswas SS, Awal SK. Rhino-orbital mucormycosis in COVID-19 patients—a new threat? Egypt J Radiol Nucl Med 2021;52:152

15. Patil A, Mohanty HS, Kumar S, Nandikoor S, Meganathan P. Angioinvasive rhinocerebral mucormycosis with complete unilateral thrombosis of internal carotid artery-case report and review of literature. BJR Case Rep 2016;2(2):20150448

16. Lone PA, Wani NA, Jehangir M. Rhino-orbito-cerebral mucormycosis: magnetic resonance imaging. Indian J Otol 2015;21(3):215–218

17. Kilpatrick C, Tress B, King J. Computed tomography of rhinocerebral mucormycosis. Neuroradiology 1984;26(1):71–73

18. Patel DD, Adke S, Badhe PV, Lamture S, Marfatia H, Mhatre P. COVID-19 associated rhino-orbito-cerebral mucormycosis: imaging spectrum and clinico-radiological correlation—a single centre experience. Clin Imaging 2022;82:172–178

19. Centeno RS, Bentson JR, Mancuso AA. CT scanning in rhinocerebral mucormycosis and aspergillosis. Radiology 1981;140(2):383–389

20. Press GA, Weindling SM, Hesselink JR, Ochi JW, Harris JP. Rhinocerebral mucormycosis: MR manifestations. J Comput Assist Tomogr 1988;12(5):744–749

3B

Diagnostic Utility of Multidetector Computed Tomography Scan versus Cone Beam Computed Tomography Scan in Rhino-Orbito-Cerebral Mucormycosis

Chapter 3B

Diagnostic Utility of Multidetector Computed Tomography Scan versus Cone Beam Computed Tomography Scan in Rhino-Orbito-Cerebral Mucormycosis

S. K. Priyadarshini and P. Subramanian

Introduction

Imaging studies are inevitable in the diagnosis and management of mucormycosis and both magnetic resonance imaging (MRI) and computed tomography (CT) scans are useful. The aggressive, fulminating, and angioinvasive spread of the disease necessitates rapid and accurate diagnosis and initiation of treatment for better prognosis.[1] Empirical antifungal therapy can be started in clinically suspected cases with substantiating imaging evidence of rhino-orbito-cerebral mucormycosis (ROCM)[2] as even a 1-week delay in treatment raises the mortality from 35 to 66%.[3] MRI exquisitely depicts and delineates the extent and progress of ROCM with the soft-tissue details and bone involvement. Diagnosis can be more precise with combination imaging with multidetector computed tomography (MDCT) and (or) cone beam computed tomography (CBCT) since subtle erosions, especially in early or recurrent disease, are not well appreciated in MRI and therefore may be easily missed or overlooked by utilizing MRI alone.

MDCT versus CBCT

MDCT and CBCT scans are valuable in mucormycosis to demonstrate bony involvement. MDCT uses a fan beam to acquire the considered volume by a rotating gantry where the patient is moved at a constant speed and data are acquired in multiple axial sections followed by multiplanar reformation, whereas CBCT utilizes a conical beam to acquire the entire dataset in a single gantry rotation. Thus, the volumetric dataset that is produced in MDCT has anisotropic voxels with voxel surfaces as small as 0.625 mm[2] with a depth of 1 to 2 mm, whereas CBCT produces isotropic voxels ranging from 0.4 to 0.09 mm[4,5] with resultant high spatial resolution as compared to MDCT.[6] CBCT has excellent spatial resolution that is extremely useful in picking up early bone changes and subtle bone erosions especially in dentoalveolar and palatal involvement, but the contrast resolution of CBCT is

very poor, thus providing images with only the bony details. With 35% lesser radiation dose and quick scanning time than conventional CT head scan,[7,8] CBCT is a good choice for combined imaging with MDCT/MRI for ROCM. Most of the CBCT machines available in the market require the patient in the sitting or standing position for the scanning procedure. The minimum slice thickness of conventional CT head scan is 0.625 mm depending on the machine, whereas CBCT has resolution as low as 0.15 mm, which attributes to superior delineation of adjacent structures by CBCT. The major limitation of CBCT is the increased noise with the resultant grainy images providing poor contrast resolution than conventional CT scan images. There is barely any noise in MDCT machines due to the high milliampere (mA) and negligible scattered radiation by effective collimation.[9] MDCT scans have unparalleled image quality with bone and soft-tissue window settings offering bone and soft-tissue details with contrast enhancement characteristics. Three-dimensional (3D) volumetric rendering is possible in both CT and CBCT scans, but not in MRI.

MDCT is superior in depicting fine bony structures such as lamina papyracea, cribriform lamina, orbital floor, and infundibular complex along with soft tissue.[10] All the paranasal sinuses and their walls are clearly visualized in CBCT as well. However, the fine and thin bony landmarks especially the medial wall of the orbit may not be visualized as accurately as in MDCT especially when associated with significant mucosal thickening. This makes interpretation of thinning/erosions of the delicate structures using CBCT scan difficult (**Figs. 3B.1** and **3B.2**). A detailed evaluation of the paranasal sinuses, nasal cavity, orbits, skull base, and brain is possible with conventional CT in bone and soft-tissue window settings. The maximum field of view that is available in most of the CBCT machines does not include the entire skull and may cover only up to the frontal sinus. Unlike MDCT in which bone and surrounding soft tissue is visualized (**Figs. 3B.3–3B.5**), only the bony details can be assessed in CBCT (**Fig. 3B.6**). Nonenhanced CT depicts soft-tissue

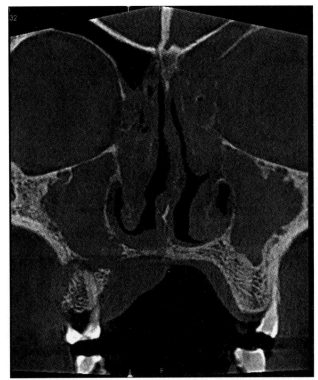

Fig. 3B.1 Cone beam computed tomography (CBCT) slice showing mucosal thickening of bilateral maxillary, ethmoid sinuses, and left frontal sinus with destruction of the right maxillary alveolus and medial wall of the left orbit.

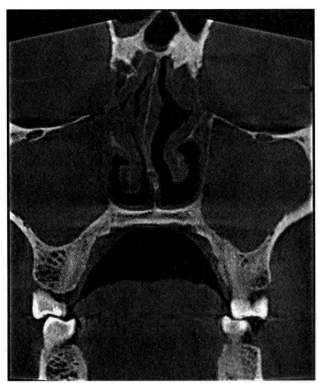

Fig. 3B.2 Cone beam computed tomography (CBCT) image showing significant mucosal thickening of the bilateral maxillary and right ethmoid sinus. Note the medial wall of the bilateral orbits were intact but not well appreciated in this section.

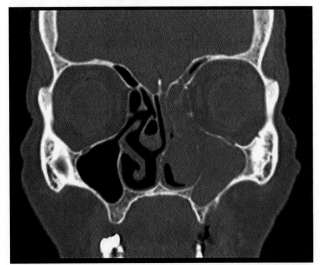

Fig. 3B.3 Multidetector computed tomography (MDCT)—bone window—images show mucosal thickening in the left maxillary sinus, nasal cavity, ethmoid sinus, and frontal sinus with erosions of the left side nasal turbinates, osteomeatal unit, and medial wall of the left maxillary sinus.

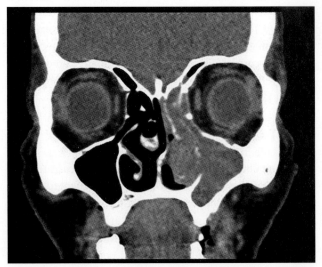

Fig. 3B.4 Multidetector computed tomography (MDCT)—soft-tissue window: Extraocular muscles appear intact. No intraorbital soft-tissue component or subperiosteal collections are seen.

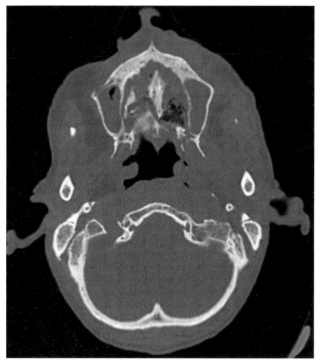

Fig. 3B.5 Multidetector computed tomography (MDCT) axial slice depicting bony destruction involving bilateral hard palate with air pockets. Bony erosions are also seen in the pterygoid hamulus and the medial pterygoid plate on the left side.

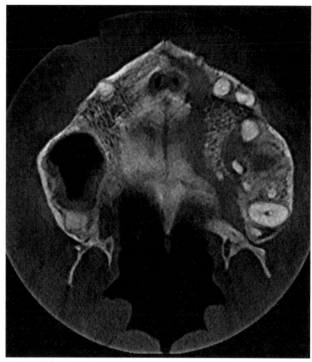

Fig. 3B.6 Cone beam computed tomography (CBCT) axial section shows bony destruction involving the entire left side hard palate.

thickening within the paranasal sinuses and nasal cavity and thinning and erosions of the nasal and sinus walls, turbinates, cribriform plate, medial wall and floor of the orbits, sphenoid bone, greater and lesser wings of the sphenoid, floor of the sella, basi-occiput, clivus, and skull base involvement. Disease from the sphenoid sinus may spread directly to the skull base and cavernous sinus. Moreover, involvement of the posterior ethmoid and sphenoid sinus carries an increased risk of intracranial extension.[11] Disease of the frontal sinus may also result in intracranial spread with involvement of the frontal and parietal bone. The soft-tissue details such as subdural collection, leptomeningeal thickening, subgaleal collections, retroantral, facial, orbital, and premaxillary fat stranding can be visualized even in pre-/noncontrast CT scan (**Fig. 3B.7**) but not in CBCT. Although bone erosions and destruction may be a feature of advanced disease, the subtle erosions in rapid spread of disease may not be evident on CT images.[12] Contrast-enhanced CT (CECT) is particularly useful in the cases without MRI to depict parasellar and cavernous sinus involvement and in demonstrating vascular and intracranial complications such as occlusion, stenosis, and thrombus of the internal carotid artery and mycotic aneurysms.[13] With the excellent bone details and nonenhancing soft tissue denoting devitalized tissue, CECT best aids in presurgical planning. However, when CECT is contraindicated, MRI with noncontrast CT will be useful.

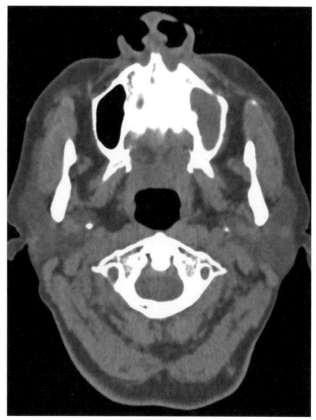

Fig. 3B.7 Premaxillary fat stranding appreciated in multidetector computed tomography (MDCT) soft-tissue window.

Evaluation of Dentoalveolar Component

The dentoalveolar component is best visualized and evaluated in CBCT than in MDCT (**Fig. 3B.8**). The hypodense areas and alteration in the trabecular pattern of bone denoting early osteomyelitic changes, erosions of the buccal and palatal cortical plates, hard palate, sinus and nasal floor, and unhealed extraction sockets are clearly depicted in CBCT. Sometimes it may be difficult to differentiate chronic periodontitis with tooth mobility from early rhinomaxillary disease prior to radiological presentation of bony changes involving the maxillary alveolus in CBCT sections; however, clinical features and marrow edema in MRI should help in the diagnosis. Early osteomyelitic changes present as alteration/decrease/loss of trabecular pattern with distinct tiny hypodense areas within the alveolar bone with/without intact cortical bone (**Fig. 3B.9**). As the disease progresses, there is irregular moth-eaten appearance of alveolar bone loss (**Fig. 3B.10**), erosion of buccal and palatal cortices (**Figs. 3B.11** and **3B.12**), and destruction of alveolar bone with sequestrum formation. On the other hand, in chronic periodontitis, we see interproximal crestal bone loss, blunting of the alveolar crest, horizontal or vertical (angular) defects involving the furcation of multirooted teeth, resorption, and loss of the cortical plates (**Fig. 3B.13**). The bone loss in periodontitis has smooth margins, whereas an irregular pattern is seen in osteomyelitis. The early and subtle bony changes in early and recurrent disease are detected best in CBCT rather than MDCT.

3D Reformatting in MDCT and CBCT

3D images are obtained in both MDCT and CBCT. 3D images with surface rendition of anatomy are executed with the help of incorporated software that scans each CT slice in case of MDCT and the volume data in case of CBCT to create a 3D image. The quality of 3D image in MDCT is superior to that in CBCT due to their differences in inherent acquisition and reconstruction of data. Artifacts due to dense materials in the region of scan are reflected in 3D-reconstructed images, which are unavoidable in both the modalities and may be reduced but cannot be eliminated. The surface renditions of 3D images provide excellent details of the bony erosions, destruction, exact size and shape of bone fragments, and bone defects (**Figs. 3B.14–3B.18**). 3D-reconstructed images are not diagnostic but aids the surgeons in presurgical evaluation and treatment planning.[14] Both MDCT and CBCT images are acquired in the digital imaging and communication in medicine (DICOM) format, which are easily transferred for conversion to the stereolithography (STL) file format for planning, evaluation, and 3D printing for maxillofacial reconstruction. MDCT is the preferred imaging modality when planning for maxillofacial reconstruction as it offers bone and soft-tissue features of the entire skull with superior image quality.

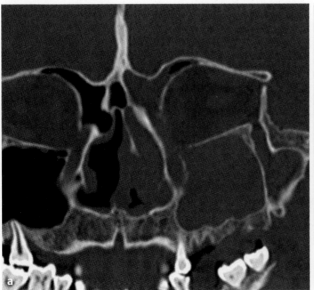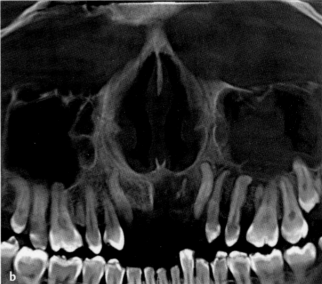

Fig. 3B.8 Comparative panoramic section of **(a)** multidetector computed tomography (MDCT) and **(b)** cone beam computed tomography (CBCT) of two different cases. Note the detailed depiction of trabecular pattern and areas of bone destruction of maxillary alveolar bone extending from the central incisor to the first molar on the left side in CBCT.

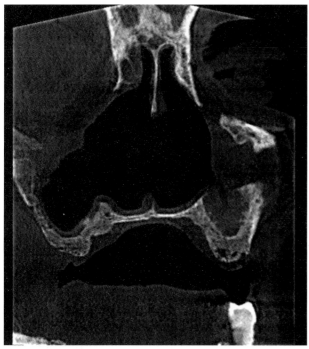

Fig. 3B.9 Osteomyelitic changes seen in the left maxillary alveolus at the crestal and subcrestal levels in a case with recurrence.

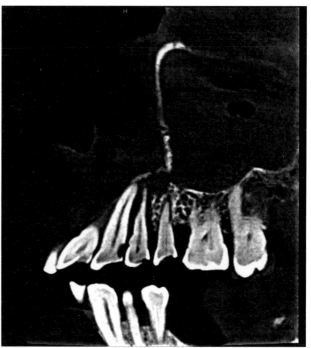

Fig. 3B.10 Cone beam computed tomography (CBCT) section of post-COVID-19 mucormycosis patient with osteomyelitis. There is alveolar bone destruction in the left canine and premolar regions with erosion of the anterior wall of the left maxillary sinus.

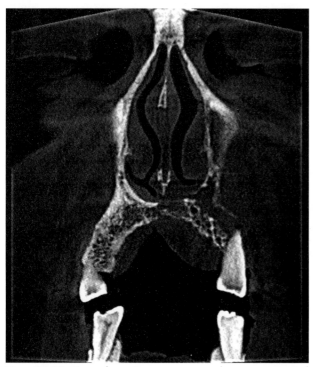

Fig. 3B.11 Coronal section on cone beam computed tomography (CBCT) showing features of osteomyelitis with alveolar destruction in left premolar region and erosion of buccal cortical bone. Thinning and erosion of lateral wall of nose is also noted on the left side.

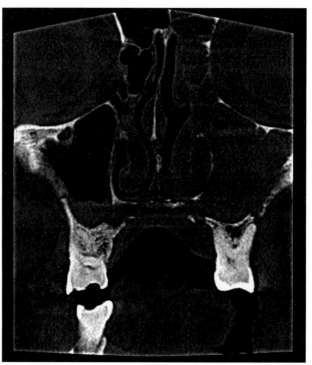

Fig. 3B.12 Coronal cone beam computed tomography (CBCT) slice depicting bilateral destruction of the hard palate. Also seen are significant mucosal thickening of the left maxillary and ethmoid sinuses with destruction of the medial wall of the left maxillary sinus.

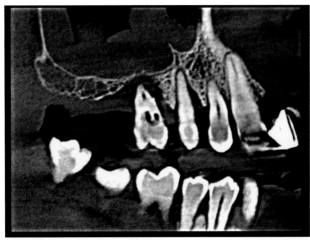

Fig. 3B.13 Sagittal cone beam computed tomography (CBCT) image of chronic periodontitis seen as severe alveolar bone loss in the right premolar and the first molar.

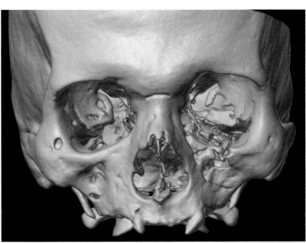

Fig. 3B.14 Anterior view of volume-rendered 3D multi-detector computed tomography (MDCT) image illustrating bony destruction of the floor of the orbit and anterior wall of the maxillary sinus on the left side.

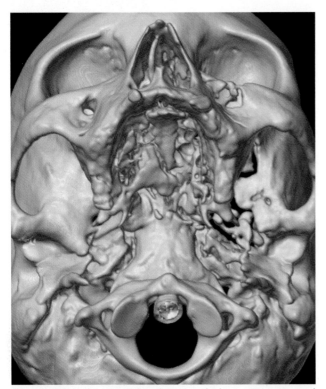

Fig. 3B.15 Volume-rendered 3D multidetector computed tomography (MDCT) image showing erosion of bilateral hard palate.

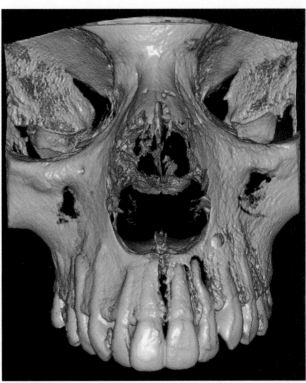

Fig. 3B.16 Volume-rendered 3D cone beam computed tomography (CBCT) image showing destruction of the anterior maxillary alveolus on the left side involving the central and lateral incisors.

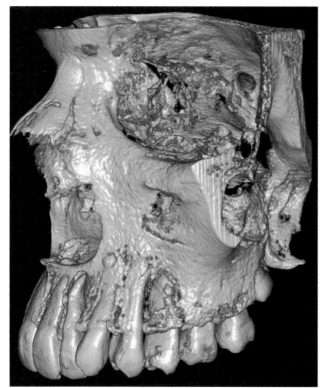

Fig. 3B.17 Left lateral view of volume-rendered 3D cone beam computed tomography (CBCT) image showing destruction of alveolar bone involving the canine and premolars.

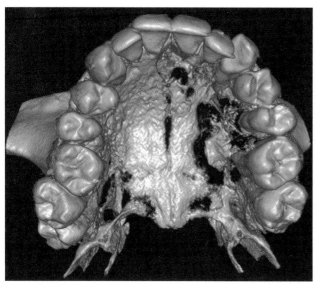

Fig. 3B.18 Volume-rendered 3D cone beam computed tomography (CBCT) image illustrating the destruction of the left side hard palate.

Conclusion

MDCT is ideal for depicting the bony involvement and erosions in ROCM, and CECT is the next best alternative if MRI is contraindicated. CBCT is the best imaging choice to be combined with MRI and for follow-up scans in localized (rhinomaxillary) disease involving the maxilla, hard palate, dentoalveolar component, and nasal cavity without orbital or intracranial extension.

References

1. Karadeniz Uğurlu Ş, Selim S, Kopar A, Songu M. Rhino-orbital mucormycosis: Clinical findings and treatment outcomes of four cases. Turk J Ophthalmol 2015;45(4):169–174

2. Honavar SG. Code mucor: guidelines for the diagnosis, staging and management of rhino-orbito-cerebral mucormycosis in the setting of COVID-19. Indian J Ophthalmol 2021;69(6):1361–1365

3. Werthman-Ehrenreich A. Mucormycosis with orbital compartment syndrome in a patient with COVID-19. Am J Emerg Med 2021;42:264.e5–264.e8

4. Izzetti R, Gaeta R, Caramella D, Giuffra V. Cone-beam computed tomography vs. multi-slice computed tomography in paleoimaging: where we stand. Homo 2020;71(1):63–72

5. Venkatesh E, Elluru SV. Cone beam computed tomography: basics and applications in dentistry. J Istanb Univ Fac Dent 2017;51(3, Suppl 1):S102–S121

6. Lechuga L, Weidlich GA. Cone beam CT vs. fan beam CT: a comparison of image quality and dose delivered between two differing CT imaging modalities. Cureus 2016;8(9):e778

7. Kim S, Yoshizumi TT, Toncheva G, Yoo S, Yin F-F. Comparison of radiation doses between cone beam CT and multi detector CT: TLD measurements. Radiat Prot Dosimetry 2008;132(3):339–345

8. Pauwels R, Araki K, Siewerdsen JH, Thongvigitmanee SS. Technical aspects of dental CBCT: state of the art. Dentomaxillofac Radiol 2015;44(1):20140224

9. Jaju P, Jain M, Singh A, Gupta A. Artefacts in cone beam CT. Open J Stomatol 2013;3:292–297

10. Hamza A, Ishfaq Q, Afzal A, et al. Evaluation of fungal sinusitis on computed tomography and its correlation with endoscopy and histopathology findings. Eur J Health Sci 2019;4(2):12–19

11. Mathur S, Karimi A, Mafee MF. Acute optic nerve infarction demonstrated by diffusion-weighted imaging in a case of rhinocerebral mucormycosis. AJNR Am J Neuroradiol 2007;28(3):489–490

12. Desai SM, Gujarathi-Saraf A, Agarwal EA. Imaging findings using a combined MRI/CT protocol to identify the "entire iceberg" in post-COVID-19 mucormycosis presenting clinically as only "the tip." Clin Radiol 2021;76(10):784.e27–784.e33

13. Manchanda S, Semalti K, Bhalla AS, Thakar A, Sikka K, Verma H. Revisiting rhino-orbito-cerebral acute invasive fungal sinusitis in the era of COVID-19: pictorial review. Emerg Radiol 2021;28(6):1063–1072

14. Ram MS, Joshi M, Debnath J, Khanna SK. 3 dimensional CT. Med J Armed Forces India 1998;54(3):239–242

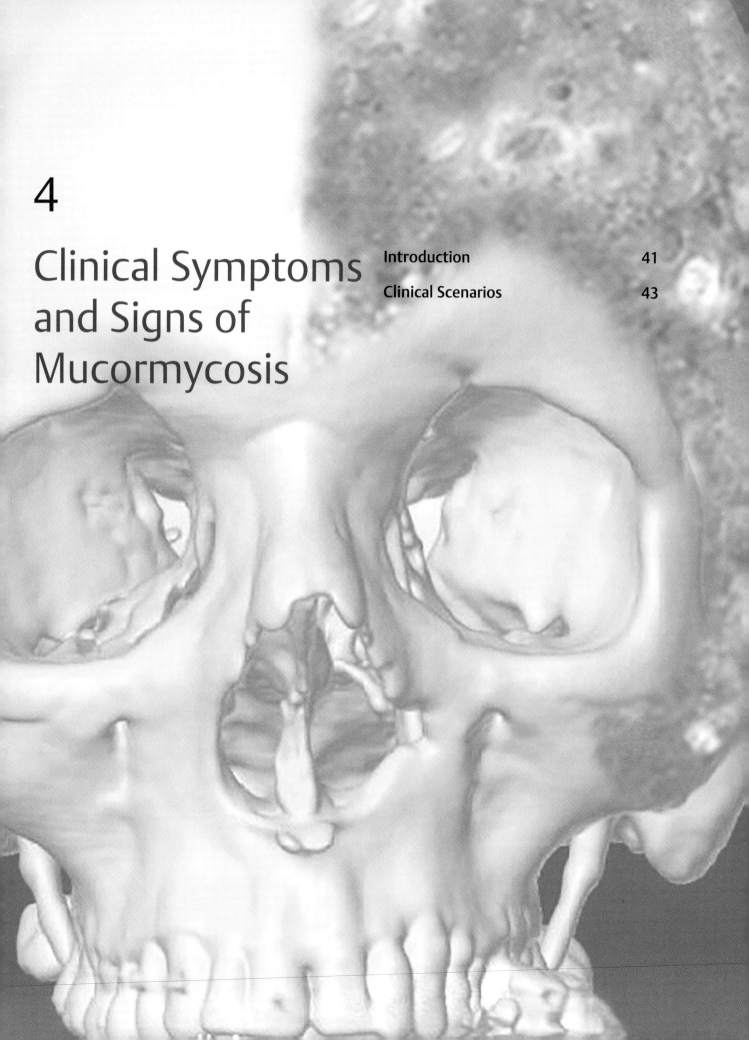

4

Clinical Symptoms and Signs of Mucormycosis

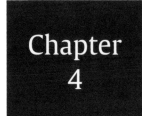

Chapter 4

Clinical Symptoms and Signs of Mucormycosis

Narayanan Janakiram, Sathyanarayanan Janakiram, Ashritha M.C.V., Lekshmy R. Kurup, and Harshita Singh

Introduction

Rhino-orbito-cerebral mucormycosis (ROCM) is a fulminant infection that typically commences from the nasal mucosa and extends into the paranasal sinuses (PNSs), orbit, palate, intracranial structures, and neck spaces.[1] In the authors' series of 193 patients, ROCM was noted more in males (65%) than in females with a mean age of 51 ± 12 years.

Mucor is an angiotropic fungus that has a predilection for internal elastic lamina of the blood vessels, especially the arteries, and it eventually invades the lymphatics and veins. The fungus directly involves blood vessels by inducing arteritis and thrombotic vascular occlusions, which result in ischemia, coagulative and hemorrhagic necrosis, ischemic infarction, endothelial venous damage, aneurysms and pseudoaneurysms, and gangrene; however, it generally results in little inflammation. When present, the inflammation occurs in a diffusive manner as a spreading, necrotizing reaction that is coupled with mycotic aneurysms. The organism thrives in this matrix of dead organic tissue and continues to spread by direct extension along injured blood vessels.[2,3]

Mucormycosis grows and spreads via three primary mechanisms: Soft-tissue invasion, angioinvasion, and perineural invasion.[4] These processes create a devastating effect on local tissue as the *mucor* invades the lumen of blood vessels and adheres to the internal elastic lamina. Its broad, nonseptate hyphae block the lumen and interrupt perfusion, causing thrombosis, infarction, and rapid tissue necrosis accelerated by various fungal proteases, lipases, and mycotoxins.[5-7] The mechanism of perineural invasion accounts for the spread of infection that can occur further away from the primary site of infection, such as through the trigeminal ganglion.[4]

The signs and symptoms of the disease can be segregated depending upon the stage of the disease into nasal, sinonasal, orbital, oral, and cerebral.

In the acute phase, ROCM presentation is similar to sinusitis.[8] Low-grade fever, mild headache, facial pain and swelling, nasal congestion, nasal discharge, and nasal and palatal ulceration are the most common initial clinical features.[9] Most common early symptoms are nasal blockade and discharge, which are due to fungal sinusitis. The nasal discharge

in particular was seen to be foul smelling in about 41.4% of cases in the authors' series. Headache (80.8%) and fever (24.9%) were due to sinusitis and septicemia, respectively. Epistaxis was noted as a primary symptom among 14.5% of patients. Further spread of infection causes increase in facial pain due to angioinvasion and perineural invasion, mainly in those cases involving infraorbital nerve.[10] Perineural spread may also be attributed to the loss of olfaction wherein the olfactory nerve is involved. In the authors' case series, facial pain was experienced by about 76.2% (*n* = 147) of patients and anosmia was noted in 13% of individuals. Facial nerve palsy was also a presentation of post-COVID-19 mucormycosis due to perineural spread and via the vidian canal in sinonasal mucormycosis. At the author's center, about four patients presented with facial nerve palsy as part of initial clinical presentation.

In authors' experience, change in the normal appearance of the nasal mucosa was the most consistent finding in the nasal endoscopy. The main clinical findings included the black necrotic eschar tissue with underlying purulent exudates with an unpleasant odor. The presence of white discoloration indicates tissue ischemia, which was secondary to angiocentric invasion. Angioinvasion further leads to tissue infarction and massive necrosis with bone destruction. This explains the black discoloration of the mucosa seen in this disease.[11]

In patients with high index of suspicion, while performing nasal endoscopy one should carefully inspect the common sites for fungal debris, which includes the middle turbinate (43%), septum (10%), palate (30%), and inferior turbinate (17%). If there is decreased mucosal bleeding and/or absence of sensation in these areas, it may be considered a sign of fungal disease. At the authors' center, decreased bleeding was present in 15% and loss of sensation, that is, facial numbness, in 14% of patients.

Once the fungal elements invade the sinuses, especially the ethmoidal sinus, it provides a pathway for spreading the disease into the orbit. Involvement of the orbit occurs through the lamina papyracea. Fat stranding, edema, and loss of muscle plane were seen in almost all the patients in whom the orbit was involved. Involvement of the orbit can also happen via the nasolacrimal duct.[12] In the authors' series, there have been cases of orbital involvement even without involvement of the nose and PNS. This was mainly seen in secondary cases.

The fungus first involves the muscles and the contents of the orbit causing orbital cellulitis.[13] Orbital cellulitis was the most common orbital complication, seen in about 37% of cases in the authors' series.

The presentation of orbital cellulitis may be varied. Lid and periorbital swelling, fungal eyelid abscesses, chemosis, and corneal edema were the common presentations noticed in the cases with orbital cellulitis. The most important distinguishing feature of orbital cellulitis is the presence of ophthalmoplegia, painful eye movement, and/or proptosis. Ophthalmoplegia can happen because of two reasons: either through direct involvement of muscles of the orbit by the disease, which is through angioinvasion, or through perineural invasion of the nerves supplying these muscles.[14] At the authors' center, three patients presented with complete ophthalmoplegia at the initial presentation.

The next symptom noticed was diplopia. The etiology was similar to ophthalmoplegia. The most commonly involved muscle was the medial rectus.[15]

The fungus spreading more posteriorly can lead to orbital apex syndrome, which involves multiple cranial neuropathies with associated optic nerve dysfunction. In most cases, orbital apex syndrome is associated with superior orbital fissure involvement or cavernous sinus involvement. The cranial nerves passing through these structures can cause variable symptoms when involved.

The main symptoms seen in the involvement of the posterior part of the orbit are blurring of vision or partial or complete loss of vision depending upon the degree of optic nerve involvement; ptosis due to cranial nerve III involvement; diplopia due to cranial nerve III or VI involvement; ophthalmoplegia due to invasion of cranial nerves III, IV, and VI; sensory loss to the corresponding areas of the cornea and face; increased retrobulbar pressure; loss of tone in the eyeball; and proptosis due to venous congestion in cases of cavernous thrombosis.[15] Among all 193 patients, total distribution of orbital symptoms was as follows: Orbital swelling (53%), ptosis (52%), orbital pain (29%), loss of vision (16.5%), proptosis (11%), epiphora (8%), and diplopia(5%).

A major complication of ROCM is blindness, which can be attributed to both angiomatous and perineural spread. Angioinvasion can cause a central retinal artery or ophthalmic artery infarct, which in turn leads to partial or complete loss of vision; it may also be direct perineural invasion of the optic nerve. At the author's center, about 10 patients had loss of vision as initial presentation.

The disease can either spread from the nose and the orbit to the brain or form skip lesion and involve the brain directly, which is predominantly seen in revision cases. In the authors' experience, of 64 revision cases, 13 showed the above-mentioned pattern of spread.

In cerebral involvement of mucormycosis, intracranial spread occurs via one of the following routes[16–18]:

- Ophthalmic artery.
- *Superior orbital fissure*: Spread via this route may cause sinus thrombosis and internal carotid artery thrombotic occlusion.
- *Cribriform plate*: The spread of the infection to the frontal lobes and to the cavernous sinus occurs via perivascular and perineural channels through the cribriform plate and the orbital apex, respectively.

The main areas of cerebral involvement seen were the temporal and frontal lobes due to direct spread from emissary veins or cavernous sinus.[19] The angioinvasion leads to the formation of intravascular thrombi leading to ischemia and infarction of the brain, including the cerebrum, cerebellum, and brainstem. Diffuse vasculitis causes aneurysm due to weakening of the blood vessel walls. Rupture of the aneurysms causes hematoma formation in subarachnoid and subdural regions and intracranial hemorrhages. The intracranial involvement is depicted by signs of cavernous sinus thrombosis, lethargy, slurred speech, cranial neuropathies, altered mentation, and focal seizures. Diffuse vasculitis in ROCM may lead to meningitis. Brain abscess formation has been evident in chronic cases of ROCM leading to hemiplegia. At the author's center, the order of neurological symptoms experienced by patients were as follows: headache (80%), fever (24.9%), delirium (7.3%), vomiting (7.3%), and seizures (1%). Out of all, 32 patients presented with intracerebral disease, 9 patients with cavernous sinus thrombosis, and one patient with superior orbital apex syndrome.

Another important feature seen in post-COVID-19 mucormycosis was the involvement of bone, mainly the frontal bones and the maxilla. This is mainly due to angioinvasion forming thrombi, which occlude the arterioles supplying the marrow of these bones. It can be seen as a visible swelling or a bony defect that can be seen outside, due to erosion of the involved part. In the authors' experience, 16 patients developed frontal bone erosion with extensive disease. Almost all individuals witnessed involvement of the maxilla in all forms of ROCM and palatal mucormycosis.

Further spread via soft tissue from the bone can result in cutaneous involvement. This is usually seen in very advanced cases. Small erythematous nodules, which were ulcerative and painless, were seen in most cases. Further involvement led to black discoloration and skin necrosis. Out of the 193 patients, only 4 patients who were severely immunocompromised developed cutaneous mucormycosis with advance disease.

Clinical Scenarios

Case 1: A 55-year-old, post-COVID-19 diabetic male presented with right-sided facial swelling and facial pain associated with headache, 15 days following treatment of COVID-19 infection. He did not give history of treatment with steroids or oxygen. On evaluation, MRI of the nose and PNSs with the orbit and brain (postcontrast T1W FS [fat suppressed] and T2W FS) revealed mucosal thickening in the right maxillary sinus with T2 hypointensities, suggestive of fungal infection. Also enhancing soft tissue in the right retromaxillary region abutting the pterygoid muscle was noted. After thorough preoperative evaluation and glycemic control, he underwent a right endoscopic modified Denker's (EMD) procedure with disease clearance from the right infratemporal fossa. Postoperatively, the patient's symptoms reduced and he was discharged on intravenous amphotericin-B. The preoperative disease extent and postoperative clearance are depicted in MR images in **Figs. 4.1** and **4.2**.

Case 2: A 55-year-old, post-COVID-19 diabetic lady presented with left-sided facial pain and ptosis of the left eye, 1 week following the treatment of COVID-19 infection. Vision was unaffected in both eyes. No history of treatment with steroids or oxygen was given. On evaluation, MRI of the nose

and PNSs with the orbit and brain (postcontrast T1W FS and T2W FS) revealed mucosal thickening in the bilateral ethmoidal sinuses with erosion of the left lamina papyracea and inflammation of the medial orbital muscles. She underwent a left EMD with left medial orbital decompression and transcutaneous retro-orbital amphotericin-B. Postoperatively, the patient's left eye ptosis recovered and she was discharged on intravenous amphotericin-B. The preoperative picture, MRI, and postoperative picture are depicted in **Fig. 4.3**.

Case 3: A 45-year-old, post-COVID-19 diabetic female patient presented with severe swelling, pain, proptosis, and loss of vision in the right eye with purulent discharge. She gave history of treatment with intravenous dexamethasone for 1 week during the treatment for COVID-19 infection. The patient also complained of severe frontal headache. On evaluation, MRI of the PNS with the orbit and brain (postcontrast T1W FS and T2W FS) showed severe soft-tissue edema around the right eye with evidence of abscess formation causing proptosis. Orbital muscles appeared edematous and inflamed, and erosion of the lamina papyracea was noted. T2 hypointense shadows were noted in the frontal sinus. She underwent a right eye exenteration and bilateral Draf IIB procedure. The patient improved clinically and was discharged on intravenous amphotericin-B.

Preoperative and postoperative clinical pictures and preoperative MRI are depicted in **Fig. 4.4**.

Case 4: A 43-year-old, post-COVID-19 diabetic woman presented with left-sided headache, toothache, facial swelling,

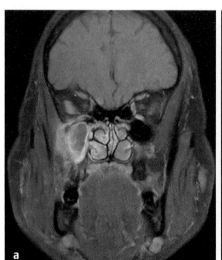 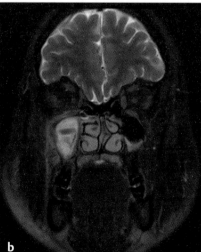 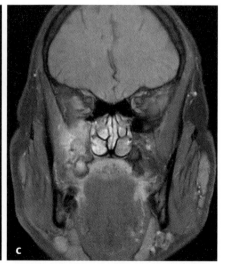

Fig. 4.1 (a) Coronal T1-weighted (T1W) short tau inversion recovery (STIR) postcontrast magnetic resonance imaging (MRI) showing right maxillary sinusitis with T1 nonenhancing areas with surrounding soft-tissue edema. **(b)** Coronal T2-weighted (T2W) STIR image showing right maxillary sinusitis with clear-cut T2 hypointense area suggestive of invasive fungal sinusitis. **(c)** Coronal T1W postcontrast MRI showing the right infratemporal fossa (ITF) hypointense areas surrounded by enhancing soft tissue suggestive of viable inflammatory tissue.

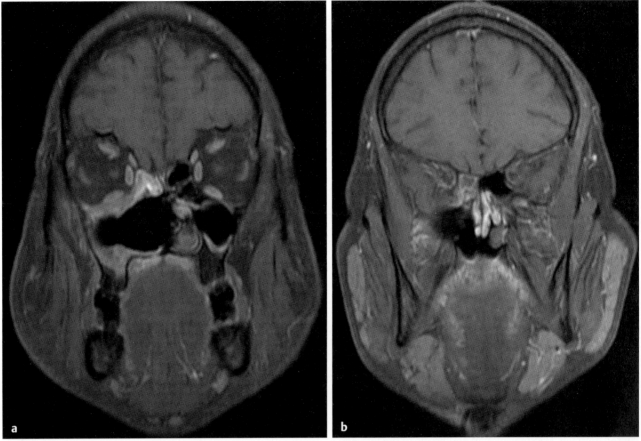

Fig. 4.2 **(a)** Coronal T1-weighted (T1W) short tau inversion recovery (STIR) noncontrast postoperative magnetic resonance imaging (MRI) showing right Denker's cavity with no evidence of disease. **(b)** Coronal T1W STIR noncontrast postoperative MRI showing complete disease clearance from the right infratemporal fossa (ITF).

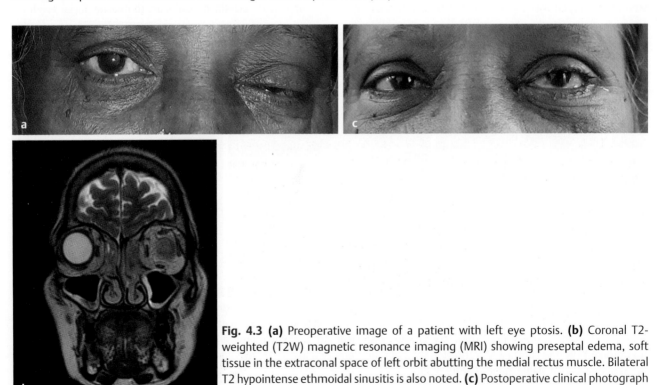

Fig. 4.3 **(a)** Preoperative image of a patient with left eye ptosis. **(b)** Coronal T2-weighted (T2W) magnetic resonance imaging (MRI) showing preseptal edema, soft tissue in the extraconal space of left orbit abutting the medial rectus muscle. Bilateral T2 hypointense ethmoidal sinusitis is also noted. **(c)** Postoperative clinical photograph of the same patient. Note that the left eye proptosis has recovered

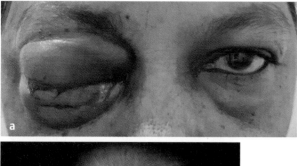
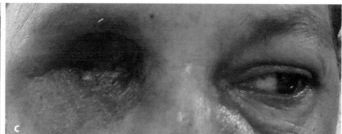
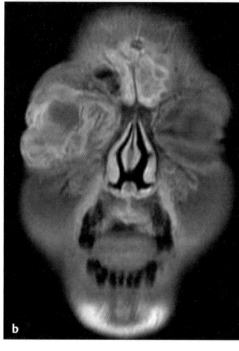

Fig. 4.4 **(a)** Preoperative image of a patient with right eye proptosis, edema, and loss of vision. **(b)** Coronal T1-weighted (T1W) magnetic resonance imaging (MRI) showing erosion of the right medial orbital wall with abscess formation infiltrating the intraconal and extraconal spaces, causing severe proptosis and periorbital edema. **(c)** Postoperative clinical photograph of the same patient, following right eye exenteration.

and facial pain. She was treated with inhalational oxygen by mask for 1 week during treatment for COVID-19 infection. The patient was diagnosed with post-COVID-19 mucormycosis and was operated at an outside hospital twice (details not available). On evaluation, MRI of the PNS with the orbit and brain (postcontrast T1W FS and T2W FS) showed left premaxillary soft-tissue edema with left alveolar cortical erosion. The bilateral maxillary sinus showed mucosal thickening. Reduced uptake of contrast in the region of the left pterygoid wedge and the greater wing of the sphenoid (GWS) was noted along with fat stranding of the left infratemporal fossa. The patient underwent a bilateral EMD procedure with left transpterygoid drilling and disease clearance from the left GWS. Left-sided sublabial palatectomy with preservation of palatal mucosa was done. Pre- and postoperative MRI with postoperative clinical image is depicted in **Fig. 4.5**. Note that the left EMD with partial palatectomy has caused a cosmetic deformity on the left side for the patient.

Case 5: A 43-year-old, post-COVID-19 diabetic male patient presented with complaints of loosening of teeth in the left upper jaw, palatal ulcer, toothache, and left-sided facial pain. Symptoms commenced 20 days after treatment for COVID-19

infection. He gave history of treatment with intravenous methyl prednisolone and inhalational oxygen. The patient was diagnosed with post-COVID-19 mucormycosis and was operated at an outside hospital twice (palatal debridement with endoscopic sinus surgery) and treated with a cumulative dose of 6 g of liposomal amphotericin-B. On evaluation, MRI of the PNS with the orbit and brain (postcontrast T1W FS and T2W FS) showed gross erosion of the left half of the alveolar bone with inflammatory edema of the left premaxillary soft tissues. T1W hypointensity was noted in bilateral pterygoid wedges, and bony erosion was seen in the clival cortex. The patient underwent left EMD procedure with dissection of the infratemporal fossa, and transclival and transpterygoid drilling with clearance of the bony disease from the left GWS. Left sublabial palatectomy with debridement of the palatal mucosa was also done. He underwent a wide middle meatal antrostomy and complete sphenoethmoidectomy on the right side. The patient was discharged in a stable condition and he received 2 g of liposomal amphotericin-B in the post-op period under strict monitoring of renal parameters. Preoperative MRI, clinical photograph, and postoperative MRI showing complete disease clearance are shown in **Fig. 4.6**.

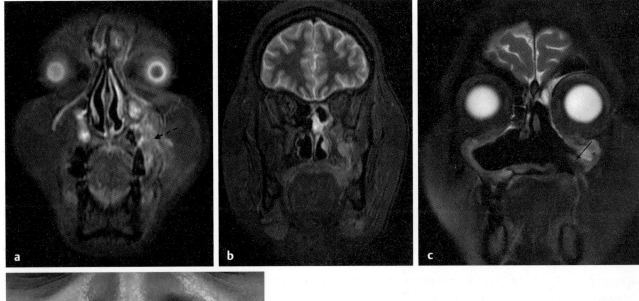

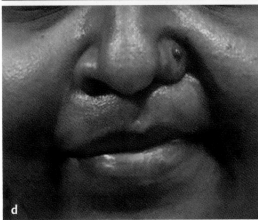

Fig. 4.5 (a) Coronal T1-weighted (T1W) magnetic resonance imaging (MRI) showing the left maxillary sinusitis eroding the left alveolar surface of the maxilla (*broken arrow*) with mixed signal intensity of soft tissue and inflammation of the left premaxilla. Hypointense shadows are noted in the frontal sinus. **(b)** Coronal T2-weighted (T2W) MRI showing reduced uptake in the region of the left pterygoid wedge along with fat stranding of the left infratemporal fossa (ITF). **(c)** Postoperative T2W MRI showing bilateral Denker's cavity. Note the left palatal defect. **(d)** Postoperative clinical photograph of the patient. Note the cosmetic deformity at the left ala.

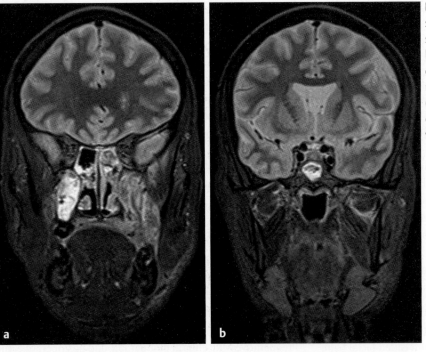

Fig. 4.6 (a) Coronal T2-weighted (T2W) short tau inversion recovery (STIR) image showing bilateral maxillary sinusitis with hypointense areas in the left maxilla eroding the alveolar surface of the maxilla, with premaxillary inflammation. **(b)** Coronal T2W STIR image showing osteonecrosis of bilateral pterygoid wedge and clivus. *(Continued)*

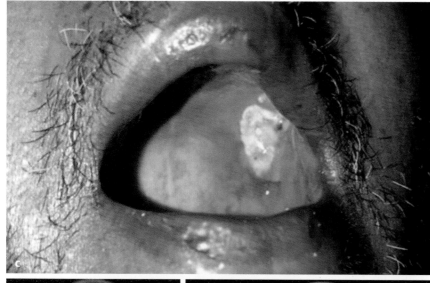

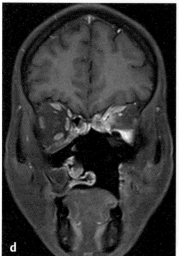
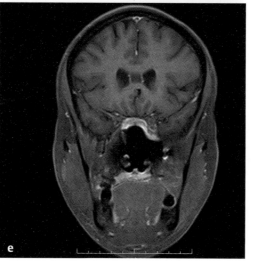

Fig. 4.6 *(Continued)* **(c)** Clinical photograph of a patient showing necrosis of palatal mucosa on the left side. **(d)** Coronal T1-weighted (T1W) postoperative magnetic resonance imaging (MRI) image showing left Denker's cavity. Note the gross palatal defect. No evidence of disease is noted. **(e)** Coronal T1W postoperative MR image showing clearance of bilateral infratemporal fossa (ITF), pterygoid wedge, and left greater wing of the sphenoid (GWS).

Case 6: A 61-year-old, post-COVID-19 diabetic male patient presented with complaints of complete ptosis of the left eye associated with headache. There was no history of loss of vision. He was under home isolation during the period of COVID-19 infection, and was not treated with oral or intravenous steroids. On evaluation, MRI of the PNS with the orbit and brain (postcontrast T1W FS and T2W FS) showed bilateral pan sinusitis with T2W hypointensity. Homogenous enhancement was noted in the orbital muscles at the orbital apex along with perineural inflammation along the optic nerve, suggestive of superior orbital fissure syndrome. The patient underwent a bilateral EMD with bilateral complete sphenoethmoidectomy, right transpterygoid drilling, and clearance of the right superior orbital fissure. The patient improved clinically in the immediate postoperative period, but ptosis did not recover. Preoperative clinical photograph and MR image are shown in **Fig. 4.7**.

Case 7: A 49-year-old, post-COVID-19 diabetic man who was diagnosed with mucormycosis, and operated in an outside hospital thrice for the same (functional endoscopic sinus surgery [FESS] and right lateral rhinotomy), presented to us with complaints of right-sided facial swelling, facial pain, and intractable headache. A cumulative dose of 7 g of liposomal amphotericin was given to him previously. On evaluation, MRI of the PNS with the orbit and brain (postcontrast T1W FS and T2W FS) showed involvement of the right maxilla, GWS, lateral wall, medial wall and inferior wall of the right orbit, right temporal fossa, temporalis muscle, zygoma, and sphenoid sinus. Multidetector computed tomography (MDCT) of the PNS with 3D facial reconstruction showed extensive erosion of the right floor of the orbit, zygoma, remnant maxilla, pterygoid wedge, and GWS. The patient underwent right EMD procedure, right endoscopic completion maxillectomy, transpterygoid drilling, and clearance of

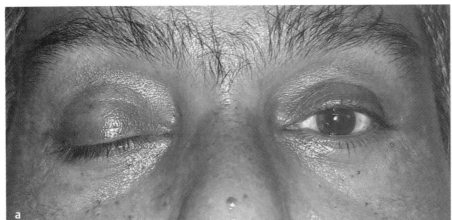

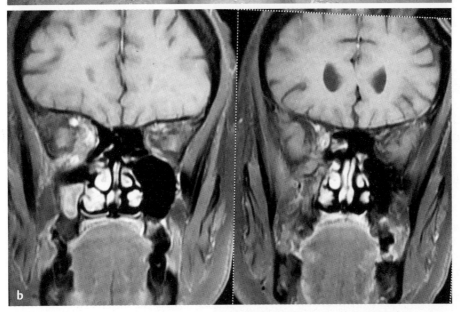

Fig. 4.7 (a) Clinical photograph of a patient showing right eye ptosis (ophthalmoplegia). **(b)** Coronal T1-weighted (T1W) short tau inversion recovery (STIR) image showing homogenous enhancement in the orbital muscles at the orbital cone along with perineural inflammation along the optic nerve.

the pterygoid wedge and GWS. The V2 and V3 branches of the trigeminal nerve and vidian nerve were found necrosed and was resected. A right hemicoronal incision was made, the right temporalis muscle was debrided partially, and the right lateral orbital wall was cleared. He also underwent a right temporalis muscle flap rotation to close the defect in the right lateral orbital wall and zygoma. The patient was treated postoperatively with 3.5 g of intravenous liposomal amphotericin-B. He improved clinically and was discharged in a stable condition. Preoperative clinical photograph of the patient, MRI, MDCT, and postoperative MRI showing complete clearance are shown in **Fig. 4.8**.

Case 8: A 39-year-old, post-COVID-19 non-diabetic man who was diagnosed to have sinonasal mucormycosis presented to us with complaints of midline frontal swelling, severe headache, and facial puffiness. He had undergone a

surgery elsewhere (endoscopic sinonasal debridement). The patient was treated with remdesivir, intravenous methyl prednisolone, and inhalational oxygen during treatment for COVID-19 infection. On evaluation, MRI of the PNS with the orbit and brain (postcontrast T1W FS and T2W FS) showed gross involvement of the left pterygoid wedge, GWS, and infratemporal fossa with extensive cortical bony erosion of both anterior and posterior frontal tables. MDCT also showed evidence of frontal table necrosis, with erosion of the GWS. He underwent a left EMD procedure with transpterygoid drilling and clearance of the GWS. This was followed by a bi-coronal approach and complete drilling and clearance of frontal tables. The underlying anterior cranial dura appeared normal after clearance of diseased bone. Preoperative clinical photographs with MRI and MDCT are depicted in **Fig. 4.9**.

A clinical photograph of a patient with cutaneous mucormycosis is depicted in **Fig. 4.10**.

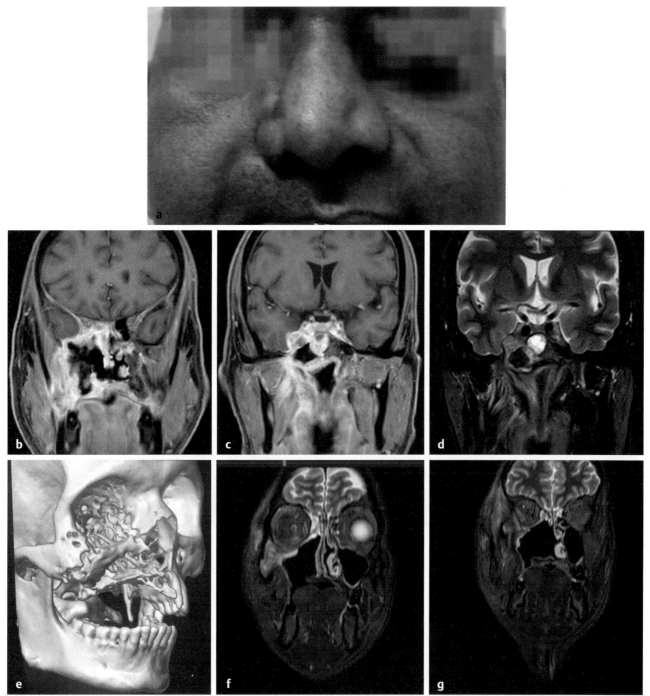

Fig. 4.8 **(a)** Clinical photograph of a patient showing right lateral rhinotomy scar. **(b)** Coronal T1-weighted (T1W) MRI short tau inversion recovery (STIR) image showing postoperative changes in the right maxilla with right palatal defect. **(c)** Coronal T1W STIR image showing osteonecrosis of the right pterygoid wedge with hyperintensities involving the clivus and bilateral paraclival carotid arteries. **(d)** Coronal T2-weighted (T2W) STIR image showing gross osteonecrotic focus at the right pterygoid wedge. **(e)** Multidetector computed tomography (MDCT) paranasal sinus (PNS) with 3D CT reconstruction showing extensive destruction of the floor of the orbit, zygoma, pterygoid wedge, and lateral orbital wall. **(f)** Coronal T2W STIR postoperative magnetic resonance imaging (MRI) showing right Denker's cavity with no evidence of disease. Note the right temporalis muscle rotation flap. **(g)** Coronal T2W STIR postoperative MRI showing surgical defect in the region of the zygoma, temporal fossa, and lateral orbital wall.

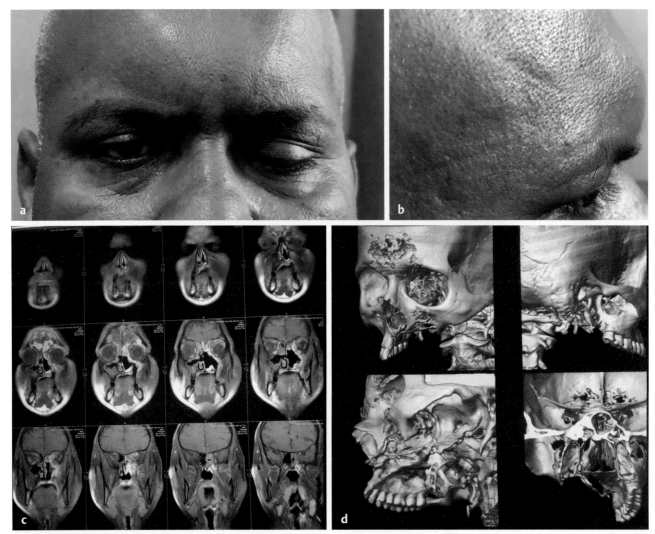

Fig. 4.9 (a) Preoperative clinical photograph of a patient showing frontal swelling. **(b)** Lateral view of the patient showing marked frontal swelling. **(c)** Coronal T1-weighted (T1W) images showing marked frontal hypointense shadows suggestive of invasive fungal sinusitis with erosion of the frontal tables and crista galli. **(d)** Multidetector computed tomography (MDCT) paranasal sinus (PNS) with 3D CT reconstruction showing extensive destruction of the frontal tables.

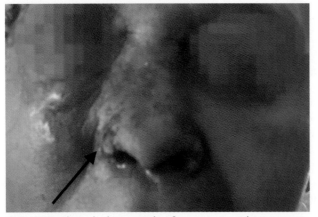

Fig. 4.10 Clinical photograph of a patient with cutaneous mucormycosis.

References

1. Onerci M, Gürsel B, Hosal S, Gülekon N, Gököz A. Rhinocerebral mucormycosis with extension to the cavernous sinus. A case report. Rhinology 1991;29(4):321–324

2. Schwartz JN, Donnelly EH, Klintworth GK. Ocular and orbital phycomycosis. Surv Ophthalmol 1977;22(1):3–28

3. Agrawal R, Yeldandi A, Savas H, Parekh ND, Lombardi PJ, Hart EM. Pulmonary mucormycosis: risk factors, radiologic findings, and pathologic correlation. Radiographics 2020; 40(3):656–666

4. Sravani T, Uppin SG, Uppin MS, Sundaram C. Rhinocerebral mucormycosis: pathology revisited with emphasis on perineural spread. Neurol India 2014;62(4):383–386

5. González Martín-Moro J, López-Arcas Calleja JM, Burgueño García M, Cebrián Carretero JL, García Rodríguez J. Rhinoorbitocerebral mucormycosis: a case report and literature review. Med Oral Patol Oral Cir Bucal 2008;13(12): E792–E795

6. Teixeira CA, Medeiros PB, Leushner P, Almeida F. Rhinocerebral mucormycosis: literature review apropos of a rare entity. BMJ Case Rep 2013;2013:bcr 2012008552

7. Shatriah I, Mohd-Amin N, Tuan-Jaafar TN, Khanna RK, Yunus R, Madhavan M. Rhino-orbito-cerebral mucormycosis in an immunocompetent patient: case report and review of literature. Middle East Afr J Ophthalmol 2012;19(2): 258–261

8. Sen M, Lahane S, Lahane TP, Parekh R, Honavar SG. Mucor in a viral land: a tale of two pathogens. Indian J Ophthalmol 2021;69(2):244–252

9. Swain SK. Sinonasal mucormycosis with an unusual involvement of palate. Apollo Medicine. 2022;19(3):177–179

10. Hada M, Gupta P, Bagarhatta M, et al. Orbital magnetic resonance imaging profile and clinicoradiological correlation in COVID-19-associated rhino-orbital-cerebral mucormycosis: a single-center study of 270 patients from North India. Indian J Ophthalmol 2022;70(2):641–648

11. Lunge SB, Sajjan V, Pandit AM, Patil VB. Rhinocerebrocutaneous mucormycosis caused by *Mucor* species: a rare causation. Indian Dermatol Online J 2015;6(3):189–192

12. Kashkouli MB, Abdolalizadeh P, Oghazian M, Hadi Y, Karimi N, Ghazizadeh M. Outcomes and factors affecting them in patients with rhino-orbito-cerebral mucormycosis. Br J Ophthalmol 2019;103(10):1460–1465

13. Gappy C, Archer SM, Barza M. Orbital cellulitis. UpToDate. Accessed November 17, 2016 at http://www.uptodate com/contents/orbitalcellulitis. 2013

14. Rapidis AD. Orbitomaxillary mucormycosis (zygomycosis) and the surgical approach to treatment: perspectives from a maxillofacial surgeon. Clin Microbiol Infect 2009; 15(Suppl 5):98–102

15. Gamaletsou MN, Sipsas NV, Roilides E, Walsh TJ. Rhino-orbital-cerebral mucormycosis. Curr Infect Dis Rep 2012; 14(4):423–434

16. Turunc T, Demiroglu YZ, Aliskan H, Colakoglu S, Arslan H. Eleven cases of mucormycosis with atypical clinical manifestations in diabetic patients. Diabetes Res Clin Pract 2008; 82(2):203–208

17. Thajeb P, Thajeb T, Dai D. Fatal strokes in patients with rhino-orbito-cerebral mucormycosis and associated vasculopathy. Scand J Infect Dis 2004;36(9):643–648

18. Ma J, Jia R, Li J, et al. Retrospective clinical study of eighty-one cases of intracranial mucormycosis. J Glob Infect Dis 2015;7(4):143–150

19. Mantadakis E, Samonis G. Clinical presentation of zygomycosis. Clin Microbiol Infect 2009;15(Suppl 5):15–20

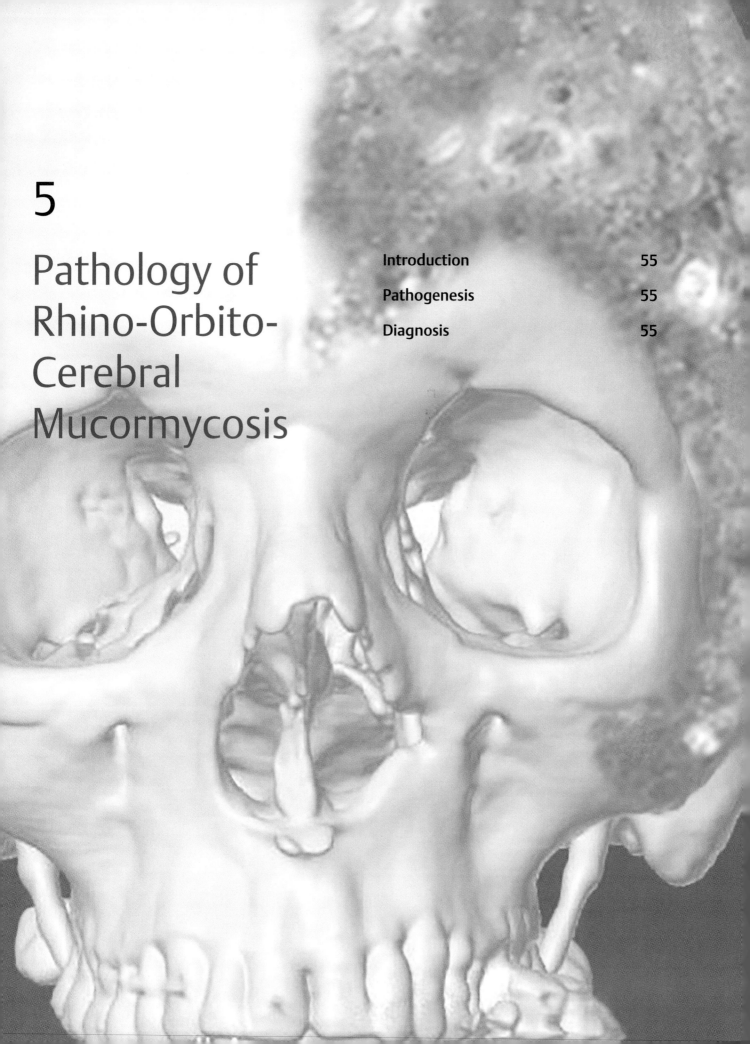

5

Pathology of Rhino-Orbito-Cerebral Mucormycosis

Chapter 5

Pathology of Rhino-Orbito-Cerebral Mucormycosis

Rath P.K. and Lekshmy R. Kurup

Introduction

Rhino-orbito-cerebral mucormycosis is a potentially lethal infection, which has been on rise in the current post-COVID-19 scenario, especially in immunocompromised individuals. In addition to the low oxygen concentration, poor glycemic control, compromised airway, and high serum ferritin level add to the morbidity.

Pathogenesis

Mucor is a fungus which is omnipresent and does not affect or invade the tissues of normal individuals.

Patients who are at high risk to develop invasive mucormycosis are[1]:

- Patients with underlying cancer or on anticancer chemotherapy both causing immunosuppression.
- Patients with HIV/AIDS.
- Patients who have diabetes or undergoing dialysis for chronic renal failure.
- Patients on immunosuppressive therapy—organ transplanted cases or patients with autoimmune disorders.
- Patients with severe malnutrition and hypoproteinemia as in cirrhosis and hepatic/renal failure.

Entry of Organism

The entry of fungus is via inhalation, traumatic inoculation, or ingestion, of which inhalation is the most common. It does not cause infection in an immunocompetent person. However, in an immunocompromised patient, inhaled mucor enters the nasal cavity in a spore form and in an acidic medium with low oxygen concentration the spores germinate into hyphae. The neutrophils available locally are less effective against the hyphae and without any resistance the hyphae grow into the tissues specifically targeting the blood vessels causing endothelial damage forming multiple thrombi and obstructing the blood flow causing severe ischemic necrosis of the arterial supply distally. Interactions between cells lining the blood vessels and the fungi form a key step in the pathogenesis of the disease.[2] This further increases hypoxia favoring more branching of hyphae and unchecked growth of mucor which enters the bone marrow spaces. The involvement of ethmoid sinus leads to orbital involvement, and intracranial extension occurs when cribriform plate and perivascular channels are involved.[3]

The following factors in host favor the growth of the fungus: Ketoreductase enzyme which assists the fungus in utilizing ketone bodies to grow in acidic environment, decreased inflammatory response due to immunocompromised state, and rhizoferrin produced by the fungus which helps in its iron-binding capacity.[4]

Diagnosis

To reach a conclusive diagnosis, fungal hyphae need to be directly identified under microscope or the organism must be isolated in culture of tissue specimen. Biopsy or tissue sampling of the patient must be done by the clinician for the following:

- Microscopy (fungal smear).
- Fungal culture.
- Frozen sections.
- Histopathology.
- Routine/Microwave processing.
- Molecular study.

Diagnostic Tests

Microscopy

Direct microscopy in a clinical setting allows a clinician the advantage of rapid diagnosis if the fungal load is adequate. Mucorales hyphae are easy to find; they are aseptate with thin irregular borders and obtuse angle branching or pauciseptate. A rapid presumptive diagnosis with potassium hydroxide (KOH) mount allows early commencement of antifungal therapy and therefore can be lifesaving.[5]

Fungal smear for KOH mount (procedure): Tissue sample (transported in saline) may be obtained by nasal endoscopy or from a palatal or nasal smear. Specimen is placed on a glass slide and 20% KOH is added on it and a cover glass is placed. Excess solution is blotted, and the specimen is examined under microscope in low power and, if fungi is suspected, changed to high power magnification (400X).[6] The appearance of the fungi is as depicted in **Fig. 5.1.**

Various other microscopic techniques may be used to identify fungi in culture medium. But these are time

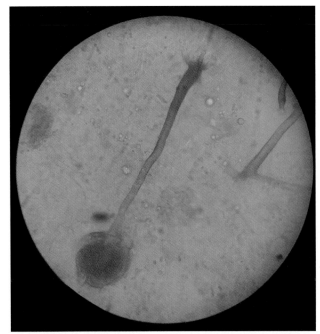

Fig. 5.1 Potassium hydroxide (KOH) wet mount showing the presence of fungal hyphae.

consuming since they require the growth of fungus in the culture initially.

Lactophenol cotton blue (LPCB) is one such staining reagent. It has three components, namely, lactic acid which conserves the fungal architecture, phenol which is a disinfectant, and cotton blue which gives the blue color to the fungi. The fungal element from culture is gently teased into a thin preparation using a nichrome inoculating wire and then placed on a glass slide and a drop of LPCB is added over it.[7] Microscopic appearance of the fungus is shown in **Fig. 5.2**.

Fungal Culture

Mucorales grow swiftly and abundantly on Sabouraud dextrose agar (SDA) and potato dextrose agar at 25 to 30°C. A micro-aerophilic environment enhances growth because it simulates infarcted tissue. These fungal elements are easily bruised because of the brittle aseptate hyphae, which explains the negative culture report but positive histopathological study. The distinctive structures for species identification are presence of sporangiophores, shape of columella, presence or absence of apophysis and rhizoids, and shape and size of zygospores.[8] The appearance on culture is depicted in **Fig. 5.3**. The authors would like to ascertain that the clinicians should always communicate with the microbiologists and inform they are expecting a fungal growth, lest the growth might be discarded as a contaminant.

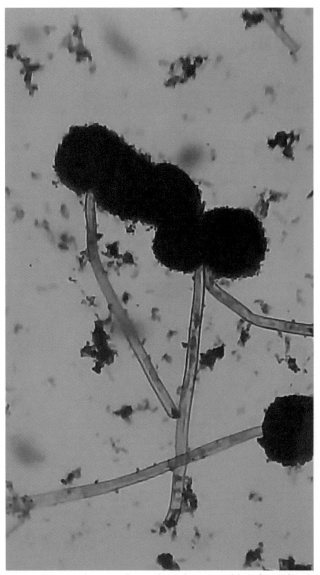

Fig. 5.2 Fungal stain (lactophenol cotton blue [LPCB]) on cultured growth showing fungal hyphae (400X magnification).

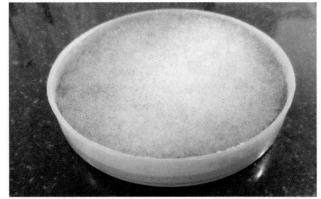

Fig. 5.3 Cotton wool white colonies of mucor grown in Sabouraud dextrose agar (SDA).

Frozen Section

This is a specific and sensitive modality for intraoperative confirmation of the disease and helps in deciding resection margins.[9] Tissue from suspected areas including bone should be sent for frozen sectioning which can give a positive report within 30 minutes (**Fig. 5.4**). This allows radical surgical excision and is time saving. Frozen section report is always confirmed by histopathological studies.

Histopathology

Tissues biopsied from sinonasal areas would invariably show presence of marked necrosis and characteristic features of angioinvasion with mucosal ulceration and exudates with sheets of polymorphs and lymphocytes (**Fig. 5.5**). There may or may not be presence of epithelioid cell granulomas with multinucleated giant cells (seen in chronic forms). Fungal hyphae may be easily identified at low power magnification, but to confirm the branching pattern high power magnification is used. Mucorales have typical aseptate or pauciseptate broad papery hyphae with irregular borders and obtuse angle branching. The fungal hyphae characteristically have an affinity to invade blood vessels and thereby tend to obstruct blood flow and cause ischemic necrosis involving all the tissues (**Fig. 5.6a, b**). They also invade the woven bone and grow within the marrow spaces. The authors have noticed on multiple occasions when they had failed to demonstrate fungi in the sinuses and turbinate but found them invariably within the marrow spaces. This finding was most often seen in patients previously treated with amphotericin-B (**Fig. 5.7a, b**).

Special stains like Gomori's methenamine silver (GMS) highlights the fungus very well in the tissue sections (**Figs. 5.8a, b** and **5.9**). GMS stain is the ideal choice on a tissue section, although the routine hematoxylin and eosin stain can pick up the fungi easily. Sometimes intracellular fungi inside the giant cells are not demonstrable by routine sections.

Periodic acid Schiff (PAS) staining is yet another stain that was used previously, but it is no more in use at our center.

Microwave Processing

Using the microwave oven, the tissue processing time of 16 hours is reduced to just 2 hours, followed by blocking and cutting sections for routine histopathological examination. Advantage is rapid report availability, and the blocks and slides can be archived and documented. This is used when frozen section facility is not available, but the surgeon still needs a rapid diagnosis.

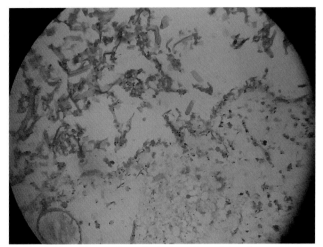

Fig. 5.4 Frozen section depicting fungal hyphae within a blood vessel.

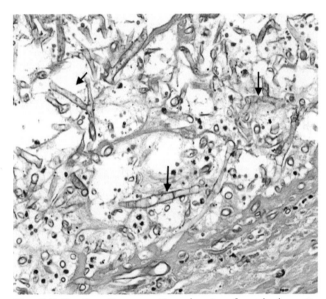

Fig. 5.5 Routine tissue section showing fungal elements (*black arrows*) under 400X magnification using hematoxylin and eosin (H&E) stain.

Molecular Studies

All the mucorales share a common DNA, the detection of which can lead to the molecular diagnosis of zygomycosis. These molecular studies have upgraded the diagnosis and management of this angioinvasive fungal disease.

A study published by Hata et al describes the innovative real-time polymerase chain reaction (RT-PCR) test for the detection of Zygomycets in culture and tissue specimens.[10] The sensitivity and specificity of the test in formalin fixed tissues were 56 and 100%, respectively. The total turnaround time of the test was 4 hours.

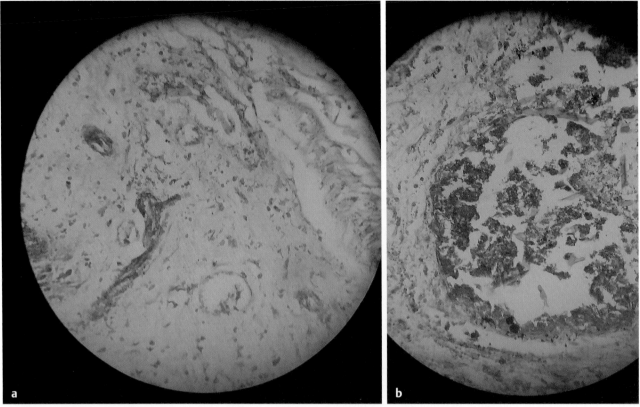

Fig. 5.6 (a, b) Blood vessels invaded by fungal hyphae (100X and 400X magnification, respectively).

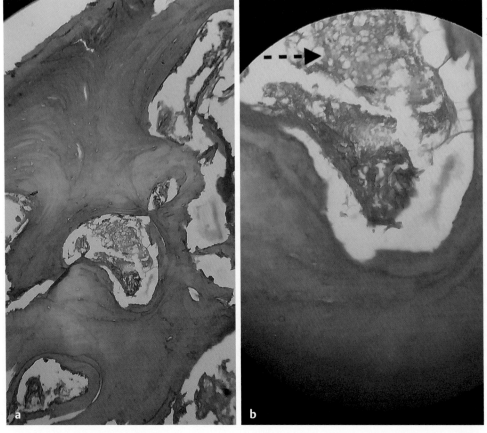

Fig. 5.7 (a, b) Bony trabeculae with marrow spaces. Note the necrosed marrow (black arrow) with fungal infiltration (magnification 100X and 400X, respectively).

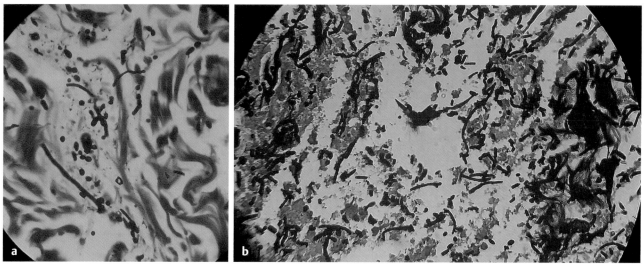

Fig. 5.8 (a, b) Fungal stain (Gomori's methenamine silver [GMS]) on tissue sections showing fungal hyphae (400X).

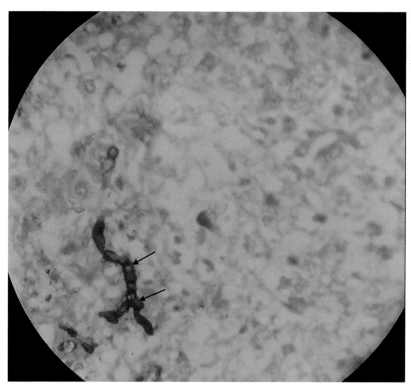

Fig. 5.9 Fungal stain (Gomori's methenamine silver [GMS]) showing fungal hyphae. Note the irregular fragile borders (*black arrows*) of the fungus.

The fresh tissues or formalin fixed paraffinized tissues can be processed for identification of the specific mucor DNA by amplifying it million-fold, making it easier to diagnose when the fungi are absent in the smears or are less in number in the superficial tissues. A cycle threshold (Ct) value of < 35 is taken as positive for detection of mucor DNA. **Fig. 5.10** shows the presence of mucor DNA which has been amplified along with positive control.

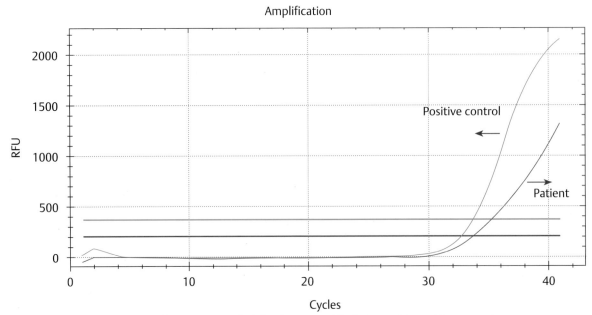

Fig. 5.10 Study showing presence of mucor DNA which has been amplified along with positive control.

References

1. Sharma A, Goel A. Mucormycosis: risk factors, diagnosis, treatments, and challenges during COVID-19 pandemic. Folia Microbiol (Praha) 2022;67(3):363–387

2. Baldin C, Ibrahim AS. Molecular mechanisms of mucormycosis—the bitter and the sweet. PLoS Pathog 2017;13(8):e1006408

3. Singh VP, Bansal C, Kaintura M. Sinonasal mucormycosis: A to Z. Indian J Otolaryngol Head Neck Surg 2019;71(3, Suppl 3):1962–1971

4. Ibrahim AS, Spellberg B, Walsh TJ, Kontoyiannis DP. Pathogenesis of mucormycosis. Clin Infect Dis 2012; 54(Suppl 1):S16–S22

5. Mohanty A, Gupta P, Arathi K, et al. Evaluation of direct examination, culture, and histopathology in the diagnosis of mucormycosis: reiterating the role of KOH mount for early diagnosis. Cureus 2021;13(11):e19455

6. Ponka D, Baddar F. Microscopic potassium hydroxide preparation. Can Fam Physician 2014;60(1):57

7. Koneman EW, Allen SD, Janda WM, Schreckenberger PC, Winn WC. Diagnostic microbiology. The nonfermentative gram-negative bacilli. Philedelphia: Lippincott-Raven Publishers. 1997:253-320

8. Lackner M, Caramalho R, Lass-Flörl C. Laboratory diagnosis of mucormycosis: current status and future perspectives. Future Microbiol 2014;9(5):683–695

9. Hofman V, Castillo L, Bétis F, Guevara N, Gari-Toussaint M, Hofman P. Usefulness of frozen section in rhinocerebral mucormycosis diagnosis and management. Pathology 2003;35(3):212–216

10. Hata DJ, Buckwalter SP, Pritt BS, Roberts GD, Wengenack NL. Real-time PCR method for detection of zygomycetes. J Clin Microbiol 2008;46(7):2353–2358

6

Orbitotomy and Other Orbital Interventions in Rhino-Orbito-Cerebral Mucormycosis

Chapter 6

Orbitotomy and Other Orbital Interventions in Rhino-Orbito-Cerebral Mucormycosis

Raghuraj Hegde and Akshay Gopinathan Nair

Introduction

Mucormycosis is known to be a life-threatening fungal infection caused by the opportunistic fungi, belonging to the order Mucorales. Mucormycosis is pathognomically angioinvasive and is seen primarily in patients with uncontrolled diabetes mellitus (DM). Other predisposing conditions include systemic corticosteroid and other immunosuppressive drug therapy, generalized immunodeficiency, hematological malignancies, post–stem cell and solid organ transplantation, solid organ malignancies, and iron overload, among others.[1] In 2021, India saw an exponential rise in the incidence of rhino-orbito-cerebral mucormycosis (ROCM), especially in patients with a history of recent infection of coronavirus disease 2019 (COVID-19).[2–5] The number of COVID-19-associated mucormycosis (CAM) was very high in India in the period from September to December 2020 and from April to August 2021. Large case series and reports on CAM have been published describing the clinical features, management, and outcomes of CAM with up to 6 months of follow-up in survivors.[6–8] The second wave of the COVID-19 pandemic in India caused a huge surge in mucormycosis in many Indian hospitals.[9]

Outcomes can be improved manifold by early diagnosis. Early diagnosis can be achieved by better awareness among the public regarding symptoms and high index of suspicion regarding clinical signs among physicians. Once diagnosis is confirmed by appropriate modalities, initiation of surgical and medical treatments by a multidisciplinary team can be started, thereby reducing both morbidity and mortality.[1,10] It has been the experience of the authors that the formation of a mucormycosis team consisting of different subspecialties gives the best outcomes for patients suffering from this disease. This chapter will highlight the orbital aspects of ROCM and role of an orbital surgeon in the multidisciplinary mucormycosis team.

Clinical Features

The initial symptoms of mucormycosis usually start with symptoms that are consistent with acute or chronic sinusitis: Nasal stuffiness, nasal discharge (blood), blood-tinged mucous discharge, rhinorrhea, headaches, fever, and malaise. Orbital involvement is indicated with signs of preseptal cellulitis (eyelid edema/ecchymoses, periorbital tissue swelling, and conjunctival congestion). Postseptal orbital involvement is inflammatory changes like conjunctival chemosis, proptosis, extraocular muscle restriction, cranial neuropathies (namely, CNs III, V-1, V-2, and/or VI secondary to cavernous sinus involvement/thrombosis and sometimes even CN VII), and loss of vision (CN II: compressive and vascular causes). Extraocular motility is more indicative of orbital involvement than loss of vision as vision loss can also be due to vascular causes (central retinal arterial occlusion [CRAO], central retinal venous occlusion [CRVO], and ophthalmic artery occlusion [OAO]). Involvement of the contralateral eye can be a sign that cavernous sinus is involved. Subsequent development of other neurological signs such as cognitive behavioral changes, seizures, or other focal neurological deficits may be an indication of intracranial extension of the infection[1,10,11] (**Table 6.1**).

Pathways of Spread of Mucormycosis into Orbit

Typically, the fungal spores are inhaled into the nasal cavity and paranasal sinuses. Following this, the fungi cause necrotizing vasculitis of the nasal mucosa and adjoining sinuses. This typically is seen as patches of necrosis in the nose, which can rapidly extend into adjacent structures. This occurs due to perivascular infection, perineural disease spread, or direct invasion by the fungi into the surrounding soft tissue, causing suppurative arteritis, vascular thrombosis, and eventual infarction.[12,13]

This direct extension of the disease across anatomical spaces is by bone destruction, by spreading across natural bony defects, along natural pathways such as the nasolacrimal ducts, lymphatics, and neurovascular bundles.[14] It was traditionally thought that ROCM spreads from the nose into the paranasal sinuses and then medially into the orbit, then gradually extending into the orbital apex, followed by intracranial spread.[11] This is, however, an oversimplified

Table 6.1 Clinical features of mucormycosis

Nasal and sinus	Ophthalmic	Neurological
Nasal stuffiness Nasal discharge: Mucoid, purulent, blood tinged, and black Epistaxis Foul smell Nasal mucosal erythema, purple or bluish discoloration, ischemia, and eschar	Eyelid and facial edema Eyelid or periocular discoloration: Purple or bluish or black eschar Chemosis Proptosis Sudden ptosis Sudden loss of vision: Direct optic nerve compression, vascular: CRAO, CRVO, and OAO Ocular motility restrictions: Mild restriction to total external ophthalmoplegia	Facial pain: Orbit, paranasal sinus, dental, and headache Facial paresthesia, anesthesia in areas supplied by sensory cranial nerve V: Infraorbital anesthesia particularly common Altered sensorium Isolated or multiple cranial nerve palsies: II–VII

Abbreviations: CRAO, central retinal arterial occlusion; CRVO, central retinal venous occlusion; OAO, ophthalmic artery occlusion.

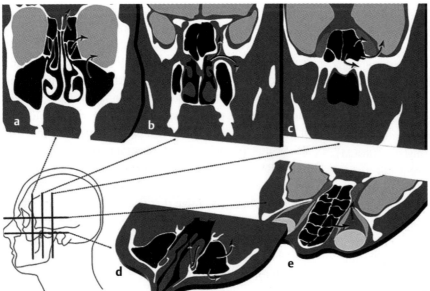

Fig. 6.1 Pathways of spread of mucormycosis to and from the orbit. **(a)** Direct spread from the ethmoid and maxillary sinuses into the orbit or intracranial compartment. **(b)** The pterygopalatine fossa is the bridge at the skull base, where nasal pathology spreads into the infratemporal fossa, into the orbit and cavernous sinus. **(c)** Sphenoid sinus disease may extend into the cavernous sinus, brain, and skull base. **(d)** The disease may extend from the maxillary sinus into the facial and retroantral soft tissue and also along the nasolacrimal duct. **(e)** Intraorbital disease may spread into the orbital apex and cavernous sinus. (Reproduced with permission from Sreshta et al.[14])

schema as newer evidence has shown that there are multiple anatomical routes of spread of the disease. There have been cases where the nasal mucosa appears healthy, and the sinuses show radiological evidence of disease. Therefore, the routes of spread of ROCM (**Fig. 6.1**) can be summarized as follows[14,15]:

- Direct spread from the ethmoid and maxillary sinuses into the orbit or intracranial compartment.
- Spread from the pterygopalatine fossa in the infratemporal fossa and the cavernous sinus, or into the inferior orbital fissure and the orbit.
- Extension of the disease from the sphenoid sinus into the adjoining structures such as the cavernous sinus, brain, and skull base.
- Spread from the maxillary sinus into facial tissue planes, retroantral soft tissue, and along the nasolacrimal duct and subsequently into the orbit.
- Orbital disease extends posteriorly to involve the orbital apex, the cavernous sinus, and the intracranial space.

Role of Imaging in Decision-Making

The role of imaging in the management of mucormycosis is extremely important. As discussed earlier, the disease essentially begins in the nasal cavity and the paranasal sinuses, and gradually spreads into the orbit and the intracranial space. Therefore, aggressive endoscopic debridement of the nasal and the paranasal sinuses is crucial along with control of diabetes, administration of systemic antifungal medication, and reversal of immunosuppression. However, once the disease has spread into the orbit, surgical intervention is often needed. The different treatment strategies for the management of orbital extension of mucormycosis include orbital debridement, orbital exenteration, and transcutaneous retrobulbar amphotericin-B (TRAMB) injections.[16] Other used treatment modalities include local irrigation of the affected sites with amphotericin-B (AMB) and surgical packing of the orbit and the sinuses with amphotericin-B-soaked gauze.[16]

It is here that imaging plays a significant role because it is through the interpretation of the radiological investigations that the clinician can decide which treatment modality is indicated in that case. The most commonly employed investigations for assessment and management of patients with ROCM are magnetic resonance imaging (MRI) and computed tomography (CT) scans of the orbit, brain, and paranasal sinuses. CT scan helps assess the bony anatomy as well as the integrity of the orbital structures such as the globe and extraocular muscles. CT scans, however, cannot differentiate between viable and necrotic/devitalized tissue within the orbit. Therefore, MRI with contrast remains the radiological investigation of choice in ROCM.[14]

Typically in the orbit, mucormycosis affects the extraconal space first and then involves the extraocular muscles. As a result, there is inflammation, hyperemia, and congestion in the extraocular muscles. On MRI, this is seen as increase in size of the extraocular muscles along with contrast enhancement as a result of the inflammatory changes and hyperemia. Therefore, when contrast enhancement of the extraocular muscle is seen, it indicates that the contrast material injected intravenously is reaching the site that is visualized on the scan; therefore, the intravenous AMB that is given to treat the patient would also reach the involved site. As the disease progresses, angioinvasion and subsequent occlusive thrombosis of the involved blood vessel occur. This is seen radiologically as loss of contrast enhancement. If the contrast material is not able to reach the site as seen on the scans, it is unlikely that the intravenous drug would also be able to reach the site. This indicates that the involved tissue is ischemic and possibly necrotic/devitalized. Therefore, the location and amount of loss of contrast enhancement decide the type of surgical intervention in cases of orbital extension of mucormycosis (**Fig. 6.2**).[14,17] Based on this, understanding of the disease or recommended indications for orbital exenteration are as follows:

- Loss of contrast enhancement over the orbital apex (**Fig. 6.3**).
- Generalized loss of contrast enhancement in the entire orbit.
- Globe distortion with the intraconal abscess.
- Perineural with diffuse intraconal involvement.

Diagnosis

In a recent editorial, Honavar has introduced the diagnostic criteria for post-COVID-19 ROCM infection. Expanding on the same, the authors looked at (1) the host factors relevant to the subset of COVID-19 and ROCM, (2) the diagnostic criteria, and (3) the mycological criteria for diagnosing possible, probable, and proven mucormycosis (**Table 6.2**).[11]

In patients with typical clinical features suggestive of ROCM, namely eyelid signs such as ptosis, periocular or facial edema, which may be associated with discoloration, proptosis, conjunctival chemosis, ophthalmoplegia, central retinal artery occlusion, panophthalmitis, and palatal eschar, the host factors, diagnostic criteria, and mycologic criteria as listed in **Table 6.2** were looked for.[1,10,11]

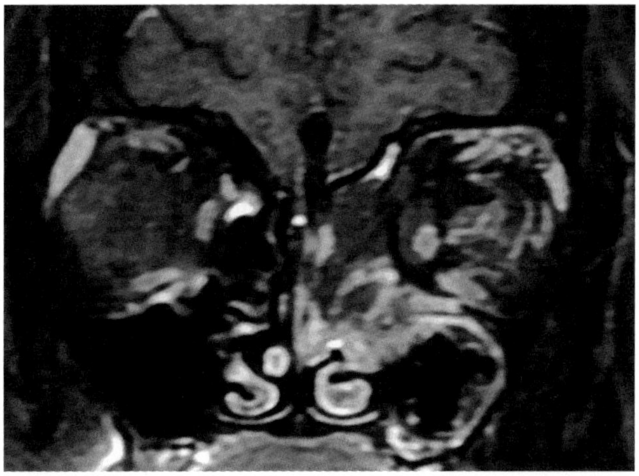

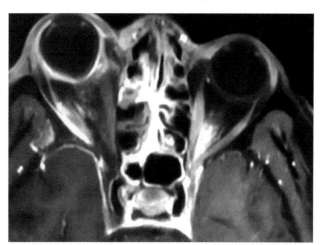

Fig. 6.2 Postcontrast T1-weighted coronal slice showing the involved left orbit. Note the black turbinate sign showing no contrast uptake. Observe the increased thickness of all the extraocular muscles as compared to the contralateral healthy side. In addition, the left medial rectus shows only a sliver of contrast uptake—indicating a *dying* muscle that has lost much of its vascularity. The diffuse intraconal perineural disease can also be seen.

Fig. 6.3 Postcontrast T1-weighted axial magnetic resonance imaging (MRI) showing a distorted globe (guitar pluck sign) and diffuse intraconal abscess. Also note the loss of contrast enhancement present on the right medial rectus (as compared to the left side) and over the apex. The patient had complete ophthalmoplegia with no perception of light. Clinically and radiologically, this would be an indication for orbital exenteration in mucormycosis.

Table 6.2 Diagnosis of post-COVID-19 ROCM infection

Host factors	Diagnostic criteria	Mycologic criteria

1. Concurrently or recently (<6 wk) treated for COVID-19
2. Treated for COVID-19 with steroids
3. Treated for COVID-19 with immunomodulators (tocilizumab)
	1. Diagnostic nasal endoscopy: Signs of nasal eschar, discoloration, and ulceration over the nasal mucosa were examined in the region of the middle turbinate, middle meatus, and the septum
	2. MRI of the orbit, paranasal sinus, and brain with gadolinium contrast was performed and fat saturation postcontrast sequences were examined
	Features evaluated were the following:
	  a. Early osseous erosion or marrow edema
	  b. Haziness of the paranasal sinuses
	  c. Soft tissue inflammation around the paranasal sinuses
	  d. Retroantral extension
	  e. Intraorbital extension
	  f. Intracranial extension
		1. Mycological evidence of mucormycosis in tissue biopsy taken during sinus debridement or from the orbital biopsy:
		  i. Direct examination of biopsy or aspirated material was performed using 10% potassium hydroxide or calcofluor white staining solution
		  ii. The specimens were inoculated on Sabouraud dextrose agar and blood agar and incubated at 37 and 25°C for up to 1 and 2 wk, respectively. Rapid growth of gray fluffy colonies was identified on conventional morphologic assessment. The growth was subcultured and reported as significant if the direct examination of the sample showed the presence of fungal filaments[15]
		2. Histopathologic evidence of mucormycosis in tissue biopsy was performed by examining for aseptate hyphae branching at wide angle and ribbonlike hyphae associated with tissue damage on slides stained by hematoxylin and eosin, periodic acid–Schiff, and Gomori's methenamine silver stains

Abbreviations: MRI, magnetic resonance imaging; ROCM, rhino-orbito-cerebral mucormycosis.

Management

General Principles

Cornely et al published the Global guideline for the diagnosis and management of mucormycosis: an initiative of the European Confederation of Medical Mycology in cooperation with the Mycoses Study Group Education and Research Consortium in 2019.[10] This global guideline is sufficiently flexible so that treatment protocols can be customized as per the resources available in every country. The first step in management is correction of metabolic derangements, which are risk factors for mucormycosis like hyperglycemia and diabetic ketoacidosis. Tapering or stoppage of corticosteroids and immunomodulators to be attempted if possible.Early surgical debridement of necrosed tissues is found to have lower mortality compared to those who did not have early debridement. There is no clear evidence regarding the extent of debridement. However, the general principle guiding this is that debridement is continued until bleeding tissue—soft as well as bony—is generally accepted. Surgical debridement brings down the fungal load in the patient as well as better perfusion of local as well as systemic antifungals. Life salvage followed by globe salvage and finally vision salvage are the general hierarchical principles considered. Medical management precedes and follows surgical management. Before any

surgery is attempted, it is important to correct metabolic derangements. Once surgical debridement is done, medical management continues postsurgery with systemic antifungals and further monitoring of metabolic parameters. The histopathological examination confirms aseptate hyphae on microscopy with stains. The end game is rehabilitation—restoring function and aesthetics of the face so that the patient can get back to his or her old life with minimal or no stigma associated with this disease.

Early surgical debridement by the surgical team is an essential primary intervention, whereas medical management of metabolic correction and antifungal medications remain the mainstay of treatment. Imaging, microbiology, and pathology are cornerstones of diagnosis. Rehabilitation remains challenging in many patients who manage to survive this very destructive disease, and best efforts can remain suboptimal.[10] **Flowchart 6.1** shows the general principles in the treatment of ROCM.

Medical Management

The first-line antifungal medication for the management of ROCM is AMB. AMB comes in three formulations and all are given by intravenous route:

- Deoxycholate AMB (D-AMB).
- Lipid emulsion AMB (LE-AMB).
- Liposomal AMB (L-AMB).

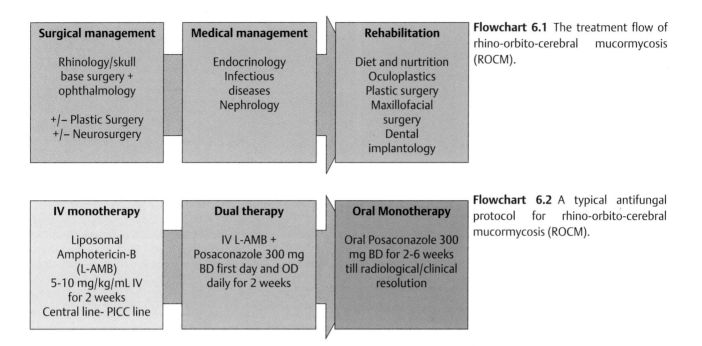

Flowchart 6.1 The treatment flow of rhino-orbito-cerebral mucormycosis (ROCM).

Flowchart 6.2 A typical antifungal protocol for rhino-orbito-cerebral mucormycosis (ROCM).

The US Food and Drug Administration (USFDA) has approved isavuconazole as the first-line antifungal medication for ROCM in renal-compromised patients. This is available in both oral and intravenous formulations.

Posaconazole is a second-line antifungal used in the treatment of ROCM and is usually used in the form of step-down treatment in the maintenance phase of the treatment. The detailed medical management has been covered in a previous chapter.[10] **Flowchart 6.2** is an example of how the antifungal treatment is done. This can be customized as per local availability of medications and patient-specific variables by the infectious diseases team.

Interventions by the Orbit Surgeon

Transcutaneous Retrobulbar Amphotericin-B

TRAMB is a minimally invasive procedure that does not need to be done in the operating room and can be performed at the bedside. Therefore, it may be done even in weak, debilitated patients who otherwise may not be fit for major surgeries, especially those under general anesthesia. TRAMB has been employed previously in sino-orbital aspergillosis with success in the past.[17,18] However, mucormycosis is a far more aggressive fungal disease.[19]

With regard to its use in mucormycosis, there have been previously published case reports that have demonstrated the benefit of TRAMB, an off-label use of AMB. It must be borne in mind that TRAMB should *not* be used as the only form of intervention in orbital mucormycosis. It should be considered only as an adjunctive therapy. All patients receiving TRAMB must receive systemic antifungal therapy, adequate reversal of DM/immunosuppression, and concurrent aggressive sinus debridement to eliminate or reduce the disease load. Possible candidates for TRAMB include patients with ROCM who have disease identified early with minimal vision loss. The selection of cases for TRAMB should be on the basis of radiologic evidence only—preferably based on the interpretation of MRI scans by an experienced radiologist.[16] As discussed earlier, the indications for orbital exenteration have been enlisted earlier.

Nair and Dave have recommended TRAMB retrobulbar injections consisting of 1 ml of 3.5 mg/mL D-AMB with antecedent retrobulbar injection of anesthetic (2% lidocaine and 0.5% bupivacaine in a 1:1 ratio). D-AMB must be reconstituted with sterile water and cannot be mixed with saline, as exposure to sodium chloride could induce precipitation.[16] In the literature, both the liposomal formulation and the deoxycholate formulation have been used in TRAMB with reported success.[20,21] In the literature, the most commonly followed regimen is three injections of TRAMB given on consecutive days. However, it is known that TRAMB can cause inflammation, and swelling with transient increase in proptosis. Therefore, it may be prudent to administer TRAMB injections on alternate days or as per the clinical condition. The area of injection should be decided on the basis of radiological involvement.[16]

The generally accepted indications for TRAMB include the following[16]:

- Contrast enhancement with increase in size of extraocular muscle(s) (**Fig. 6.4**).

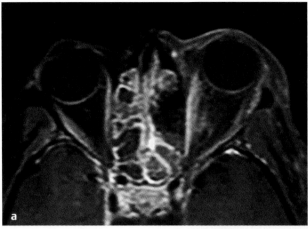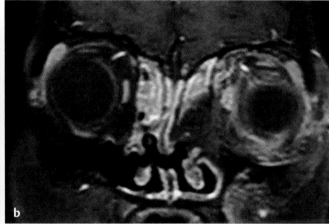

Fig. 6.4 Postcontrast T1-weighted axial **(a)** and coronal **(b)** images showing the black turbinate and thickened medial and inferior rectus. The medial rectus on the affected left side shows contrast enhancement with increase in size. The patient's vision was unaffected with limited adduction.

- Extraconal fat stranding with diffuse enhancement.
- Perineural enhancement without diffuse intraconal disease.
- Apical disease with contrast enhancement (**Fig. 6.5**).

Therefore, the presence of contrast enhancement in the orbit, by and large, suggests that vascular perfusion is present and in addition to the systemically administered AMB, adjunctive local injection can be attempted to increase the locally available drug.

Harmsen et al reported that at high concentration AMB is a cytotoxic drug. After exposure to AMB concentrations beyond 100 mg/ml for more than 1 hour, widespread cell death was seen in mouse osteoblasts and fibroblasts.[22] Among cases where TRAMB was administered in cases of mucormycosis, Safi et al reported an inflammatory response following TRAMB, which manifested as transient yellow-tinged inferior conjunctival chemosis that resolved after a week.[23] Hirabayashi et al reported that following the third injection, MRI showed increased facial and periorbital enhancement, a mild increase in inferomedial extraconal and intraconal fat stranding and episcleral enhancement—which was likely caused by the retrobulbar injection.[24] Brodie et al reported a case where the patient developed orbital compartment syndrome with extremely high intraocular pressure and vision deterioration immediately following TRAMB injection. A lateral canthotomy and cantholysis had to be performed to relieve the condition.[25]

In the authors' own experience, TRAMB has shown good outcomes in select patients. **Fig. 6.6** shows a patient whose orbital disease improved substantially with just two injections of TRAMB.

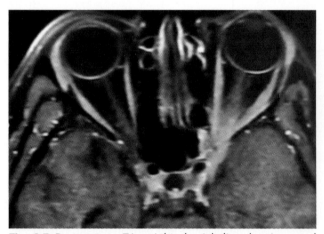

Fig. 6.5 Postcontrast T1-weighted axial slice showing good contrast uptake in all extraocular muscles with the presence of apical disease component.

Exploratory Orbitotomy with Surgical Debridement of Necrotic Tissues

One of the biggest learnings by the authors treating patients suffering from CAM is the very important role timely exploratory orbitotomies and debridement of devitalized tissues can play to save the globe, vision, and sometimes even life. In limited involvement of the orbit in ROCM, limited surgical debridement of the orbit in lieu of the radical measure like orbital exenteration has been reported in the literature.[13,26,27] However, there have been only a few case reports and limited case series to appreciate the value of exploratory orbitotomy in the management of ROCM. Since ROCM was formerly a very rare entity, the intermediate interventions mentioned

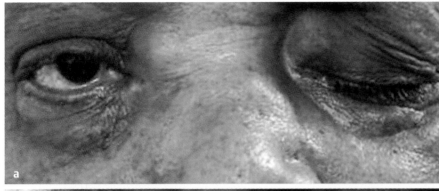

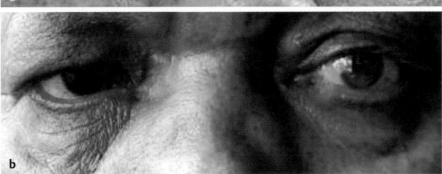

Fig. 6.6 Clinical pictures showing functional improvement after trans-cutaneous retrobulbar amphotericin-B (TRAMB). **(a)** Left orbital cellulitis, proptosis, external ophthalmoplegia, and complete ptosis. **(b)** Reduction in inflammatory changes, proptosis, and ocular movements and complete resolution of left eye ptosis.

in these case reports did not have enough power to support or reject them. The mucormycosis epidemic within the COVID-19 pandemic characterized by the exponential rise in ROCM in the setting of COVID-19 infections provided a deluge of cases with early orbital involvement which needed surgical debridement short of exenteration. The high number of cases in a short duration of time started causing shortages of AMB, the first-line medical treatment for mucormycosis.[28] There were severe shortages in supply of all three formulations: D-AMB, LE-AMB, and L-AMB. The shortages prompted the mucormycosis treating teams in various cities to be more aggressive in surgical debridement so as to buy time while the supply of AMB improved. This also prompted many oculoplastic surgeons including the authors to entertain exploratory orbitotomy and surgical debridement of devitalized tissues into their armamentarium of surgical interventions in treating orbital mucormycosis.

Orbital involvement in mucormycosis usually affects the globe last among the orbital tissues. The order of involvement is usually periorbita facing the involved sinuses, orbital fat, extraocular muscles, orbital portions of cranial nerves II to VI, and finally the globe. Visual loss can happen with early orbital involvement and sometimes even with no orbital involvement due to vascular causes as explained in the earlier section.[29]

Exploratory orbitotomy with surgical debridement of necrotic tissues (EOSDNT) is a useful intermediate intervention in the spectrum of surgeries for orbital mucormycosis

between TRAMB and exenteration. Exploratory orbitotomies are performed in the location from which the disease spreads into the orbit from the sinuses. The spread of disease from the sinus to the orbit can be through perineural spread via the infratemporal fossa, pterygopalatine fossa, and infraorbital nerve, and through vascular channels of the ethmoidal vessels or/and by direct invasion by eroding bones of the floor and medial walls of the orbit as explained earlier in the chapter in section "Pathways of Spread of Mucormycosis into Orbit." MRI helps in identifying locations where the exploratory orbitotomies need to be performed. The indications for EOSDNT have not been adequately elucidated in the literature, but using the proof of concept used by our rhinology colleagues using functional endoscopic sinus surgery (FESS) and aggressive surgical debridement, which have been validated with from multiple adequately powered studies,[1,4,10,30] some guidelines for indications can be framed:

- Contrast enhancement of extraocular muscles with clear demarcated areas with loss of contrast in the orbital tissues indicating presence of devitalized necrotic portions within the orbit (**Fig. 6.7**).[31]
- Extraconal fat stranding with limited loss of contrast with mild to no fat stranding of the intraconal space. This indicates the globe can be salvaged[14] (**Fig. 6.8**).
- Perineural enhancement on short tau inversion recovery (STIR) sequence with no loss of contrast around the optic nerve and retrobulbar fat. This indicates that vision can be salvaged.[32]

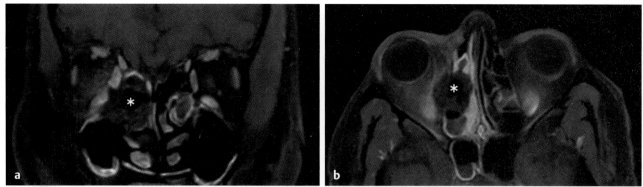

Fig. 6.7 (a, b) Contrast enhancement of the extraocular muscles with clear demarcated areas with loss of contrast in the orbital tissues indicating the presence of devitalized necrotic portions within the orbit.

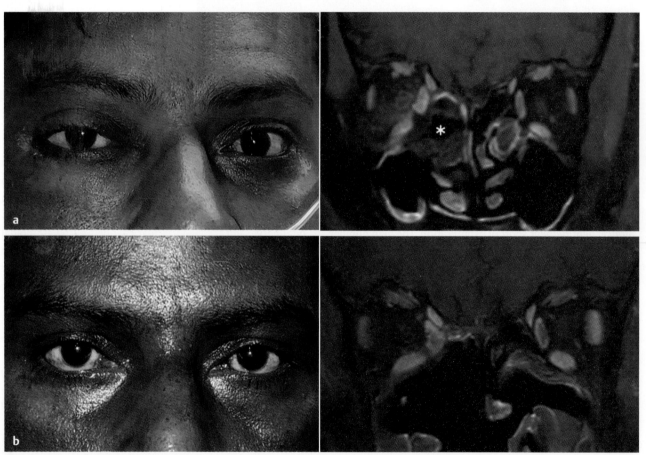

Fig. 9.8 (a) Right orbital cellulitis at presentation with necrosed tissues (*white asterisk*) indicated by contrast loss on magnetic resonance imaging (MRI) and healthy but inflamed tissue indicated by contrast enhancement on MRI. **(b)** This image shows the benefit provided by the timely orbitotomy with complete resolution of orbital cellulitis after 4 weeks of postoperative antifungal treatment.

- Thickened infraorbital nerve seen on enhanced-short tau inversion recovery (e-STIR) sequence with some perineural enhancement and areas of necrosis surrounding the thickened nerve (**Fig. 6.9**). This is one of the pathways of ROCM into the orbit. Debridement of necrotic tissues along with excision of the infraorbital nerve will stop further spread of mucormycosis into the orbit (**Fig. 6.9**).

EOSDNT has a positive effect on two counts:

- It decreases fungal load from the patient, thus reducing treatment time.
- It enhances the perfusion of systemic AMB into the surviving orbital tissue since AMB will not reach necrosed tissues.

EOSDNT provides good disease control and optimizes the medical treatment. An example is shown in **Fig. 6.8**. **Fig. 6.8a** shows right orbital cellulitis at presentation with necrosed tissues (*white asterisk*) indicated by contrast loss on MRI and healthy but inflamed tissue indicated by contrast enhancement on MRI. **Fig. 6.8b** shows the benefit provided by the timely orbitotomy with complete resolution of orbital cellulitis after 4 weeks of postoperative antifungal treatment.

In extensive orbital involvement of mucormycosis with extensive areas of necrosis, especially in the orbital apex with patients usually presenting with complete loss of vision in the affected eye and total external ophthalmoplegia, prognosis is not improved with exploratory orbitotomy and the patient can be considered a candidate for exenteration.

EOSDNT can be done along with FESS and surgical debridement by the rhinology team or as an isolated procedure after full evaluation. Once the orbital planes are dissected, the devitalized tissues are identified and debrided. The end point of the debridement is the appearance of bleeding tissues: muscle, fat, and bone.

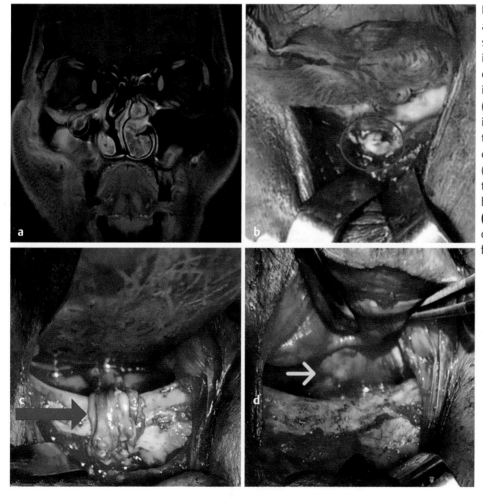

Fig. 6.9 (a) Magnetic resonance imaging (MRI) paranasal sinus (PNS) enhanced short tau inversion recovery (e-STIR) sequence showing right thickened infraorbital nerve (*red circle*). **(b)** Exposure of the necrosed infraorbital nerve at the exit in the anterior wall of the maxilla during exploratory orbitotomy (*blue circle*). **(c)** Full length of the infraorbital nerve dissected before excision (*purple arrow*). **(d)** Intraorbital involvement of mucormycosis with abscess formation (*yellow arrow*).

Orbital Exenteration

As mentioned earlier, orbital exenteration is indicated in cases of ROCM based on the radiological and clinical findings. Historically, the indications for orbital exenteration have been less specific, with some authors advocating orbital exenteration for clinical findings such as ophthalmoplegia, proptosis, cranial involvement, and ocular involvement.[30,33–37] Some authors have even reported that exenteration could increase patients' survival in the presence of intracranial spread and rapid progression.[35] However, it has also been reported that orbital exenteration, by itself, does not actually affect the patients' survival in ROCM.[38] The logical explanation for these contradictory conclusions is that orbital exenteration in these reports was performed in patients with severe disease and intracranial extension, where eliminating the disease load from the orbit may not particularly be helpful as there was always residual disease left behind.

Recent advances such as TRAMB have reduced the need for drastic surgical interventions such as orbital exenteration. Ashraf et al, in their report, employed a modified treatment ladder algorithm utilizing TRAMB injection in patients with moderate orbital disease.[39] They analyzed the outcomes of patients who were treated using this algorithm and compared it with outcomes of patients from their previous work largely as historical controls. Their outcomes showed that patients with invasive fungal rhino-orbital sinusitis with

moderate orbital disease who were treated with TRAMB (as per their algorithm) had a lower risk of exenteration and a similar risk of mortality, suggesting the potential for this minimally invasive approach.

However, when indicated, orbital exenteration performed at the right time may be lifesaving in many cases. Surgically, the technique of orbital exenteration is slightly different from the technique routinely employed for advanced periocular or orbital malignancies. If the eyelids and periocular skin are healthy, it is advisable to attempt a lid-sparing orbital exenteration and at closure, one must make sure that the orbicularis is well opposed and skin closure is not too tight (**Fig. 6.10**). As mentioned earlier, orbital apex involvement, which threatens to extend intracranially, is an indication for exenteration. Therefore, orbital apex clearance is extremely important: separate tissue specimens from the orbital apex must be sent for histopathological and microscopic examination to ensure that the last bit of tissue taken from the orbital apex does not contain fungal elements. In many cases, the medial orbital wall may appear to be thin, broken, breached, and necrotic. In these cases, it may be prudent to open up the medial orbital wall, especially simultaneous orbital exenteration and endoscopic debridement are being performed. An AMB-soaked piece of gauze roll can be placed within the orbit with the end of the roll hanging out through the gap between the sutures to be taken out 24 to 48 hours after surgery. The most common complication of orbital exenteration

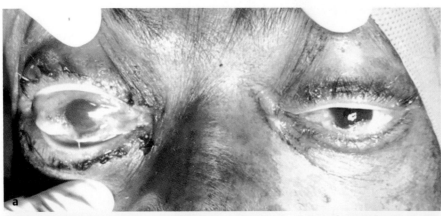

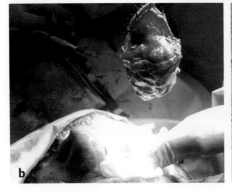
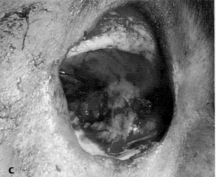

Fig. 6.10 (a) Right orbital cellulitis with proptosis, complete vision loss, and total external ophthalmoplegia. **(b)** Exenteration of the right orbit. **(c)** Left postexenteration socket.

for mucormycosis is flap necrosis or gaping of the skin wound. If the wound gape is small and easily closed without too much tension, then it can be attempted; however, they tend to progressively enlarge and therefore conservative management is advised. A split-skin graft may be placed to the orbital cavity only after complete disease clearance, which may be months after surgery. In case a large bony socket has been left behind, daily dressing with AMB and/or povidone–iodine solution is advisable.

Rehabilitation

- Eyelid and orbital reconstruction.
- Correction of lid malpositions.
- Strabismus correction.
- Microvascular free flaps and grafting.
- Socket reconstruction with exenteration prosthesis fitting (**Fig. 6.11**).

Recurrence and Late Sequelae

Recurrence of mucormycosis can occur if there is inadequate initial surgical debridement and/or suboptimal dosage and duration of both first- and second-line systemic antifungal medication. Recurrences can occur if systemic antifungals are held back due to metabolic derangements or poor nephrological status. In the case of recurrence, the treatment protocols remain the same as in the primary disease: surgical debridement, correction of metabolic factors, and adequate long-term systemic antifungal medication.[40]

The authors have been observing late sequelae occurring during and after treatment of mucormycosis, which cannot be directly attributed to the fungal disease—cardiovascular events like cardiac arrests, pulmonary embolism, and strokes.[41] There have been a few cases of reactivation of dormant pulmonary tuberculosis and possibly immune-mediated unexplained inflammatory episodes in the eyes, head, and neck region.[42]

Remarkably among the late sequelae are secondary bacterial infections by low-virulent bacteria and sometimes sterile abscess in the face and other parts of the body. CT (**Fig. 6.12**) and MRI (**Fig. 6.13**) are diagnostic modalities to detect what appears to be suppurative osteomyelitis. There have been few reports of these types of late sequelae in earlier studies.[43,44] The etiology of osteomyelitis is not clearly known but is hypothesized to be due to vascular compromise leading to avascular necrosis of the bone earlier involved with mucormycosis disease. Treatment is by abscess drainage and debridement of any residual necrosed tissues.[45] The histopathology/microbiological identification of viable aseptate hyphae is not always present, giving more credence to the hypothesis that this sequela is caused by vascular compromise rather than by the recurrence of mucormycosis.[46]

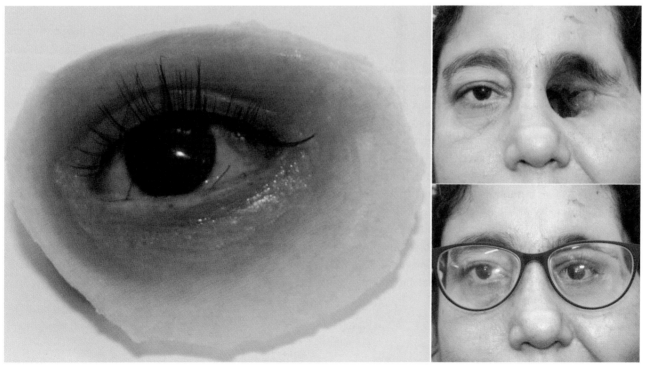

Fig. 6.11 Customized silicone exenteration prosthesis providing good cosmetic rehabilitation in a patient with a left exenterated socket.

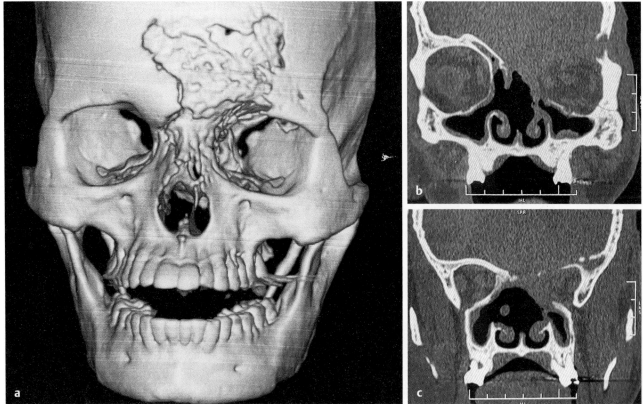

Fig. 6.12 Computed tomography (CT) scan showing osteomyelitic changes in a previously involved location in a patient who had completed the full antifungal medication regimen. **(a)** 3D reconstructed CT Image showing osteomyelitic changes in the left frontal bone. **(b, c)** Coronal sections (bone windows) showing bony defect of the orbital roof and medial wall including the skull base due to the osteomyelitis.

Conclusion

Public awareness of this disease resulting in early presentation followed by prompt attention to warning signs and symptoms by physicians having a high index of clinical suspicion and direct tissue biopsy on suspicion can help achieve early diagnosis and better outcomes. Diagnosis is supported by imaging, and contrast-enhanced MRI scan is preferred over CT scan. Early aggressive surgical debridement should be done. The extent of surgical debridement should balance the morbidity and mutilation on one side against possible mortality from this devastating disease on the other side.[13] Surgery should quickly be followed by correction of metabolic factors with concomitant initiation of full-dose AMB while awaiting the results of culture and histopathology.

The challenges in treatment of this rapidly progressive disease lie in identification of indications for FESS, TRAMB, EOSDNT, orbital exenteration, and meticulous postsurgical medical management. Long-term antifungal treatment with monitored step-down to oral antifungals is continued until clinical and radiological resolution is achieved. The outcome of ROCM in the setting of COVID-19 needs to be optimized with a multidisciplinary mucormycosis team who respect a protocol-based strategy. This is the key to success. Resolution of the disease is not the end of the treatment journey. Adequate rehabilitation is very important to rid the patient of stigma of the disease as well as to assimilate the patient back to society. Orbital exenteration prosthesis is a good measure for both aesthetic and psychological rehabilitation of the patients.[47,48]

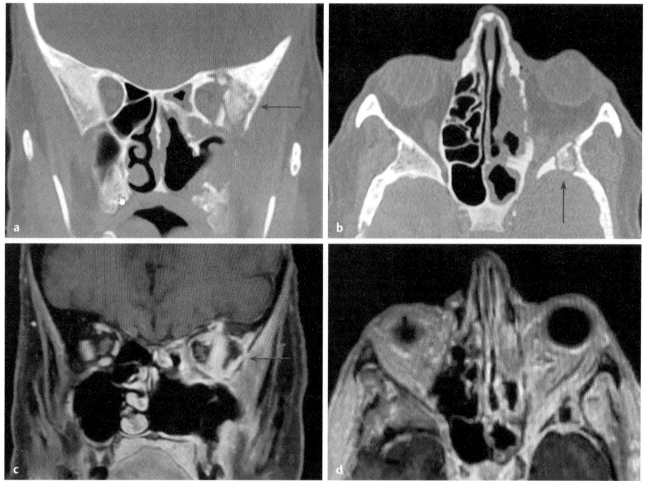

Fig. 6.13 Left lateral orbital wall osteomyelitis, bone necrosis, and abscess formation involving the greater wing of the sphenoid bone: the skull base (*red arrow*). **(a)** Computed tomography (CT) scan coronal view. **(b)** CT scan axial view. **(c)** Magnetic resonance imaging (MRI) scan coronal view. **(d)** MRI scan axial view.

References

1. Skiada A, Pavleas I, Drogari-Apiranthitou M. Epidemiology and diagnosis of mucormycosis: an update. J Fungi (Basel) 2020;6(4):265

2. Sen M, Lahane S, Lahane TP, Parekh R, Honavar SG. Mucor in a viral land: a tale of two pathogens. Indian J Ophthalmol 2021;69(2):244–252

3. Sarkar S, Gokhale T, Choudhury SS, Deb AK. COVID-19 and orbital mucormycosis. Indian J Ophthalmol 2021;69(4):1002–1004

4. Moorthy A, Gaikwad R, Krishna S, et al. SARS-CoV-2, uncontrolled diabetes and corticosteroids: an unholy trinity in invasive fungal infections of the maxillofacial region? A retrospective, multi-centric analysis. J Maxillofac Oral Surg 2021;20(3):418–425

5. Ravani SA, Agrawal GA, Leuva PA, Modi PH, Amin KD. Rise of the phoenix: mucormycosis in COVID-19 times. Indian J Ophthalmol 2021;69(6):1563–1568

6. Dave TV, Gopinathan Nair A, Hegde R, et al. Clinical presentations, management and outcomes of rhino-orbital-cerebral mucormycosis (ROCM) following COVID-19: a multi-centric study. Ophthal Plast Reconstr Surg 2021;37(5):488–495

7. Sen M, Honavar SG, Sharma N, Sachdev MS. COVID-19 and eye: a review of ophthalmic manifestations of COVID-19. Indian J Ophthalmol 2021;69(3):488–509

8. Arora S, Hemmige VS, Mandke C, et al; Mycotic Infections in COVID-19 (MUNCO) Network. Online registry of COVID-19-associated mucormycosis cases, India, 2021. Emerg Infect Dis 2021;27(11):2963–2965

9. Mucormycosis: the "black fungus" maiming Covid patients in India. BBC News. May 9, 2021. Accessed December 12, 2021 at: https://www.bbc.com/news/world-asia-india-57027829

10. Cornely OA, Alastruey-Izquierdo A, Arenz D, et al; Mucormycosis ECMM MSG Global Guideline Writing Group. Global guideline for the diagnosis and management of mucormycosis: an initiative of the European Confederation of Medical Mycology in cooperation with the Mycoses Study Group Education and Research Consortium. Lancet Infect Dis 2019;19(12):e405–e421

11. Honavar SG. Code mucor: guidelines for the diagnosis, staging and management of rhino-orbito-cerebral mucormycosis in the setting of COVID-19. Indian J Ophthalmol 2021;69(6): 1361–1365

12. Parsi K, Itgampalli RK, Vittal R, Kumar A. Perineural spread of rhino-orbitocerebral mucormycosis caused by *Apophysomyces elegans*. Ann Indian Acad Neurol 2013; 16(3):414–417

13. Kohn R, Hepler R. Management of limited rhino-orbital mucormycosis without exenteration. Ophthalmology 1985; 92(10):1440–1444

14. Sreshta K, Dave TV, Varma DR, et al. Magnetic resonance imaging in rhino-orbital-cerebral mucormycosis. Indian J Ophthalmol 2021;69(7):1915–1927

15. Hosseini SMS, Borghei P. Rhinocerebral mucormycosis: pathways of spread. Eur Arch Otorhinolaryngol 2005; 262(11):932–938

16. Nair AG, Dave TV. Transcutaneous retrobulbar injection of amphotericin B in rhino-orbital-cerebral mucormycosis: a review. Orbit 2022;41(3):275–286

17. Kalin-Hajdu E, Hirabayashi KE, Vagefi MR, Kersten RC. Invasive fungal sinusitis: treatment of the orbit. Curr Opin Ophthalmol 2017;28(5):522–533

18. Mainville N, Jordan DR. Orbital apergillosis treated with retrobulbar amphotericin B. Orbit 2012;31(1):15–17

19. Trief D, Gray ST, Jakobiec FA, et al. Invasive fungal disease of the sinus and orbit: a comparison between mucormycosis and *Aspergillus*. Br J Ophthalmol 2016;100(2):184–188

20. Mekonnen ZK, Ashraf DC, Jankowski T, et al. Acute invasive rhino-orbital mucormycosis in a patient with COVID-19-associated acute respiratory distress syndrome. Ophthal Plast Reconstr Surg 2021;37(2):e40–e80

21. Bayram N, Ozsaygılı C, Sav H, et al. Susceptibility of severe COVID-19 patients to rhino-orbital mucormycosis fungal infection in different clinical manifestations. Jpn J Ophthalmol 2021;65(4):515–525

22. Harmsen S, McLaren AC, Pauken C, McLemore R. Amphotericin B is cytotoxic at locally delivered concentrations. Clin Orthop Relat Res 2011;469(11):3016–3021

23. Safi M, Ang MJ, Patel P, Silkiss RZ. Rhino-orbital-cerebral mucormycosis (ROCM) and associated cerebritis treated with adjuvant retrobulbar amphotericin B. Am J Ophthalmol Case Rep 2020;19:100771

24. Hirabayashi KE, Kalin-Hajdu E, Brodie FL, Kersten RC, Russell MS, Vagefi MR. Retrobulbar injection of amphotericin B for orbital mucormycosis. Ophthal Plast Reconstr Surg 2017;33(4):e94–e97

25. Brodie FL, Kalin-Hajdu E, Kuo DS, Hirabayashi KE, Vagefi R, Kersten RC. Orbital compartment syndrome following retrobulbar injection of amphotericin B for invasive fungal disease. Am J Ophthalmol Case Rep 2016;1:8–10

26. Langford JD, McCartney DL, Wang RC. Frozen section: guided surgical debridement for management of rhino-orbital mucormycosis. Am J Ophthalmol 1997;124(2):265–267

27. Joos ZP, Patel BCK. Intraorbital irrigation of amphotericin B in the treatment of rhino-orbital mucormycosis. Ophthal Plast Reconstr Surg 2017;33(1):e13–e16

28. Arun AB, Hasan MM, Rackimuthu S, Ullah I, Mir T, Saha A. Antifungal drug shortage in India amid an increase in invasive fungal functions during the coronavirus disease 2019 (COVID-19) pandemic. Infect Control Hosp Epidemiol 2021:1–2

29. Wipf JE, Paauw DS. Ophthalmologic emergencies in the patient with diabetes. Endocrinol Metab Clin North Am 2000;29(4):813–829

30. Kursun E, Turunc T, Demiroglu YZ, Alışkan HE, Arslan AH. Evaluation of 28 cases of mucormycosis. Mycoses 2015; 58(2):82–87

31. Desai SM, Gujarathi-Saraf A, Agarwal EA. Imaging findings using a combined MRI/CT protocol to identify the "entire iceberg" in post-COVID-19 mucormycosis presenting clinically as only "the tip." Clin Radiol 2021;76(10):784.e27–784.e33

32. Kanda T, Miyazaki A, Zeng F, et al. Magnetic resonance imaging of intraocular optic nerve disorders: review article. Pol J Radiol 2020;85(1):e67–e81

33. Peterson KL, Wang M, Canalis RF, Abemayor E. Rhinocerebral mucormycosis: evolution of the disease and treatment options. Laryngoscope 1997;107(7):855–862

34. Ketenci I, Unlü Y, Kaya H, et al. Rhinocerebral mucormycosis: experience in 14 patients. J Laryngol Otol 2011;125(8):e3

35. Jung SH, Kim SW, Park CS, et al. Rhinocerebral mucormycosis: consideration of prognostic factors and treatment modality. Auris Nasus Larynx 2009;36(3):274–279

36. Reed C, Bryant R, Ibrahim AS, et al. Combination polyene-caspofungin treatment of rhino-orbital-cerebral mucormycosis. Clin Infect Dis 2008;47(3):364–371

37. Dhiwakar M, Thakar A, Bahadur S. Improving outcomes in rhinocerebral mucormycosis: early diagnostic pointers and prognostic factors. J Laryngol Otol 2003;117(11): 861–865

38. Kashkouli MB, Abdolalizadeh P, Oghazian M, Hadi Y, Karimi N, Ghazizadeh M. Outcomes and factors affecting them in patients with rhino-orbito-cerebral mucormycosis. Br J Ophthalmol 2019;103(10):1460–1465

39. Ashraf DC, Idowu OO, Hirabayashi KE, et al. Outcomes of a modified treatment ladder algorithm using retrobulbar amphotericin B for invasive fungal rhino-orbital sinusitis. Am J Ophthalmol 2022;237:299–309

40. Pasternak M, Olszanecki R. Mucormycosis in head and neck area: the emerging health problem in COVID-19 pandemic. The perspective of a dental practitioner. Folia Med Cracov 2021;61(2):117–127

41. Thajeb P, Thajeb T, Dai D. Fatal strokes in patients with rhino-orbito-cerebral mucormycosis and associated vasculopathy. Scand J Infect Dis 2004;36(9):643–648

42. Maniglia AJ, Goodwin WJ, Arnold JE, Ganz E. Intracranial abscesses secondary to nasal, sinus, and orbital infections in adults and children. Arch Otolaryngol Head Neck Surg 1989;115(12):1424–1429

43. Pandey A, Bansal V, Asthana AK, Trivedi V, Madan M, Das A. Maxillary osteomyelitis by mucormycosis: report of four cases. Int J Infect Dis 2011;15(1):e66–e69

44. Mengji AK, Yaga US, Gollamudi N, Prakash B, Rajashekar E. Mucormycosis in a surgical defect masquerading as osteomyelitis: a case report and review of literature. Pan Afr Med J 2016;23(16):16

45. Mendhe D, Wankhede P, Wanjari M, Alwadkar S. Mucormycotic osteomyelitis of maxilla post-COVID patient: a case report. Pan Afr Med J 2021;39:275

46. Selvamani M, Donoghue M, Bharani S, Madhushankari GS. Mucormycosis causing maxillary osteomyelitis. J Nat Sci Biol Med 2015;6(2):456–459

47. Kaur H, Nanda A, Verma M, Mutneja P, Koli D, Bhardwaj S. Prosthetic rehabilitation of resected orbit in a case of mucormycosis. J Indian Prosthodont Soc 2018;18(4):364–369

48. Sendul SY, Yildiz AM, Yildiz AA, Akbas E. Osseointegrated implants for orbito-facial prostheses: common complications and solutions. J Craniofac Surg 2021;32(5):1770–1774

7

Orbital Exenteration in Rhino-Orbito-Cerebral Mucormycosis

Chapter 7

Orbital Exenteration in Rhino-Orbito-Cerebral Mucormycosis

Renuka Bradoo

Introduction

Rhino-orbito-cerebral mucormycosis (ROCM) is a relatively uncommon, rapidly progressive, angioinvasive, often fatal, opportunistic fungal infection.[1,2] It has both contiguous as well as noncontiguous vascular spread involving the nose, paranasal sinuses, orbit, and brain.

There is a three-pronged approach to its management:

- Rapid reversal of predisposing comorbidity, for example, diabetic ketoacidosis.
- Aggressive surgical debridement of all involved tissues.
- Medical treatment with amphotericin-B; posaconazole and isavuconazole are second-line drugs.

The most critical decision in the management of ROCM is whether the orbit should be exenterated.[3] The Sion Hospital Scoring System (SHSS) has been devised to aid the surgeons (ENT and oculoplastic) to take a rational and evidence-based decision on orbital exenteration.[4]

Management

Early mucormycosis requires a high index of suspicion for diagnosis. Routine history taking must include enquiry into any premorbid conditions. Clinical examination includes a diagnostic nasal endoscopy and tissue from the suspected area being sent for microscopic examination on potassium hydroxide (KOH) mount, culture, and histopathology.[2] Of these, histopathological presence of fungal hyphae in the tissue is the most conclusive evidence. An ophthalmic reference for orbital involvement and a medical reference for predisposing conditions and neurological examination are undertaken. This is followed by radiological investigations. Computed tomography (CT) of paranasal sinuses (PNS) (plain and contrast) scan is done for all patients in order to have a road map during surgery. Magnetic resonance imaging (MRI) of brain with contrast with orbital cuts is also done to rule out intracranial or orbital spread of the disease. Ophthalmoscopy should be performed in all the patients.

Medical Therapy

The first drug of choice is liposomal amphotericin-B which is given 5 to 10 mg intravenously in 100 mL of 5% dextrose, preceded and followed by 500 mL normal saline to maintain hydration. If it is not available or there are financial constraints, then amphotericin-B deoxycholate injection is given intravenously after an initial test dose of 20 mg. Dosage of amphotericin-B is 1 mg/kg/day with hydration and continued till a total dose of 2 to 3 g is administered. Daily intake/output ratio is calculated with monitoring of blood sugar, serum creatinine, urea, sodium, potassium, and magnesium levels along with complete blood count twice a week. Patients are also encouraged to have 2 to 3 L of oral fluids along with coconut water. Any ion deficit should be corrected promptly. In case of rising levels of blood urea nitrogen (BUN) or serum creatinine, the drug should be stopped for a few days till the levels normalize. Amphotericin-B is to be given for a minimum of 4 weeks followed by a step-down treatment (oral isavuconazole 200 mg thrice a day on days 1 and 2, and 200 mg once a day from day 3, or oral posaconazole 300 mg twice a day on day 1 followed by 300 mg once a day from day 2) for at least 3 to 6 months or a minimum of 6 weeks following clinical regression and radiological regression or stabilization.[5]

The surgical management of sinonasal mucormycosis is critical. Surgical debridement of all the necrosed tissue needs to be carried out including the infratemporal fossa, premaxillary tissue, and palate, whenever involved. However, when the orbit is involved, the decision-making is not as clearly defined. Vision is arguably the most important special sense. Psychosocial problems associated with orbital exenteration need to be considered as well. The decision to either preserve the eye or exenterate it as a part of surgical debridement must be taken jointly by the otolaryngologists and the ophthalmologists. Thus, the decision must be a close balance between preserving the eye and preventing further intracranial spread and eventually death.

Indications for Orbital Exenteration

The role of imaging in the management of mucormycosis is extremely important. As discussed earlier the disease essentially begins in the nose and the paranasal sinuses, and gradually spreads into the orbit and the intracranial space. Therefore, aggressive endoscopic debridement of the nose and the paranasal sinuses is crucial along with control of diabetes, administration of systematic antifungal medication, and reversal of the immunosuppressive condition. However, once the disease has spread into the orbit, surgical intervention is often needed. The different treatment strategies for the management of orbital extension of mucormycosis include orbital debridement, orbital exenteration, and transcutaneous retrobulbar amphotericin-B (TRAMB) injections.[6] Other treatment modalities include local irrigation of the affected sites with amphotericin-B and surgical packing of the orbit and the sinuses with amphotericin-B-soaked gauze.[6]

Mucormycosis typically involves the extraconal space first and then spreads to involve the extraocular muscles. As a result, there is inflammation, followed by hyperemia and congestion within the extraocular muscles. On MRI, this is seen as increase in the thickness of extraocular muscles along with contrast enhancement as a result of the inflammatory changes and hyperemia. Thus, on MRI scan, contrast enhancement of the extraocular muscle indicates that the contrast material, which is injected intravenously, is reaching it; therefore, intravenous (IV) amphotericin-B would also reach the involved site. As the disease progresses, angioinvasion and subsequent occlusive thrombosis of the involved blood vessel occur which are seen radiologically as loss of contrast enhancement. This means that if the contrast material is not able to reach the site as seen radiologically, it is unlikely that the IV drug would also be able to reach the site. This indicates that the involved tissue is ischemic and possibly necrotic/devitalized. Therefore, the location and amount of loss of contrast enhancement decide the type of surgical intervention in cases of orbital extension of mucormycosis.[7] Based on this understanding of the disease, recommended indications for orbital exenteration are as follows:

- Loss of contrast enhancement over the orbital apex.
- Generalized loss of contrast enhancement in entire orbit.
- Globe distortion with intraconal abscess.
- Perineural spread with diffuse intraconal involvement.

Orbital Exenteration

Orbital exenteration is performed under general anesthesia. A lid-sparing orbital exenteration is preferred in cases when it is possible to salvage the lids. A tarsorrhaphy is done and a skin incision is made 4 mm from the lid margin all around the lid margin. Subsequently, dissection is done in the suborbicularis plane up to the orbital rim superiorly and inferiorly. The periosteum is exposed, and a periosteal incision is made 4 mm from the orbital rim. The periosteum is elevated, and subperiosteal dissection is done into the orbit. The supraorbital, supratrochlear, and infraorbital neurovascular bundles are structures of importance that need to be cut. The lacrimal sac, zygomatic-temporal vessels, and zygomatic-facial

vessels are cut. Medially, the anterior ethmoidal artery and posterior ethmoidal arteries are identified and cauterized. After reaching the posterior-most part of the orbit and lifting the periosteum, superior orbital fissure and inferior orbital fissure are identified and cauterized. Optic nerve is identified and sharply cut. Finally, the orbital contents, namely, the globe, the extraocular muscles, and the optic nerve, are exenterated. Tissue at the orbital apex is also cleared to ensure no residual infective tissue is left behind. The specimen (orbital tissues and eyeball) is sent for histopathological examination and microbiological assessment. The orbital cavity is washed with povidone-iodine solution. The skin is closed in layers without too much tension across the wound. A medial window of about 5 mm may be kept open for pack removal and examination postoperatively via endoscope. The orbit can be reconstructed with a prosthetic eye 3 to 4 months after cure of disease. A galeal frontalis-pericranial flap from the midforehead region can also be used for the reconstruction of the orbit.

Endoscopic Orbital Debridement

This is a newer concept where the medial and inferior parts of the orbit are debrided via the transnasal route. It offers the advantage that the uninvolved superior and lateral periorbita along with the globe can be preserved. However, this is a young concept and has a steep learning curve.

Sion Hospital Scoring System (SHSS)

A scoring system has been developed by a team of skilled otorhinolaryngologists and ophthalmologists with prior experience in managing mucormycosis. The Sion Hospital Scoring System is an accurate and promising system to solve the dilemma that is associated with orbital exenteration in ROCM.[4]

The aims of this scoring system are:
- To lay out the indications of orbital exenteration in patients with ROCM.
- To provide a system that predicts the stage at which exenteration needs to be carried out.

The scoring system is based on three main criteria (**Table 7.1**):
- Clinical signs.
- Ophthalmological signs.
- Imaging.

The score is calculated in the following way:
- 1 point = Mild symptoms/signs.
- 2 points = Moderate symptoms/signs.
- 3 points = Severe symptoms/signs.

Table 7.1 The Sion Hospital Scoring System
A. Clinical Signs

	0	2	3
Vision	Normal or same as prior to other symptoms	Decreased vision after developing other symptoms	Total blindness
Pupil	Normal	RAPD	Fixed
Ocular motility	Normal	Extraocular muscle palsy/Diplopia	Fixed eyeball
Proptosis	Absent	-	Present
Intracranial spread	Normal	Headache, projectile vomiting, confusion	Altered consciousness, pulsatile exophthalmos, coma

B. Ophthalmological Signs

Fundus changes	Points
Normal	0
Cotton wool spots	1
Congested tortuous retinal blood vessels	2
Optic disc edema	2
Central retinal vein occlusion	2
Central retinal artery occlusion	2
Retinal detachment	2
Choroidal folds	2
Optic disc pallor	2
Total	15

C. Imaging

Orbital involvement by the disease (globe/muscles/fat)	3
Intracranial spread/superior orbital fissure/inferior orbital fissure involvement	3
Optic neuritis	3
Sphenoid sinus involvement	2
Frontal sinus involvement	1
Ethmoidal sinus involvement	1
Infratemporal fossa involvement	1
Maxillary sinus involvement	1
Total	15

Abbreviation: RAPD, relative afferent pupillary defect.

The study was performed on 85 patients presenting with sinonasal mucormycosis at Sion Hospital from September 2020 to November 2021. All patients underwent clinical and endoscopic examination with microbiological and radiological investigations to confirm ROCM. All 85 patients underwent endoscopic sinonasal debridement and 26 patients underwent orbital surgery. A total of 20 patients were operated for orbital exenteration, while medial orbital wall debridement was done in 6 patients.

Further analysis of these 26 patients is as follows:
Of the 20 patients who underwent orbital exenteration, 18 had scored more than 23 in the SHSS and remaining 2 had scored less than 23 points (18 and 20, respectively). Their score was less in spite of extensive orbital involvement due to very minimal associated involvement of the nose, sinuses, and intracranial cavity.

Six patients had scored more than 23 with extensive involvement of the nose, sinuses, and intracranial cavity but showed limited involvement of the medial orbital fat. These patients underwent medial orbital debridement instead of orbital exenteration. Of the 59 patients who did not undergo orbital procedures, 4 had scored more than 23 points. They had significant involvement of nose and paranasal sinuses with negligible ophthalmic involvement resulting in a higher score.

According to SHSS, if the score is more than 23, then the patient can be considered for orbital exenteration. To know the clinical relevance of a scoring system, we need to know sensitivity and specificity of that system. Sensitivity is the percentage of true positivity. It is a measure of finding out the true positive mucor orbits in order to exenterate the eye. It should not miss out any positive orbits. Specificity is the percentage of true negativity. In the authors' case, it is a measure of identifying negative orbits, thus preventing unindicated orbital exenteration. In this case, SHSS has a sensitivity of 90% and a specificity of 95%. This means the scoring system is able to rule out true negatives (orbit free of mucor) and can help in saving the eye. To know the significance level of the authors' scoring system, they have applied chi-square test in 2 × 2 contingency table:

	Score > 23	Score < 23
Exenteration done	18	2
Exenteration not done	4	61

From the above, applying null hypothesis:

If we take confidence intervals of 99%, then p value comes to <0.00001, which is highly significant. Thus, after reviewing score of 85 patients prospectively, we were able to conclude that 23 points be considered as the watershed number.

Conclusion

The SHSS is an accurate and promising system to solve the dilemma that is associated with orbital exenteration in ROCM. A study with a larger group of patients or a meta-analysis would be a further area of research.

References

1. Roden MM, Zaoutis TE, Buchanan WL, et al. Epidemiology and outcome of zygomycosis: a review of 929 reported cases. Clin Infect Dis 2005;41(5):634–653

2. Petrikkos G, Skiada A, Lortholary O, Roilides E, Walsh TJ, Kontoyiannis DP. Epidemiology and clinical manifestations of mucormycosis. Clin Infect Dis 2012;54(Suppl 1):S23–S34

3. Hargrove RN, Wesley RE, Klippenstein KA, Fleming JC, Haik BG. Indications for orbital exenteration in mucormycosis. Ophthal Plast Reconstr Surg 2006;22(4):286–291

4. Shah K, Dave V, Bradoo R, Shinde C, Prathibha M. Orbital exenteration in rhino-orbito-cerebral mucormycosis: a prospective analytical study with scoring system. Indian J Otolaryngol Head Neck Surg 2019;71(2):259–265

5. Honavar SG. Code mucor: guidelines for the diagnosis, staging and management of rhino-orbito-cerebral mucormycosis in the setting of COVID-19. Indian J Ophthalmol 2021;69(6):1361–1365

6. Nair AG, Dave TV. Transcutaneous retrobulbar injection of amphotericin B in rhino-orbital-cerebral mucormycosis: a review. Orbit 2022;41(3):275–286

7. Kalin-Hajdu E, Hirabayashi KE, Vagefi MR, Kersten RC. Invasive fungal sinusitis: treatment of the orbit. Curr Opin Ophthalmol 2017;28(5):522–533

8

Dental Perspectives in COVID-19-Associated Mucormycosis

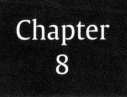

Chapter 8

Dental Perspectives in COVID-19-Associated Mucormycosis

P. Subramanian, Ashritha M.C.V., and Lekshmy R. Kurup

Introduction

Mucormycosis post-COVID-19 infection of Delta variant affects mostly the maxillary component of dentoalveolar region. Reason for this particular prediliction is unclear. The maxilla is rich in its vascular supply from multiple branches of the internal maxillary artery; hence, it rarely undergoes necrosis. However, it has been reported in multiple fungal and bacterial infections. The occurrence of palatal mucormycosis is not rare in adults. The spread of the fungus is postulated to happen in three possible modalities, namely, soft-tissue invasion, angioinvasion, and perineural invasion. In angioinvasion, the fungus invades the elastic lamina of the arteries, thus resulting in thrombosis and necrosis of the affected part. In oral cavity, angioinvasion can occur via the involvement of the greater palatine, descending palatine, and infraorbital vessels causing secondary involvement of palatal disease. Soft-tissue invasion in oral cavity can occur via the socket of freshly extracted tooth. If primary involvement of the palate is left untreated, it can result in invasion of the paranasal sinuses and orbit, and can ultimately lead to skull base osteomyelitis.

Signs and Symptoms

Patients with palatal involvement of mucormycosis can present with the following symptoms:
- Altered taste sensation in the mouth, caused due to perineural involvement of the glossopharyngeal nerve directly and pterygopalatine ganglion through the vidian nerve.
- Halitosis can occur due to purulent discharge from the palate caused from soft-tissue invasion.
- Swelling of the palatal gingiva.
- Bony invasion of mucormycosis resulting in avascular necrosis can cause mobility of the maxillary teeth and mobility of the segmental dentoalveolar bone. It can also lead to spontaneous exfoliation of the involved teeth.
- Dental pain.
- Inability to eat.
- Trismus can occur due to the involvement of muscles of mastication.

The following signs are seen in palatal involvement:
- A white necrotic ulcer without black eschar (**Fig. 8.1**).
- Infections extending from the nasal cavity to the oral cavity cause painful, black ulcerations in the hard palate, due to necrotic infarction. Ulcers also been reported on the gingivobuccal complex, alveolar ridge, and lip.[1]
- Intraoral or extraoral sinus formation.
- Periodontitis with loose teeth (**Fig. 8.2**).
- Sequestrum in the palate (**Fig. 8.3**) and maxillary alveolus.
- Formation of oroantral fistulas.[2]
- Nonhealing extraction sockets with alveolar osteitis.[2]
- Cellulitis.[2]
- Facial numbness.

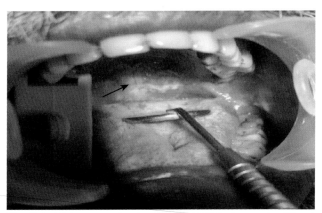

Fig. 8.1 White necrotic ulcer of palate (*black arrow*) without black eschar.

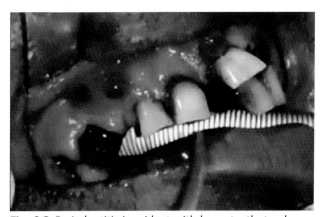

Fig. 8.2 Periodontitis is evident with loose teeth, tender on percussion.

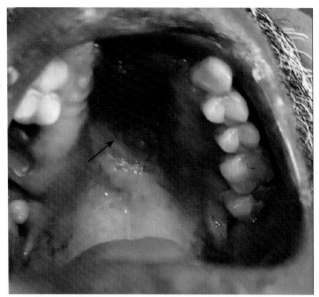

Fig. 8.3 Palatal osteomyelitis with clear demarcation of normal mucosa around.

Tissue Biopsy

Diagnosis of mucormycosis can be made on tissue sections. Microscopically involved tissues display focal areas of necrosis and hemorrhage. Demonstration of pauciseptate hyphae with wide angle branching in the presence of angioinvasion is characteristic of *Mucor* species.[2]

The tissue biopsy is usually acquired from the maxillary sinus, nasal mucosa, or palatal mucosa. Demonstration of fungal hyphae is the key to diagnosis.

Diagnostic Imaging

Diagnosis of mucormycosis is based on thorough clinical history and assessment of the underlying medical illness. Further, presence of nasal or palatal necrosis increases the probable suspicion of mucormycosis. Radiographic evaluation is the key aid. Depending on the involvement in individual cases a cone beam computed tomography (CBCT) or multidetector CT (MDCT) is added along with magnetic resonance imaging (MRI). It can help in assessing the gross bony involvement of the maxilla and frontal bone. MRI reveals the presence of bony erosions, extent of paranasal sinus involvement, orbital involvement, and intracranial spread.[3]

CBCT helps study the extent of involvement of the disease in the maxilla, nasal cavity, and alveolar apparatus. Volume-rendered images are useful in surgical planning and obturator designing. CBCT helps reveal the presence of irregular socket healing with disrupted cortical outline, which is otherwise not apparent in panoramic radiograph. Moreover, intact sinus walls in the CBCT and absence of clinical symptoms helps rule out intracranial or orbital extension of the disease.[4] CBCT is not an imaging of choice in nonambulatory cases.

However, in cases of intracranial involvement, CBCT is of limited use. In such cases, CT and MRI would give better features and soft-tissue contrast.[4] Soft-tissue infiltration with fat stranding is better diagnosed with MRI.

Management

A successful treatment of mucormycosis requires four steps[4]:
1. Prompt diagnosis.
2. Reversal of underlying predisposing risk factors.
3. Surgical debridement.
4. Antifungal therapy.

Novel therapies and treatment approaches are being explored to counter mucormycosis. But extensive surgical debridement is the mainstay of management along with antifungal treatment. Due to economic constraints and non-availability of antifungal drugs, many patients who skipped drug therapy also did reasonably well with good surgical debridement, as per the authors' experience.

Amphotericin-B deoxycholate (AmB) and its lipid formulations remain the only licensed antifungal agents for the treatment of mucormycosis. Lipid formulations of Amphotericin-B (LFABs) are significantly less nephrotoxic and can be safely administered at higher doses for a longer period than AmB.[5,6]

Blood vessel thrombosis and tissue necrosis can result in poor penetration of antifungal agents to the site of infection. Therefore, debridement of affected tissues is critical for complete eradication of disease. In a logistic regression model, surgery was found to be an independent variable for favorable outcome among patients with mucormycosis.[7]

Presentation of maxillary disease occurs in varied patterns. The palatal presentation may be as follows:
- Palate involvement without mucosal involvement.
- Palate involvement with mucosal involvement.
- Anterior palate involvement (**Figs. 8.4** and **8.5**).
- Unilateral (**Fig. 8.6** and **Fig. 8.7**) or bilateral palate involvement (**Fig. 8.8**).
- Unilateral (**Fig. 8.9**) or bilateral posterior maxillary involvement (**Fig. 8.10**).

Stage 1B cases require removal of affected bone according to the involvement by sublabial approach and degloving the mucosa. In some patients, the sublabial approach will not be adequate if the anterior maxillary involvement and dentoalveolar soft-tissue involvement are extensive, where a lip split incision extended above as lateral rhinotomy incision and classical Weber–Fergusson incision is needed. Conservative and aesthetic incisions can be given less importance as disease clearance is the priority.

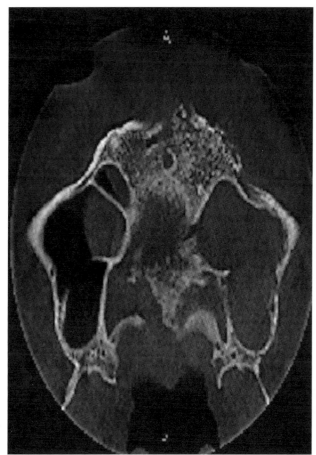

Fig. 8.4 Cone beam computed tomography (CBCT) axial view depicting anterior palatal involvement.

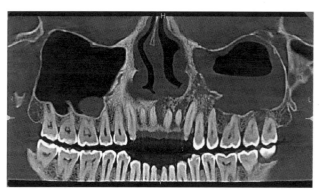

Fig. 8.5 Cone beam computed tomography (CBCT) panoramic slice showing anterior midline palatal involvement.

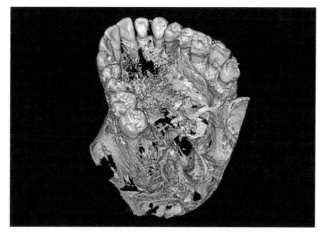

Fig. 8.6 Cone beam computed tomography (CBCT) volume-rendered image showing anterior palatal involvement.

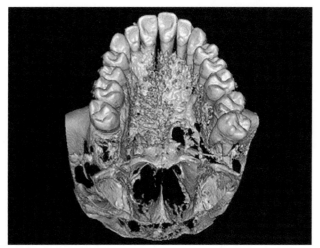

Fig. 8.7 Cone beam computed tomography (CBCT) volume-rendered image showing anterior and posterior unilateral palatal involvement.

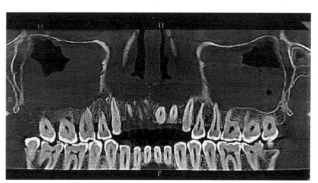

Fig. 8.8 Cone beam computed tomography (CBCT) panoramic slice showing bilateral palatal disease.

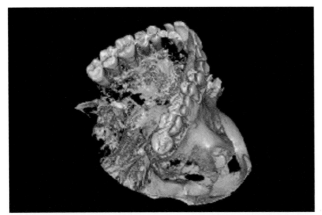

Fig. 8.9 Cone beam computed tomography (CBCT) volume-rendered image showing unilateral posterior palate with pterygoid plate erosion.

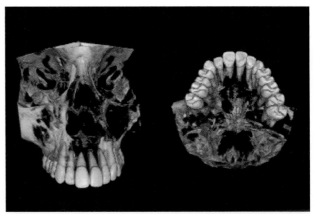

Fig. 8.10 Cone beam computed tomography (CBCT) volume-rendered image showing recurrent disease of bilateral palate. Note the post-Denker status on the left side.

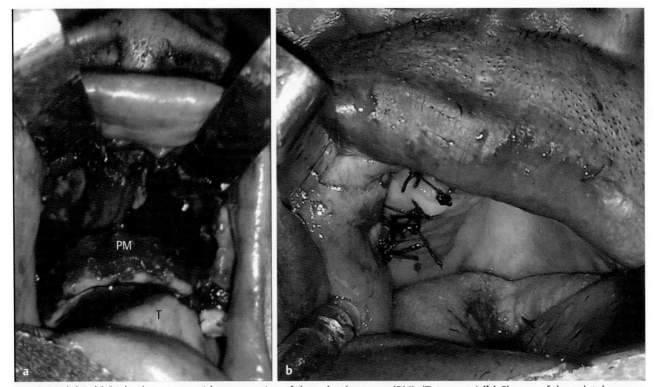

Fig. 8.11 (a) Sublabial palatectomy with preservation of the palatal mucosa (PM). (T, tongue.) **(b)** Closure of the palatal mucosa after sublabial palatectomy in a different patient.

Discrete involvement of the disease of the maxilla will not always allow a classical maxillary resection procedure. More often an extensive surgical debridement must be done till fresh bone margins are seen. Unless all necrotized bones are cleared, recurrence is expected.

Palatal surgeries are of two types:

- Mucosa preserving.
- Nonmucosa preserving.

Preservation of the palatal mucosa helps in primary closure and avoids oronasal or oroantral fistula (**Fig. 8.11**). This helps in early rehabilitation, swallowing, and speech.

If defect in the palate ensues after debridement or if the maxilla is lost, an obturator in the postoperative period is mandatory. All mobile teeth with remnant alveolus are removed and only very firm teeth with healthy bony support are spared (**Fig. 8.12**). These remaining teeth can support

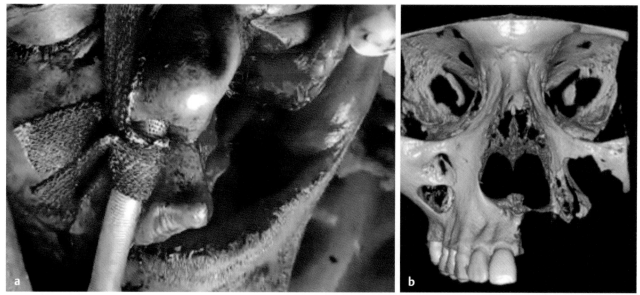

Fig. 8.12 (a) Lateral rhinotomy and resection of the left palate with the mucosa. Note the defect. **(b)** Cone beam computed tomography (CBCT) volume-rendered image showing the postoperative defect.

prosthesis or obturator in improving the quality of life for the patient.

Extensive radical surgical debridement is the key for the best chance of controlling this infection along with all classical resection procedures routinely practiced in the maxilla.

An "aggressive–conservative" approach has been discussed, in which intraoperative frozen sections are used to delineate the margins of infected tissues.

Postsurgical Rehabilitation

Prosthetic rehabilitation is advised for rehabilitation of hard and soft palate defects. Maxillary obturators are used for hard palate defects, pharyngeal obturators are used for soft palate defects, and maxillopharyngeal obturators are used for defects including both the structures. This prosthetic rehabilitation helps restore aesthetic and functional capabilities such as restoration of teeth, speech, oral food intake, and deglutition by recreation of an anatomical barrier between the oral and nasal cavities.

Depending on the duration from the date of maxillary resection, an obturator can be classified as:
- Immediate surgical obturators (feeding plates).
- Interim obturators.
- Definitive obturators.

Immediate Surgical Obturators

Patients undergo a preoperative prosthetic evaluation and a surgical impression is made, which would help in

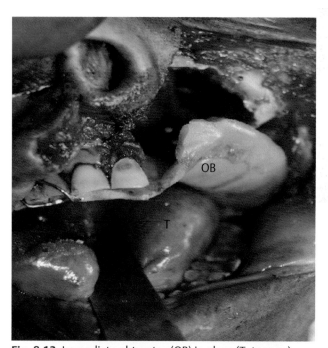

Fig. 8.13 Immediate obturator (OB) in place (T, tongue).

construction of an immediate surgical obturator. This obturator is placed just after the surgery and is mainly used to minimize postoperative complications (**Fig. 8.13**). It helps protect the surgical site from soiling and contamination, promotes postoperative oral hygiene, restores normal diet and speech, supports soft tissue, reduces disfigurement and contracture, reproduces palatal anatomy, and protects the surgical site from trauma. They can also be used to correct the contour of the lips and cheeks.[8,9]

Interim Obturator

Around 1 month postsurgery, an interim or temporary obturator is made using a postsurgical impression cast.[10] The addition of teeth in the obturator is limited to satisfying aesthetic needs and aiding speech. The bulb part of the obturator extends into the defect and accommodates it, which provides a hermetic seal. This obturator is used until the healing process is complete. This stage can last anywhere between 2 and 24 months.

Definitive Obturator

The definitive obturator is fabricated from a postsurgical maxillary cast approximately 6 months after surgery, once the surgical site healing is complete, and alterations of dimensions are less likely (**Fig. 8.14**). This obturator has a metal framework that supports the teeth and the hollow bulb, by acting as the palate.[10]

Cast Partial Prosthesis

This type of prosthesis serves as the best treatment modality in hemimaxillectomy cases or in cases with firm, retained teeth. Cast partial dentures are more comfortable, durable, biocompatible, with enhanced longevity, stability, and aesthetics in comparison to resin-based prosthesis.[11]

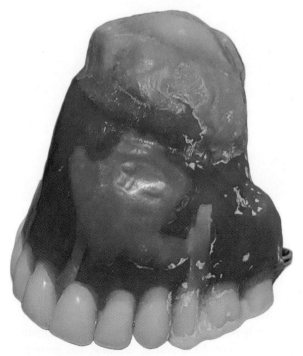

Fig. 8.14 Permanent obturator.

CAD-CAM and SLS Technology

The computer-aided design and computer-aided manufacturing (CAD-CAM) technology and selective laser sintering (SLS) technology are also used in the fabrication of prosthesis for maxillofacial defects. The SLS technique has advantages of improved mechanical properties. Its patient compliance rate in terms of cleaning of the prosthesis, speech, mastication, and reduced manufacturing time is significant. Another added advantage is the availability of saved data for future prosthesis manipulation.[12]

Zygomatic Implants

In bilateral hemimaxillectomy cases, zygomatic implants can be a solution due to the lack of maxillary bony support for prosthetic rehabilitation, especially when the entire palatal mucosa is preserved. It involves placement of implants into the disease-free zygomatic complex, which is then loaded with a dental prosthesis. It requires the use of CBCT to assess the quality of bone and to plan the placement of implants. Zygoma implant reconstruction of acquired maxillary defects is a safe, predictable, aesthetically satisfying and cost-effective treatment modality.[13]

References

1. Jones AC, Bentsen TY, Freedman PD. Mucormycosis of the oral cavity. Oral Surg Oral Med Oral Pathol 1993;75(4):455–460

2. Ribes JA, Vanover-Sams CL, Baker DJ. Zygomycetes in human disease. Clin Microbiol Rev 2000;13(2):236–301

3. Shastry SP, Murthy PS, Jyotsna TR, Kumar NN. Cone beam computed tomography: a diagnostic aid in rhinomaxillary mucormycosis following tooth extraction in patient with diabetes mellitus. J Indian Acad Oral Med Radiol 2020;32: 60

4. Spellberg B, Edwards J Jr, Ibrahim A. Novel perspectives on mucormycosis: pathophysiology, presentation, and management. Clin Microbiol Rev 2005;18(3):556–569

5. Reed C, Bryant R, Ibrahim AS, et al. Combination polyene-caspofungin treatment of rhino-orbital-cerebral mucormycosis. Clin Infect Dis 2008;47(3):364–371

6. Walsh TJ, Finberg RW, Arndt C, et al; National Institute of Allergy and Infectious Diseases Mycoses Study Group. Liposomal amphotericin B for empirical therapy in patients with persistent fever and neutropenia. N Engl J Med 1999;340(10):764–771

7. Roden MM, Zaoutis TE, Buchanan WL, et al. Epidemiology and outcome of zygomycosis: a review of 929 reported cases. Clin Infect Dis 2005;41(5):634–653

8. Andrades P, Militsakh O, Hanasono MM, Rieger J, Rosenthal EL. Current strategies in reconstruction of maxillectomy defects. Arch Otolaryngol Head Neck Surg 2011;137(8):806–812

9. Shambharkar VI, Puri SB, Patil PG. A simple technique to fabricate a surgical obturator restoring the defect in original anatomical form. J Adv Prosthodont 2011;3(2):106–109

10. Singh M, Bhushan A, Kumar N, Chand S. Obturator prosthesis for hemimaxillectomy patients. Natl J Maxillofac Surg 2013;4(1):117–120

11. Bocari G, Hysenaj N, Bocari A. The advantages of partial dentures made of cast framework cr-co toward those made of resin based dentures. Int J Dent Sci Res 2014;2:32–35

12. Soltanzadeh P, Su JM, Habibabadi SR, Kattadiyil MT. Obturator fabrication incorporating computer-aided design and 3-dimensional printing technology: a clinical report. J Prosthet Dent 2019;121(4):694–697

13. Vega L, Strait R, Ames TE. Bar-retained zygomatic implant overdenture as a first line of treatment. Compendium. 2022;43(7)

9

Anesthetic Challenges in Post-COVID-19 Mucormycosis

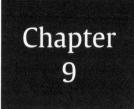

Chapter 9

Anesthetic Challenges in Post-COVID-19 Mucormycosis

Muralidhar Thodebhavi, Ganga Kamath Kudva, Sampath Chandra Prasad Rao, Balamurugan Chinnasamy, and Chinta Sangeetha Mahalakshmi

Introduction

Mucormycosis, a rare angioinvasive disease, is a serious opportunistic fungal infection. It spreads rapidly to cause tissue infarction and necrosis in post-COVID-19 patients. The most common form of mucormycosis is the rhino-orbito-cerebral (ROC) presentation.[1] With a high mortality rate, death may occur within several days to few weeks, despite administration of appropriate treatment. Early identification, reversal of underlying risk factors, timely and thorough surgical debridement of infected tissue, and prompt administration of systemic antifungal medications are all essential components of successful care of mucormycosis. Considering these factors, perioperative care plays a vital role in defining outcomes. A thorough preoperative evaluation, organized anesthetic plan, and good postoperative care help reduce morbidity and mortality.

Anesthetic Considerations

With the current rise in post-COVID-19 mucormycosis cases, anesthesiologists everywhere must stay prepared to manage this poorly understood disease population for elective or emergency surgery. The anesthetic outcome in these patients might be affected by a cadre of variables, such as post-COVID-19 systemic sequelae such as persistent pulmonary dysfunction, adrenal suppression, cardiac dysfunction, difficult airway due to mucormycosis, and deleterious effects of amphotericin-B (AmB).

These individuals are at risk of post-COVID-19 sepsis and a host of other consequences due to the coronavirus' dysregulated innate immune response, ciliary dysfunction, cytokine storm, and microvascular coagulation.

Preoperative Phase

Mucormycosis may affect multiple organ systems leading to hemodynamic instability. Multiple factors must be considered for preoperative optimization of the patient before surgery:

- **Coexisting diseases:** COVID-19 infection status and associated comorbidities such as uncontrolled diabetes mellitus, cerebrovascular disease, acute kidney injury, and pneumonia must be assessed. Complete cardiac assessment including echocardiography for preoperative workup is advisable as stress cardiomyopathy and myocardial injury have been observed with coronavirus infection.[2] It is important to also keep in mind the possibility of thromboembolic phenomena due to the hypercoagulable state brought on by COVID-19 infection.[3] An in-depth history of prolonged or inadvertent use of corticosteroids must be obtained as it may cause adrenal suppression causing perioperative hypotension. Therefore, in these patients, a stress dose of corticosteroids should be taken into consideration. Otherwise, more common causes of persistent hypotension should be ruled out.[4]

- **Preoperative assessment:** All cases must undergo complete blood count, renal function tests, liver function tests, blood sugars, and an electrocardiogram. COVID-19 patients can have restrictive lung disease, impaired gas exchange secondary to lung damage, and residual effects of myocardial injury. As such, high-resolution computed tomography (HRCT) of the chest, arterial blood gas analysis, pulmonary function test (PFT), and echocardiography should be considered based on the severity of the illness.

- **Effect of mucormycosis on the airway:** Difficulty in mask ventilation and endotracheal intubation should be anticipated in these patients. It is due to epiglottitis, sub- and supraglottic edema with fungal debris, restricted mouth opening, palatal perforations, oro-antral fistulas, and crusts in the nose. Proptosis, facial swelling, and wounds in the perioral area due to the use of ill-fitting/tight-fitting noninvasive ventilation masks during COVID-19 treatment can also hinder ventilation. A detailed examination of the airway along with plans for its management should be considered.

- **Preoptimization:** Patients should be optimized for the following conditions:
  - *Anemia*: These patients might present with anemia related to the usage of AmB or due to blood loss secondary to tissue necrosis. The emergency nature of surgical management precludes preoperative correction of anemia in many cases. These cases

should be managed with judicious intraoperative correction of anemia.

> *Sepsis*: Patients should be managed according to the guidelines for sepsis management. Large-bore intravenous access should be established (subclavian vein). The need for invasive lines should be based on the severity of the illness. A central venous access should be established if there is a need for inotropic support. Due to its proximity to the infected site, the internal jugular vein is not the primary choice for central venous cannulation.[5]

> *Adrenal suppression*: Prolonged use of corticosteroids during COVID-19 illness can lead to adrenal suppression. A detailed history regarding steroid usage should be obtained. Stress dose of corticosteroids should be given perioperatively.

> *Chest optimization*: Preexisting pulmonary diseases are increasingly encountered in these patients. Hence, meticulous workup and care are required to reduce the postoperative pulmonary complications. Preoperative spirometry and chest X-ray are useful in assessing the risk factors. Recent research on post-COVID-19 patients has revealed persistent breathlessness and deranged PFTs that are suggestive of restrictive lung disease.[6] A detailed respiratory assessment with PFTs and chest X-ray is recommended. For cases requiring emergency surgery, risk stratification and postoperative ventilatory management should be planned.

- **Anxiety:** Treatment of ROC mucormycosis (ROCM) is aggressive and prolonged. It may lead to cosmetic deformity, apprehension, and emotional instability causing patients to develop severe anxiety. Therefore, the administration of preoperative anxiolytic medications is of prime importance for perioperative anesthetic management of the patients.[7]

- **Effect of amphotericin on various systems:** Systemic AmB that is used in the treatment of mucormycosis is known to cause nephrotoxicity. Other side effects include fever, hypokalemia, hypomagnesemia, hypotension, shivering, and dyspnoea. Therefore, it is essential to achieve hemodynamic stability during the perioperative phase. Regular measurement of arterial blood gas values and intermittent biochemical analyses are essential for anesthetic management of the patients in terms of metabolic condition, fluid–electrolyte balance, and coagulopathy.[8]

Intraoperative Phase

Induction

The main challenge for an anesthesiologist during induction is the difficult airway in these cases. A definitive airway such as an endotracheal tube or tracheostomy is essential. Laryngeal mucormycosis although rare can cause cartilage necrosis and airway obstruction. The diagnostic modality of choice for major airway involvement is rigid bronchoscopy. In such cases, rigid bronchoscopy may reveal granulation tissue and gray–white mucoid material with typically edematous and necrotic appearance of involved airway. Invasive fungal infection may also appear as an endobronchial mass.[6]

An obstructed airway above the glottis warrants an awake tracheostomy. In order to minimize myopathy-induced hyperkalemia, succinylcholine use should be avoided in patients recovering from a prolonged COVID-19 illness.[9] The anesthesiologist should have access to a prearranged difficult airway trolley.[2,3]

Awake fiberoptic intubation (AFOI) is the method of choice to intubate in the cases where mask ventilation and conventional intubation are deemed difficult. This is best employed in the cases where the pathology is in the upper airway above the larynx, and it is outside the airway.

Monitoring should include electrocardiogram, pulse oximetry, arterial blood pressure, capnography, temperature (rectal probe), and central venous pressure. The severity of the illness and the extensive nature of the operation will decide the choice of invasive monitoring.

Maintenance

- **Choice of anesthetic agent:** Several volatile anesthetic drugs are reported to show antibacterial and antifungal activity in various in vitro studies. Due to its property of halting fungal growth, isoflurane can be the preferred inhalational anesthetic agent in vitro.[4] But there is little to no evidence on ideal intravenous and inhaled anesthetic agents for progressive active fungal infections like mucormycosis.

- **Hemodynamic stability and maintenance phase:** In mucormycosis patients, adequate fluid replacement and inotropes for maintaining hemodynamic stability are required. Blood transfusion should be considered based on the extent of surgery, preoperative anemia, and hemodynamic status.

Extubation

The key to efficient airway management is preparedness. Thus, an extubation strategy should be chalked out beforehand for every patient. Extubation is essentially an elective procedure. The goal is to ensure uninterrupted oxygen supply to the patient's lungs, avoid airway stimulation of any kind, and have a backup plan that would allow ventilation and reintubation with minimum difficulty and delay should the extubation fail.[9]

Consider tracheostomy if there is failed reintubation or laryngeal edema with an obstructed airway due to laryngeal pathology.

Postoperative Period

Due to the presence of comorbidities, post-COVID-19 respiratory problems, and airway-related issues, these patients may need postoperative intensive care unit (ICU) care and monitoring.

- **Observations and red flag signs:** Close monitoring of parameters such as level of consciousness, heart rate, respiratory rate, blood pressure, peripheral oxygen saturation, temperature, and pain score is recommended. Early detection of airway obstruction is facilitated using capnography.[10] Red flag signs to look for in this period include early airway compromises such as stridor, obstructed breathing, and those due to surgery such as airway bleeding, hematoma formation, and drain losses. Hemodynamic instability due to bleeding, ketoacidosis, electrolyte imbalance associated with multiorgan failure, and sepsis may appear in the postoperative period.
- **Respiratory management for patients with airway compromise:** Patients with airway compromise must be placed upright and administered high-flow humidified oxygen. Frequent coughing as well as deep breaths may be encouraged to clear secretions. Chest physiotherapy should be given if required. If upper respiratory obstruction/stridor develops, nebulized adrenaline (1 mg) can be used to subdue any airway edema.[9] Early mobilization of the patient, except in those with dural repair, is advisable.
- **Analgesia:** Appropriate and efficient analgesia optimizes postoperative respiratory function. Cautious titration of opioids and correspondingly effective antiemesis measures are essential.

- **Continuation of amphotericin:** Following surgical debridement, medical management is the mainstay of treatment. Medical management predominantly involves AmB. Liposomal AmB has proven to be as effective as conventional AmB with less nephrotoxicity and infusion reaction. Apart from metabolic derangements, peri-infusional events like fever, chills, sweats, and rigors are perceived to be more common with the AmB. The most common regimens included diphenhydramine, paracetamol, and heparin, given alone or in combination with other drugs. Maintaining pre- and posthydration helps in reducing renal complications.
- **Psychological counseling:** The high mortality and morbidity rate of mucormycosis impairs the psychological function and quality of life of patients. There is a need to address these issues with appropriate pharmacological and nonpharmacological management. Routine preoperative counseling should be supplemented with additional supportive psychotherapeutic sessions. Measures for occupational and vocational rehabilitation need to be taken to ensure that patients surviving mucormycosis infection continue to be functioning members of the society.[11]

Conclusion

ROCM has significantly high morbidity and mortality rates despite aggressive medical and surgical management. Therefore, the interprofessional teams must develop a strong interaction and coordination to achieve the best results for patients with ROCM. The role of an anesthetist as a perioperative physician is crucial in improving patient outcomes in this rather morbid condition.

References

1. Prakash H, Chakrabarti A. Global epidemiology of mucormycosis. J Fungi (Basel) 2019;5(1):26

2. Bjurström MF, Bodelsson M, Sturesson LW. The difficult airway trolley: a narrative review and practical guide. Anesthesiol Res Pract 2019;2019:6780254

3. Malhotra N, Bajwa SJS, Joshi M, Mehdiratta L, Kurdi M. Second wave of COVID-19 pandemic and the surge of mucormycosis: lessons learnt and future preparedness—Indian Society of Anaesthesiologists (ISA National) Advisory and Position Statement. Indian J Anaesth 2021;65(6):427–433

4. Barodka VM, Acheampong E, Powell G, et al. Antimicrobial effects of liquid anesthetic isoflurane on *Candida albicans*. J Transl Med 2006;4(1):46

5. Wali U, Balkhair A, Al-Mujaini A. Cerebro-rhino orbital mucormycosis: an update. J Infect Public Health 2012;5(2): 116–126

6. Husari AW, Jensen WA, Kirsch CM, et al. Pulmonary mucormycosis presenting as an endobronchial lesion. Chest 1994;106(6):1889–1891

7. Ahmetovic-Djug J, Hasukic S, Djug H, Hasukic B, Jahic A. Impact of preoperative anxiety in patients on hemodynamic changes and a dose of anesthetic during induction of anesthesia. Med Arh 2017;71(5):330–333

8. Kulkarni PK, Reddy NB, Shrinivas B, Takkalki VV. Anesthetic considerations in the management of mucormycosis. Int J Med Public Health 2015;5(4):387–390

9. Popat M, Mitchell V, Dravid R, Patel A, Swampillai C, Higgs A; Difficult Airway Society Extubation Guidelines Group. Difficult airway society guidelines for the management of tracheal extubation. Anaesthesia 2012;67(3):318–340

10. O'Sullivan E, Laffey J, Pandit JJ. A rude awakening after our fourth "NAP": lessons for airway management. Anaesthesia 2011;66(5):331–334

11. Singh A, Gupta A. Surviving mucormycosis: impact on psychological well-being and quality of life. Acta Scientific Otolaryngology 2021;3(7):90–92

10

Surgical Staging System of Rhino-Orbito-Cerebral Mucormycosis in the Endoscopic Era

Chapter 10

Surgical Staging System of Rhino-Orbito-Cerebral Mucormycosis in the Endoscopic Era

Narayanan Janakiram, Shilpee Bhatia Sharma, and Lekshmy R. Kurup

Introduction

Worldwide, the prevalence of zygomycosis is 0.005 to 1.7 per million population.[1] According to the latest estimates for 2019–2020, its prevalence is 80 times higher in India than in developed countries.[1] India has the second largest diabetic population in the world.[2] Diabetes mellitus remains the highest risk factor for mucormycosis in India, whereas hematological malignancy and transplants are the leading causes in developed nations.[3] With the increase in the diabetic population, mucormycosis has effaced as an immense public health challenge in low- and middle-income countries.[1]

The epidemiological evolution of mucormycosis is aided by factors such as immunomodulatory drugs, emergence of new species, and COVID-19 pneumonia. In the recent past, the Indian subcontinent has witnessed an alarming rise of mucormycosis in post-COVID-19 diabetic patients. The rhino-orbito-cerebral (ROCM) mucormycosis is one of the most common presentations with a formidable aggressive mortality rate. ROCM refers to a broad spectrum of presentations from limited sinonasal disease to orbital and intracranial extensions.

Rapid diagnosis of ROCM can be achieved with diagnostic nasal endoscopic biopsy and radio imaging modalities. Magnetic resonance imaging (MRI) is the primary tool for diagnosing, defining the disease extent, and postoperative surveillance. MRI provides more specific information about sinuses, orbit, and intracranial structures. Cone beam computed tomography (CBCT) has become a mainstay in oral and maxillofacial surgery. The signs of osteomyelitis in the frontal and maxillary sinuses were well depicted in three-dimensional multiplanar views.

The optimal management of ROCM is multidisciplinary. It consists of augmentation of the immune system, glycemic control, surgical debridement, and antifungal therapy. Surgical debridement plays a crucial role in the treatment of ROCM and extensive debridement of infected necrotic tissue significantly reduces the burden. A multitude of approaches has been described in the literature to surgically address ROCM. Endoscopic approaches to the sinonasal region and the skull base have revolutionized from radical to more conservative approaches in these complex anatomical regions.

These advances have provided the armamentarium with conservative techniques to approach orbital diseases and skull base. However, no formal guidelines have been formulated regarding the appropriate surgical approach and extent of excision.

This pandemic has enabled the authors to analyze the presentations and patterns of spread, and devise a multitude of approaches for surgical debridement of ROCM. New insights were gained regarding the possible site of infection and pathways of spread with a detailed assessment of skull base osteomyelitis, which was confirmed intraoperatively. The role of surgical management of this disease entity has evolved. After reviewing and summarizing our experience, a step-by-step algorithm was created to stratify ROCM extension into distinct subgroups with a defined surgical approach. This novel version of the staging can guide clinicians to develop treatment plans more rationally, evaluate the treatment more scientifically, and assess the prognosis more accurately.

Imaging Protocol

Radiology is an integral part of diagnosis, defining the disease extent, identifying complications, and assisting in postoperative surveillance. CT has long been considered an integral part of screening at-risk patients, despite the reported low specificity.[4] In CT, early changes cannot be differentiated from nonspecific sinusitis.[5] It shows hypoattenuating mucosal thickening and the inflammatory processes of the orbit and soft-tissue infiltration of retroantral tissue. In advanced stages of the disease, after the necrosis of the soft tissues, osseous erosions become evident.[6] Nasal septal destruction, turbinate erosions, sinus wall erosions, and reduced density of the maxillary alveolar bone around tooth sockets and hard palate due to infiltration and erosions can occur in advanced cases. MRI provides better visualization because of excellent soft-tissue contrast, especially in the case of equivocal nasal endoscopy and CT findings.

MRI depicts the involvement of the orbital soft tissue, infratemporal fossa, intracranial structures, perineural invasion, and vascular obstruction better than CT. The MRI findings in invasive ROCM include: isointense lesions relative to the brain on T1-weighted (T1W) and iso- to hyperintense on T2-weighted (T2W). The fungal elements tend to have a low intrinsic signal on T2W images. In postcontrast images, the devitalized mucosa appears as nonenhancing tissue.[7,8]

Orbital involvement can be observed as an orbital mass and/or thickening of the recti muscles and optic nerve. Cavernous sinus thrombosis usually results from the spread of infection from the orbit and appears as a filling defect within the enhancing sinus or as a lateral convexity. Other features like narrowing of the carotid artery, carotid arterial wall enhancement, and other intraparenchymal abnormalities like cerebral infarcts, empyema, and meningitis may also be seen.[9] Cerebral angiography may further reveal vascular occlusion, aneurysmal dilatation, or filling defect.[10]

Mucor eroding the walls of the sphenoid sinuses can cause osteomyelitis or necrosis of the pterygoid wedge, clivus, greater wing of the sphenoid, Meckel's cave, trigeminal nerves at their respective foramina, internal carotid artery, and sella. CT imaging may demonstrate diffuse, nonspecific prevertebral soft-tissue swelling and bony erosion at the central skull base. MRI is essential to better characterize the soft-tissue planes at the skull base. Early involvement of bone marrow is seen as a loss of normal fat signal on T1W images. The diseased marrow appears hypointense on T1W images, hyperintense on short tau inversion recovery (STIR) images, and heterogeneously enhanced on postcontrast images. Adjacent normal fat planes are obliterated with T2 hyperintense areas indicating soft-tissue edema. On postcontrast imaging, direct invasion and fungal soft tissue will not enhance; rather, the secondary inflammation will enhance. The margin of enhancement correlates with the plane of viable inflammatory tissue during surgical debridement. The most consistent MRI finding is focal or diffuse clival hypointensity on T1W images relative to normal fatty marrow.

CBCT provides the surgeon with multidimensional and multiplanar views without the financial burden and radiation exposure of conventional CT scans for a more accurate diagnosis and treatment.[11] It offers additional value in evaluating maxillary sinus and frontal sinus erosions, disruptions of the cortex, sequestrum, and alveolar dehiscences that require surgical treatment. Multidetector computed tomography (MDCT) with 3D CT facial reconstruction was done in selected patients with bone involvement to plan surgical resection and plan future reconstruction.

Newer sequences such as susceptibility-weighted imaging (SWI) and diffusion-weighted imaging (DWI) play an important role in the evaluation of intracranial complications. Hypointensity may be noted on SWI, surrounding the intraparenchymal lesions, due to microhemorrhages or mineral elements produced by invading fungi. DWI helps in identifying acute arterial territory infarcts. Also, a peripheral rim of restriction may be seen in fungal abscesses on DWI.[12]

Surgical Management

Staging System

The therapeutic approach should be multimodality and be considered on a case-by-case basis. The treatment of ROCM has been largely unchanged over the past decades, with tailored antifungal therapy, correction of medical comorbidities, cessation of immunosuppressive drugs, and surgical debridement. Surgical debridement of the affected site has been shown to contribute significantly to decreasing mortality.[13] Surgery serves an important role in debridement of the devitalized tissue, decompression of the fungal burden, and enhancement of antifungal delivery.

Surgical access to paranasal sinuses (PNS), orbit, and skull base is difficult and has traditionally been achieved using a variety of open approaches. Advancements in endoscopic instrumentation and techniques have allowed deep surgical corridors with excellent visualization in the orbit and skull base.[14,15] Designing a surgical classification system would help stratify patients and facilitate refinement in treatment planning. The application, indications, and results of these approaches could increase the understanding of disease and its management across the globe.

The senior author, based on his surgical experience and analysis of a total of 193 patients (129 primary and 64 revision cases) of ROCM, has proposed a surgical staging system based on radiological imaging and a protocol for the selection of appropriate techniques (Janakiram staging for post-COVID-19 mucormycosis [JSPM]; **Table 10.1**). Patients were staged from stage I to stage V. Each stage was subdivided according to the extent of disease.[16]

Although the host status can be complex to classify, and the prediction of hematogenous spread is difficult, this staging system has helped us in giving maximum disease clearance for the given stage. The authors would like to stress the importance of central skull base debridement for posterior disease to maximize the benefit of antifungal therapy. New diagnostic imaging, molecular technology, and pharmacological molecules have the potential for further refinements in surgical management.

The radiological distribution of patients in various stages is shown in **Table 10.2**. In primary disease, stage I (34.1%) was most common and in revision cases, stage IIIC (35.9%) was maximum. The percentage of patients with central skull base osteomyelitis (stage III) among primary cases was 36.4% and revision cases was 43.7%. It is evident that the stage III population constitutes a significant proportion of the total

Table 10.1   JSPM staging system with surgical protocol

Stage	Areas involved		Surgical approach
Stage I	**Rhino-palatal**		
Ia	Osteomeatal complex, middle turbinate, inferior turbinate, maxillary sinus, ethmoid sinus, and frontal sinus		Endoscopic medial maxillectomy and complete spheno-ethmoidectomy
	Premaxilla, PPF, and ITF		EMDA with dissection of PPF and ITF
Ib	Limited unilateral or unilateral with central palatal involvement (preserved palatal mucosa)		Sublabial segmental resection with primary closure
Stage II	**Rhino-orbital**		
IIa	Involvement of bony orbital walls: Medial and inferior orbital wall (with or without orbital fat involvement)		Endoscopic orbital decompression + TRAMB
IIb	Involvement of extraocular muscles (extraconal compartment)		Transnasal transorbital endoscopic globe and optic nerve sparing orbital debridement: With TRAMB
IIc	Involvement of posterior orbit including SOF and OA		Transpterygoid clearance with TRAMB
IId	Involvement of anterior and posterior globe		Orbital exenteration
Stage III	**Central skull base osteomyelitis**		
IIIa	Median: Pterygoid wedge, planum sphenoidale, sella, clivus, sphenoid sinus, floor and keel of the sphenoid sinus, and rostrum		Endoscopic midline trans-sphenoidal approach to clear the sella, clivus, floor and lateral recess of the sphenoid
IIIb	Paramedian: • PAC: Medial and lateral pterygoid plates, V2 branch of the trigeminal nerve, and quadrangular space • PMC: Cavernous sinus • PPC: Meckel' s cave and medial petrous		Transpterygoid supra-petrous approach to Meckel's cave and cavernous sinus
IIIc	Lateral: V3, greater wing of the sphenoid, base of the temporal lobe Lateral orbital wall and temporal fossa		Transpterygoid supra-petrous approach to the base of the temporal lobe Endoscopic + hemi-/bicoronal approach
IIId	Skin, palatal involvement with the mucosa		Transfacial approaches: Total maxillectomy with endoscopic skull base debridement
Stage IV	**Involvement of bones of cranium (ethmoid [cribriform and crista galli], frontal, parietal, zygoma, and superior orbital wall) with/without extradural abscess**		**Combined approach (endoscopic + external approach)**
IVa	Involvement of the bones of the cranium without extradural abscess	Frontal unilateral	Endoscopic + Lynch–Howarth, infra-brow approach
IVb	Involvement of the bones of the cranium with extradural abscess	Frontal bilateral Lateral orbital wall Zygoma Temporalis muscle Temporal bone Parietal bone	Endoscopic + bicoronal Incision with pericranial flap
		Ethmoid bone	Anterior craniofacial resection (ACFR)
Stage V	**Intracranial involvement**		**Endoscopic/transcranial approaches**
Va	Frontal and temporal intracranial abscess		Transnasal endoscopic approach
Vb	Intracranial: Dural involvement Pial involvement		Transnasal endoscopic + transcranial approach

Abbreviations: EMDA, endoscopic modified Denker's approach; JSPM, Janakiram staging for post-COVID-19 mucormycosis; ITF, infratemporal fossa; OA, orbital apex; PAC, paramedian anterior compartment; PMC, paramedian middle compartment; PPC, paramedian posterior compartment; PPF, pterygopalatine fossa; SOF, superior orbital fissure; TRAMB, transcutaneous retro-orbital amphotericin-B injection.

Table 10.2 Radiological distribution of patients according to JSPM

Stage	Primary (*n* = 129)	Revision (*n* = 64)
Stage I	44 (34.1%)	5 (7.8%)
Stage IIa	17 (13.2%)	1 (1.6%)
Stage IIb	2 (1.6%)	1 (1.6%)
Stage IIc	1 (0.8%)	3 (4.7%)
Stage IId	1 (0.8%)	0 (0%)
Stage IIIa	6 (4.7%)	2 (3.1%)
Stage IIIb	14 (10.9%)	3 (4.7%)
Stage IIIc	27 (20.9%)	23 (35.9%)
Stage IVa	3 (2.3%)	16 (25.0%)
Stage IVb	1 (0.8%)	2 (3.1%)
Stage Va	5 (3.9%)	2 (3.1%)
Stage Vb	8 (6.2%)	6 (9.4%)

Abbreviation: JSPM, Janakiram staging for post-COVID-19 mucormycosis.

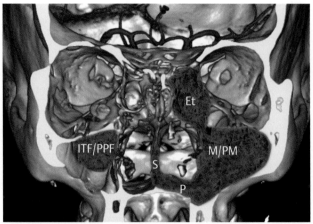

Fig. 10.1 Volume-rendered 3D multidetector computed tomography (MDCT) image of the nose and paranasal sinuses, showing pictorial depiction of stage I disease involvement. (S, nasal septum; P, palate; M, maxilla; PM, premaxilla; Et, ethmoid sinus; ITF, infratemporal fossa; PPF, pterygopalatine fossa.)

Table 10.3 Comparison of author's classification with other classifications of ROCM

Classifications	Stages	Based on	No. of patients	Central skull base debridement
Honavar[13]	1–4	Anatomical progression of ROCM	2,669	Not included
Naik and Rath[14]	ROC (1–3)	CECT/MRI	10	Not included
Metwally et al[15]	1–4	MRI	63	Not included
Soni et al[17]	I–IV	Clinical and radiological	145	Not specific
Vaid et al[18]	Mild to very severe	Radiological	65	Not included
JSPM staging	I–V	Radiological	193	Included

Abbreviations: CECT, contrast enhance computed tomography; JSPM, Janakiram staging for post-COVID-19 mucormycosis; MRI, magnetic resonance imaging; ROC, rhino-orbito-cerebral.

patient population, thereby once again marking the importance of central skull base disease clearance.

Within the staging system, the authors have classified the disease into anterior (stages I–II), posterior (stage III), and intracranial disease. Intracranial mucormycosis is divided into extradural (stage IV) and intradural (stage V). Intracranial disease is a complication of disease progression from anterior (anterior cranial base) to posterior (middle cranial base).

Residual disease was seen in 8 of 129 primary cases and in 2 of 64 revision cases. This was mostly due to patient noncompliance to amphotericin-B, deranged metabolic status, or uncontrolled diabetes.

The mortality rate was 6.2% (12 of 193). Mortality was seen more in elderly patients with associated comorbidities that presented with complications like systemic fungal disease (3 patients), multiorgan failure (3 patients), acute

myocardial infarction (2 patients), pulmonary embolism, carotid blowout, and cardiorespiratory arrest (3 patients each). This supports the fact that mucormycosis is not a localized disease and has systemic manifestations.

A pictorial representation of each stage on 3D CT is depicted in **Figs. 10.1–10.7**.

MR images of stage-wise disease and clearance are shown in **Figs. 10.8–10.17**.

A comparison between current published staging systems and the JSPM staging system is given in **Table 10.3**.

Principles of Surgical Planning

The factors critical for eradicating mucormycosis are rapid diagnosis, reversal of underlying predisposing factors, appropriate surgical debridement of infected tissues, and appropriate antifungal disease.

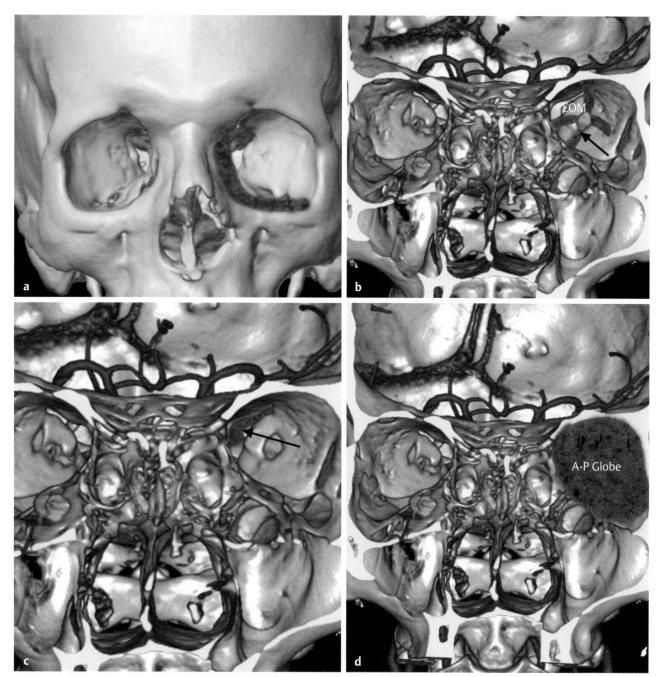

Fig. 10.2 Volume-rendered 3D multidetector computed tomography (MDCT) image of orbit, showing pictorial depiction of stage IIa to IId disease involvement. **(a)** Stage IIa: Involvement of the medial and inferior wall of the orbit. **(b)** Stage IIb: Involvement of the extraocular muscles (EOM) of the orbit (*black arrow*). **(c)** Involvement of the superior orbital fissure (*black arrow*). **(d)** Involvement of the anterior and posterior globe (A-P GLOBE).

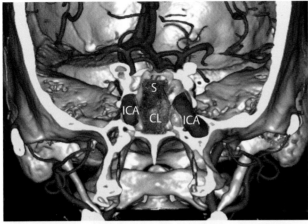

Fig. 10.3 Volume-rendered 3D multidetector computed tomography (MDCT) image at the level of the clivus (CL) showing pictorial depiction of stage IIIa involvement. Bilateral internal carotid arteries (ICA) are marked (S, sella).

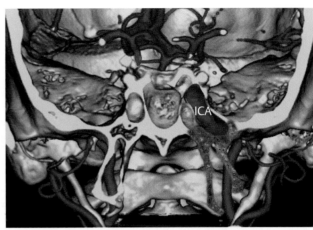

Fig. 10.4 Volume-rendered 3D multidetector computed tomography (MDCT) image at the level of the pterygoid wedge showing pictorial depiction of stage IIIb involvement. The internal carotid artery (ICA) is marked.

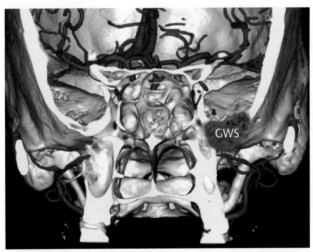

Fig. 10.5 Volume-rendered 3D multidetector computed tomography (MDCT) image at the level of the greater wing of the sphenoid (GWS) showing pictorial depiction of stage IIIc involvement.

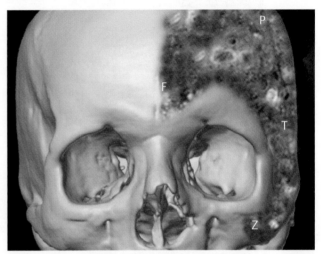

Fig. 10.6 Volume-rendered 3D multidetector computed tomography (MDCT) image showing pictorial depiction of stage IV disease involvement (F, frontal bone; P, parietal bone; T, temporal bone; Z, zygoma).

Fig. 10.7 Volume-rendered 3D multidetector computed tomography (MDCT) image at the level of the base of the temporal lobe, showing pictorial depiction of stage V disease involvement (TA, temporal lobe abscess).

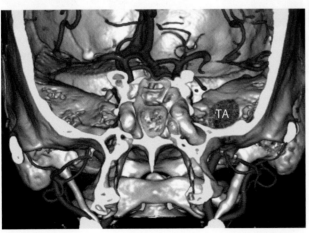

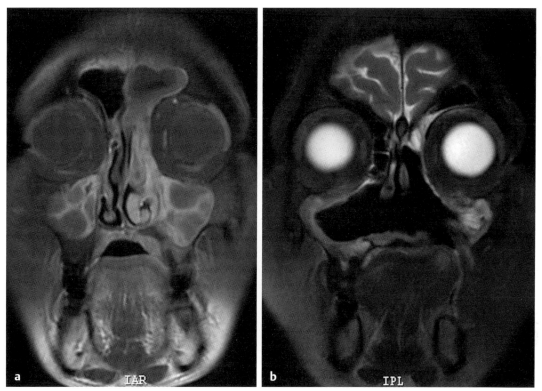

Fig. 10.8 (a) Magnetic resonance imaging (MRI) T1-weighted (T1W) postcontrast coronal image showing depiction of stage Ia disease. **(b)** MRI T2-weighted (T2W) fat-suppressed (FS) coronal image showing complete disease clearance following surgery.

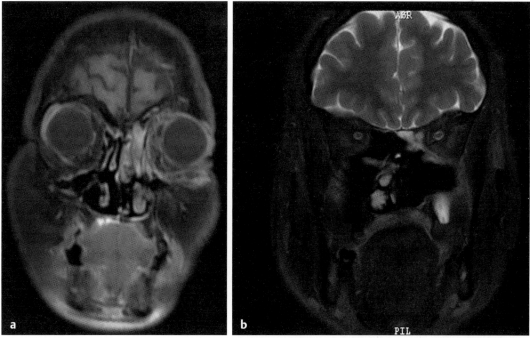

Fig. 10.9 (a) Magnetic resonance imaging (MRI) T1-weighted (T1W) postcontrast coronal image showing depiction of stage IIa disease. **(b)** MRI T2-weighted (T2W) fat-suppressed (FS) coronal image showing complete disease clearance following surgery.

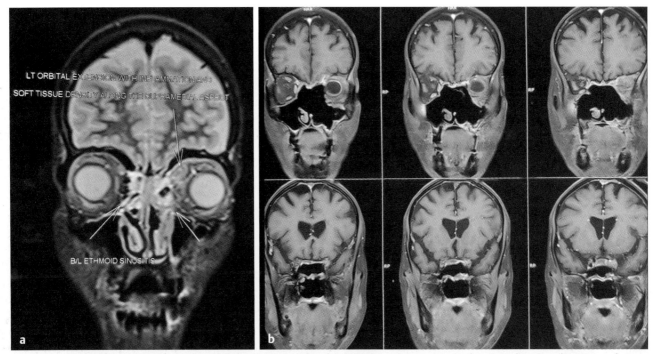

Fig. 10.10 (a) Magnetic resonance imaging (MRI) T1-weighted (T1W) postcontrast coronal image showing depiction of stage IIb disease. **(b)** MRI T1W coronal image showing complete disease clearance following surgery.

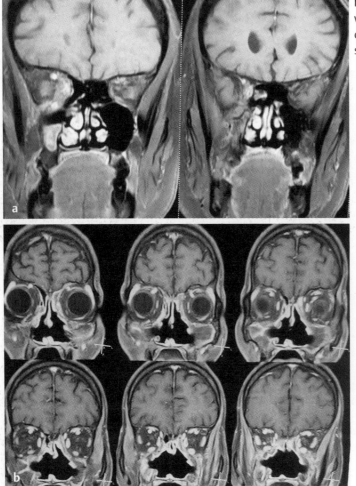

Fig. 10.11 (a) Magnetic resonance imaging (MRI) T1-weighted (T1W) postcontrast coronal image showing depiction of stage IIc disease. **(b)** MRI T1W coronal image showing complete disease clearance following surgery.

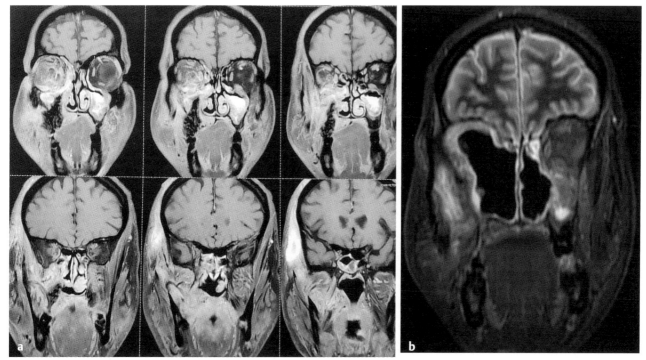

Fig. 10.12 (a) Magnetic resonance imaging (MRI) T1-weighted (T1W) postcontrast coronal image showing depiction of stage IId disease. **(b)** MRI T1W coronal image showing complete disease clearance following surgery.

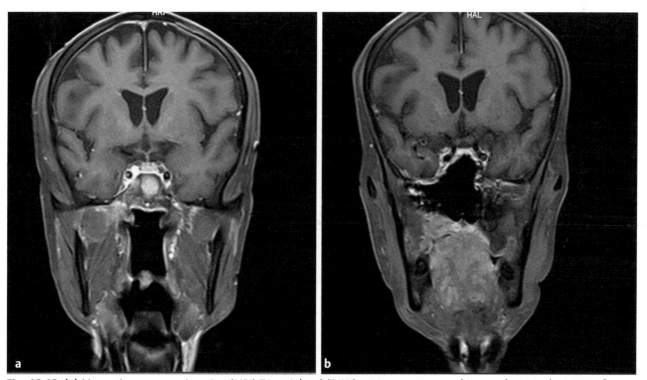

Fig. 10.13 (a) Magnetic resonance imaging (MRI) T1-weighted (T1W) postcontrast coronal image showing depiction of stage IIIa disease. **(b)** MRI T1W coronal image showing complete disease clearance following surgery.

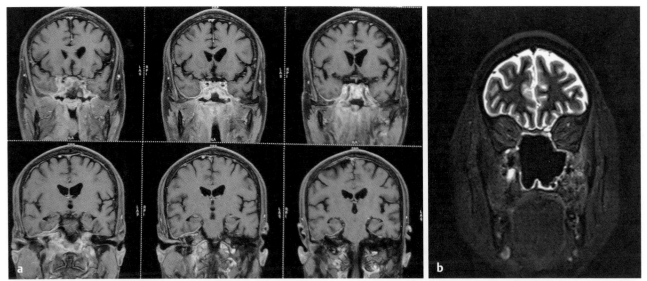

Fig. 10.14 (a) Magnetic resonance imaging (MRI) T1-weighted (T1W) postcontrast coronal image showing depiction of stage IIIb disease. **(b)** MRI T2-weighted (T2W) coronal image showing complete disease clearance following surgery.

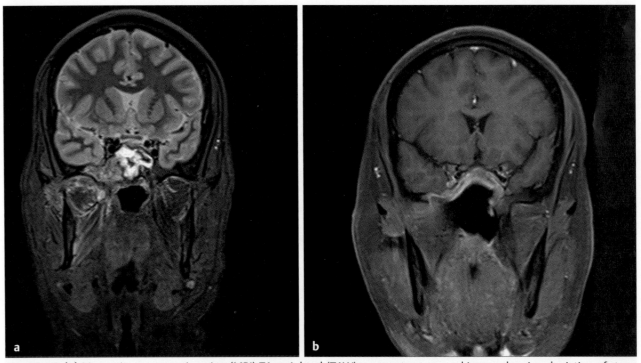

Fig. 10.15 (a) Magnetic resonance imaging (MRI) T1-weighted (T1W) postcontrast coronal image showing depiction of stage IIIc disease. **(b)** MRI T1W coronal image showing complete disease clearance following surgery.

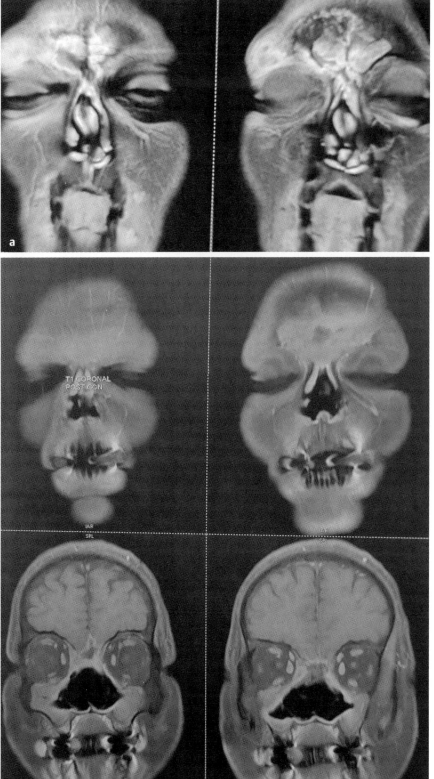

Fig. 10.16 (a) Magnetic resonance imaging (MRI) T1-weighted (T1W) postcontrast coronal image showing depiction of stage IV disease. **(b)** MRI T1W coronal image showing complete disease clearance following surgery.

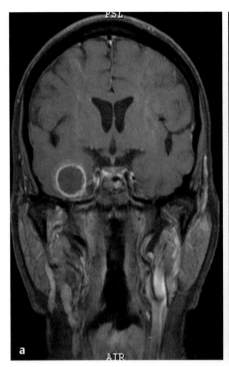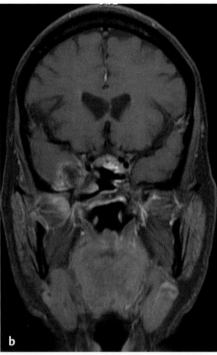

Fig. 10.17 (a) Magnetic resonance imaging (MRI) T1-weighted (T1W) postcontrast coronal image showing depiction of stage IV disease. **(b)** MRI T1W coronal image showing complete disease clearance following surgery.

Disease Mapping: Beyond Sinuses

Early diagnosis is a requisite as small focal lesions can often be surgically excised before they disseminate to critical structures. Furthermore, the initial imaging study can be negative or have subtle findings. Radiographic findings antecede clinical progression in this disease, and a negative imaging study does not provide a rationale to delay more aggressive diagnostic endoscopy with biopsy if clinical suspicion is high.

Multimodality imaging is helpful in prompting early diagnosis and aids in the selection of surgical approaches. The imaging should be performed 12 to 24 hours prior to surgery to exactly map the extent of the disease. MRI of the PNS with the brain and orbit has diagnostic superiority in early cases. The CBCT imaging is excellent for assessing dentoalveolar involvement, thus guiding dental extractions, palatal resections, and obturator designs. The cases with similar anatomical spread can be approached with endoscopic multicorridor or combined approaches for aggressive debridement.

Timing of Surgery

The highly angioinvasive nature of mucormycosis leads to ascending dissemination of infection; therefore, early surgical management should be done when feasible.[19] Surgery is independently associated with successful treatment and survival, particularly in rhino-orbital, cerebral, and pulmonary mucormycosis.[20-22] Evidence of disseminated mucormycosis,

major coagulopathy, and debilitated patients are contraindications for surgery. In case of COVID-19-positive newly diagnosed ROCM, an emergency debridement should be performed. During surgery, the use of a drill and microdebrider is avoided to reduce aerosol generation. It was noted that COVID-19-positive patients with infratemporal fossa and central skull base extension during surgery needed revision surgeries even after the completion of medical treatment.

Four-Handed Binostril Endoscopic Surgery

Endoscopic endonasal approaches are better done by a "four-handed binostril" technique, which requires two surgeons. In this technique, one surgeon holds the endoscope using the right hand and does warm saline irrigations with the left hand. The operating surgeon introduces the suction through the right nostril of the patient and the operating instrument through the left nostril. The saline irrigation keeps the tip of the endoscope clean, improves visibility, and reduces the number of times the surgeon must defog the endoscope. The scope is held at the 11 o'clock position utilizing the elasticity of the ala of the nose. This technique allows better visualization of the disease and the advantage of a panoramic view.

Several authors have argued that the mononostril technique is adequate but was contradicted by other authors stating that the binostril technique gives better surgical freedom and benefits management of hemorrhagic complications with arguably a better working space.[23,24]

Surgical Instrumentation

A battery of specialized instruments aids the surgeon in reducing the operating time and helps achieve a better outcome. It helps in identification of critical structures and removal of tumor from crowded anatomical areas. A detailed description of all the instruments the authors have used is given below.

- **Hopkin's telescope:** Harold. H. Hopkins of Imperial College of London developed the rod optic endoscope in the early 1950s. Further improvements with angled endoscopes were made by Karl Storz from Tuttlingen, Germany. The authors have used 0-degree rigid endoscopes for most part of the surgery and angled endoscopes (30 and 70 degrees) for better visualization of the frontal and maxillary sinus (**Fig. 10.18**). The 0-degree endoscope gives a panoramic view for the surgeon with better anatomical orientation. Angled endoscopes help in visualization of the corner structures of the skull base. The endoscope employs true optical media, that is, it is made of a series of glass rods and lenses, rather than using fiberoptics. The result is a crystal clear image and not a pixelated one. It also ensures better illumination, depth perception, and color contrast. The introduction of xenon light source has greatly improved the visualization. Compared to halogen light, xenon is more durable, efficient, and consumes less energy.
- **Microdebrider:** This instrument is one of the most important innovations that have been brought into the

field of rhinology. It was originally used for removing tumors around the acoustic nerve and has been used in endoscopic nasal surgeries since the early 1990s. This is a cylindrical, powered shaver with continuous suction and irrigation (**Fig. 10.19**). It allows precise resection of tissues, thus avoiding inadvertent tissue trauma. The advantages of using microdebrider are reduced blood loss, faster mucosal healing, reduced surgical time, and synechiae formation. Recent advances in this technology include 360-degree blade rotation, ability to track the tip of the instrument using navigation, and microdebrider with bipolar facilities to control bleeding.

- **Karl Storz S III Neuro drill:** This is a high-speed multifunctional motor system used in skull base surgeries. Its slender and lightweight design prevents surgical fatigue from long hours of surgery. The long handpiece with 60,000 to 100,000 revolutions per minute ensures high precision (**Fig. 10.20**). The tactile feedback from the handpiece allows the surgeon to confidently drill over critical neurovascular structures. It is enabled with a built-in irrigation system that prevents thermal damage to surrounding structures. The irrigation tip is also rotatable around the handpiece, thus facilitating the laterality while operating.
- **Camera and monitors:** All the cases were done using Karl Storz IMAGE1 S modular three-chip camera system (**Fig. 10.21**). This enables a natural viewing of the endoscopic image without altering the color. This is a three charge-coupled device (3-CCD) camera that

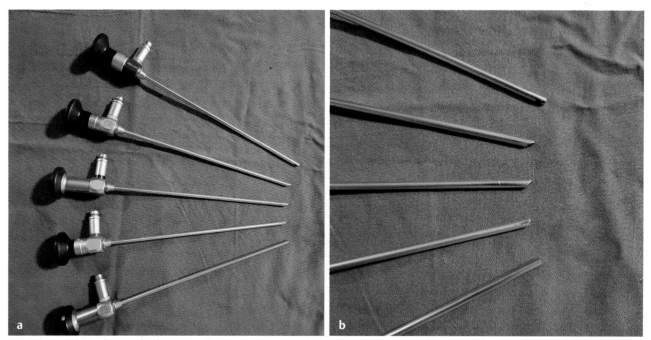

Fig. 10.18 (a) Hopkins rod telescopes: 0, 30, 45, 70, and 90 degrees. **(b)** Magnified image of the tips of all the telescopes.

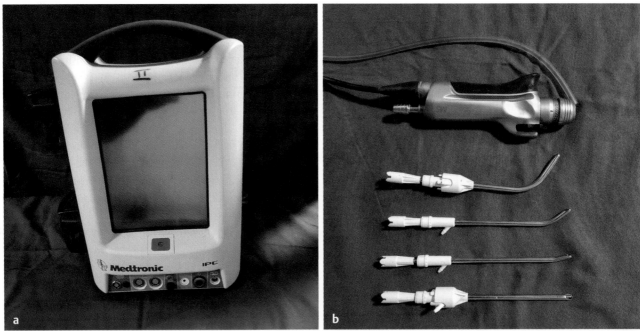

Fig. 10.19 (a) Medtronic Integrated Power Console (IPC) system microdebrider. **(b)** Straight and angled debrider blades used in the IPC system.

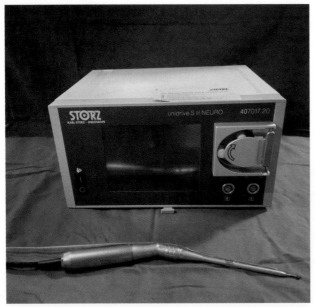

Fig. 10.20 Karl Storz UNIDRIVE S III Neuro drill with handpiece.

uses three 3 CCDs, with each device receiving filtered red, green, and blue color ranges. Compared to 1-CCD cameras, 3-CCD cameras uses full frame dichroic filters, to differentiate the three colors, resulting in greater image quality. It has a 16:9 aspect ratio; when coupled with high-definition screens, it improves visualization. Considering the advancement in technology, this camera is lightweight, which assists the maneuverability of the endoscope. The SPIES (Storz

Professional Image Enhancement System) is equipped with different modalities. The chroma mode improves the sharpness of the image; the Clara mode helps the surgeon to get a clearer visibility of the darker areas inside the image. Spectra A and B modes increase contrast and are based on color tone shift algorithms.[25]

- **Carotid microvascular Doppler:** Intraoperative endoscopic carotid doppler ultrasound is used to identify the location of the internal carotid artery and other intracranial arteries to ensure safe dissection. This instrument particularly helps in revision cases where normal anatomical landmarks are missing. It also aids in safe removal of disease in around critical vascular structures. It is a highly sensitive probe that is slender and bayonet shaped (**Fig. 10.22**). Placed perpendicular to the vessel, it enables the surgeon to hear the pulsations of the artery and thus helps trace its course, even inside a bony canal or tumor stroma.
- **Coblator:** The process of coblation was invented by Philip E. Eggers and Hira V. Thapliyal. The principle of coblation is radiofrequency energy is passed through a conductive medium like isotonic saline and thus produces a plasma field. The isotonic saline is dissociated into free sodium ions that destroy the cellular bonds causing dissociation of tissue. The temperature generated is around 60 to 70°C, thus causing minimal collateral injury.[26] Employing this technique reduces bleeding and saves operating time. The surgeon uses a sterile disposable wand for every surgery (**Fig. 10.23**).

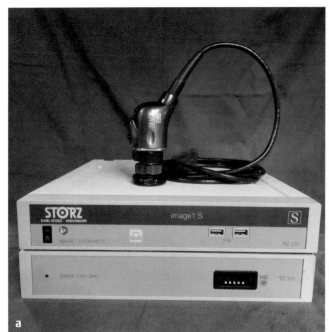
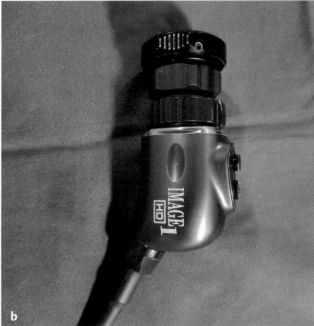

Fig. 10.21 **(a)** Karl Storz IMAGE1 S modular 3-chip camera system. **(b)** Magnified image of the camera head.

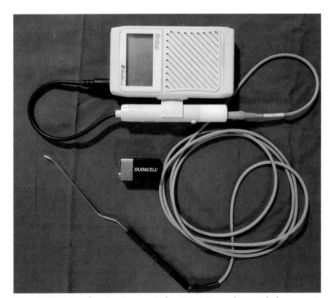

Fig. 10.22 Endoscopic carotid artery Doppler with bayonet-shaped probe and battery.

Selection of Endoscopic or Combined Approach

There is a paucity of appropriate surgical treatment paradigms for ROCM in the age of widespread endoscopic techniques. Traditional management suggested open techniques necessary in every case to debride infected tissues. The central skull base osteomyelitis associated with ROCM has received little attention. The extension of infection through contiguous planes along the skull base to the orbit and intracranial can be reduced by endoscopic radical debridement.

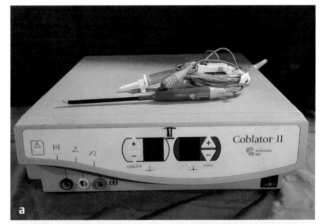
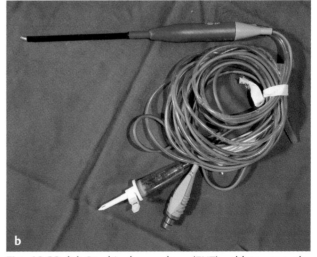

Fig. 10.23 **(a)** Otorhinolaryngology (ENT) coblator console. **(b)** Coblator wand with irrigation system.

The new technology permits detailed and magnified evaluation of deep and complex anatomical subunits in the skull base. The authors advocate that rapid advances in endoscopic skull base surgery allow surgeons to manage skull base osteomyelitis adequately to avoid intracranial morbidity and convalescence observed with open procedures. The infected caseating material of mucosa, muscle, and nerves should be removed till healthy viable tissue is noted. Thus, it is our recommendation that endoscopic evaluation should always be performed in addition to open approaches to aid in real-time decisions regarding sites for frozen biopsies and surgery extent.

Retromaxillary Window

A hallmark of mucormycosis is angioinvasion and resultant tissue necrosis. Most of the blood supply is in the pterygopalatine fossa (PPF) and infratemporal fossa (ITF). Upon endoscopic inspection, the early infected tissue may appear normal. It was noted that it was common to find retromaxillary tissue involvement without bony erosions. The debulking of infection from the retromaxillary space reduces infection through the hematogenous and contiguous planes to the palate, orbit, central skull base, and cranial nerves.

The author inspected the retroantral tissue through a window in the posterior maxillary wall. The opening was made to evaluate the appearance of the periosteum and fat. In case of decreased luster and erosions in the periosteum, fat stranding, and reduced bleeding from the lateral nasal wall, fungal invasion was suspected and debridement was done. The window was widened, and ligation of vessels was done in the PPF and ITF with debridement of muscles till normal bleeding and healthy muscles were noted. The pterygoid wedge, the V2 branch of the trigeminal nerve, and the vidian foramen were identified and the pterygoid wedge with the inferior wall of the sphenoid was drilled.

Conservative–Aggressive Approach

The appearance of tissue at endoscopy may also lag the invasion. The normal-looking mucosa from the maxillary sinus, ethmoid sinus, and sphenoid sinus should be removed and bones thoroughly inspected. There were multiple instances in the authors' experience where the sinus mucosa appeared healthy, upon removal of which clear-cut fungal bone disease was demonstrated.

Eggshell-Like Debridement

Eggshell-like debridement is a radical technique that removes nearly all cancellous bone while preserving a thin layer over the dura. This is applicable in the greater wing of the sphenoid till the temporal fossa dura, sphenoid bone till the superior orbital fissure, cavernous sinus, clivus till the posterior fossa dura and internal carotid artery, frontal sinus, and frontal lobe dura. In the skull base osteomyelitis, the spongy pneumatized trabeculated bone should be drilled till a thin healthy layer over the dura is left or till the dura is reached. This should include an adequate surgical debridement to remove all pathogens along with their biofilms and sequestra that act as a foreign material. The local soft-tissue envelope should also be debrided. In revision cases, it was noted that the bone of the clivus and the greater wing of the sphenoid formed a disconnected sequestrum with an envelope of granulation tissue. This bone was dislodged, and it was noted that vital structures like the dura and the internal carotid artery were separate, and a layer of thickened smooth mucosa was noted over them.

Medical Management

Monitoring patients for adverse events related to drug administration as well as alterations in the pharmacokinetics and pharmacodynamics of each medication resulting from interactions and underlying medical conditions is prudent for the care of these patients. The medical therapy is discussed in detail in Chapter 13.

Nutritional

In addition to medical and surgical treatment, glycemic control and nutrition are important factors for postoperative rehabilitation of ROCM. High glucose concentrations in the blood interfere with wound healing. Strict glycemic control is needed, and regular monitoring is done to avoid hyperglycemia surges. Prosthetic rehabilitation using an obturator prosthesis is essential to post palatal resection surgeries and maxillectomy. The nutritional intervention may include enteral feeding, oral supplementation, or parenteral feedings.

An individualized nutritional intervention with adequate energy and protein intake combined with tailored aerobic and strengthening exercise improved the nutritional and functional status. Nutrition should be adequate to provide sufficient protein for the growth of granulation tissue. There is no accepted standard method for nutritional assessment, but serum albumin and prealbumin levels are widely used. Albumin levels reflect long-term protein consumption, whereas prealbumin levels reflect recent protein consumption due to its short half-life. The serum levels of these hepatic proteins mainly indicate recovery from acute or chronic illnesses.[27]

Surveillance

In the postoperative period, clinical, radiological, and biochemical parameters were used to gauge and direct management of infection accurately.

The endoscopic examinations and suction clearance of the nasal cavities were done weekly. The presence of purulent discharge was noted in the early postoperative period and in patients with poor glycemic control. After the discharge was cleared, underlying tissue was examined for necrosis and osteomyelitis. In two cases, a sequestrum was noted in the posterior septum, and the greater wing of the sphenoid was removed under general anesthesia and cases were reevaluated. Pus was sent for culture, and patients were advised to do regular nasal douching with 3% saline till complete healing of cavity. It was observed that improvement in general health, nutrition, and glycemic control promoted nasal healing and recovery. Patients with steroid-induced transient hyperglycemia had recovery near normal to operated noninfected skull base cases. The mucosalization was noticed from the third month of surgery and fibrosis of the endoscopic Denker's cavity was noted after 6 months, thus indicating delayed healing in old and chronic diabetic patients.

The osteomyelitis was monitored by serial MRI scans at 1 month, 3 months, 6 months, and 1 year. A consistent, normalized value of inflammatory markers such as D-dimer, erythrocyte sedimentation rate (ESR), and C-reactive protein (CRP) for 8 to 12 weeks in asymptomatic patients was considered a biochemical indicator of disease control.

An early termination of antifungal therapy may cause relapse. Disease progression requiring repeat debridement was noted in patients who were unable to complete a course of antifungal intravenous medication.

References

1. Singh AK, Singh R, Joshi SR, Misra A. Mucormycosis in COVID-19: a systematic review of cases reported worldwide and in India. Diabetes Metab Syndr 2021;15(4):102146

2. Pradeepa R, Mohan V. Epidemiology of type 2 diabetes in India. Indian J Ophthalmol 2021;69(11):2932–2938

3. Sengupta I, Nayak T. Coincidence or reality behind mucormycosis, diabetes mellitus and Covid-19 association: a systematic review. J Mycol Med 2022;32(3):101257

4. Groppo ER, El-Sayed IH, Aiken AH, Glastonbury CM. Computed tomography and magnetic resonance imaging characteristics of acute invasive fungal sinusitis. Arch Otolaryngol Head Neck Surg 2011;137(10):1005–1010

5. Middlebrooks EH, Frost CJ, De Jesus RO, Massini TC, Schmalfuss IM, Mancuso AA. Acute invasive fungal rhinosinusitis: a comprehensive update of CT findings and design of an effective diagnostic imaging model. AJNR Am J Neuroradiol 2015;36(8):1529–1535

6. Silverman CS, Mancuso AA. Periantral soft-tissue infiltration and its relevance to the early detection of invasive fungal sinusitis: CT and MR findings. AJNR Am J Neuroradiol 1998;19(2):321–325

7. Herrera DA, Dublin AB, Ormsby EL, Aminpour S, Howell LP. Imaging findings of rhinocerebral mucormycosis. Skull Base 2009;19(2):117–125

8. Safder S, Carpenter JS, Roberts TD, Bailey N. The "black turbinate" sign: an early MR imaging finding of nasal mucormycosis. AJNR Am J Neuroradiol 2010;31(4):771–774

9. Bhatia H, Kaur R, Bedi R. MR imaging of cavernous sinus thrombosis. Eur J Radiol Open 2020;7:100226

10. Onyango JF, Kayima JK, Owen WO. Rhinocerebral mucormycosis: case report. East Afr Med J 2002;79(7):390–393

11. Li G. Patient radiation dose and protection from cone-beam computed tomography. Imaging Sci Dent 2013;43(2):63–69

12. Kondapavuluri SK, Anchala VKR, Bandlapalli S, et al. Spectrum of MR imaging findings of sinonasal mucormycosis in post COVID-19 patients. Br J Radiol 2021;94(1127):20210648

13. Honavar SG. Code mucor: guidelines for the diagnosis, staging and management of rhino-orbito-cerebral mucormycosis in the setting of COVID-19. Indian J Ophthalmol 2021; 69(6):1361–1365

14. Naik MN, Rath S. The ROC staging system for COVID-related rhino-orbital-cerebral mucormycosis. Semin Ophthalmol 2022;37(3):279–283

15. Metwally MI, Mobashir M, Sweed AH, et al. Post COVID-19 head and neck mucormycosis: MR imaging spectrum and staging. Acad Radiol 2022;29(5):674–684

16. Kurup LR, Singh H, Sharma SB, Dehgani-Mobaraki P, Zaidi AK, Janakiram N. Outcome of total surgical debridement of covid associated skull base mucormycosis based on a new surgical staging system: evidence from a cohort study. Accessed November 29, 2022; https://www.medrxiv.org/content/10.1101/2022.11.04.22281828v1

17. Soni K, Das A, Sharma V, et al. Surgical & medical management of ROCM (rhino-orbito-cerebral mucormycosis) epidemic in COVID-19 era and its outcomes - a tertiary care center experience. J Mycol Med 2022;32(2):101238

18. Vaid N, Mishra P, Gokhale N, et al. A proposed grading system and experience of COVID-19 associated rhino orbito cerebral mucormycosis from an Indian tertiary care center. Indian J Otolaryngol Head Neck Surg 2021:1–8

19. Spellberg B, Ibrahim AS. Recent advances in the treatment of mucormycosis. Curr Infect Dis Rep 2010;12(6):423–429

20. Roden MM, Zaoutis TE, Buchanan WL, et al. Epidemiology and outcome of zygomycosis: a review of 929 reported cases. Clin Infect Dis 2005;41(5):634–653

21. Kontoyiannis DP, Wessel VC, Bodey GP, Rolston KV. Zygomycosis in the 1990s in a tertiary-care cancer center. Clin Infect Dis 2000;30(6):851–856

22. Nithyanandam S, Jacob MS, Battu RR, Thomas RK, Correa MA, D'Souza O. Rhino-orbito-cerebral mucormycosis. A retrospective analysis of clinical features and treatment outcomes. Indian J Ophthalmol 2003;51(3):231–236

23. Han S, Ding X, Tie X, et al. Endoscopic endonasal transsphenoidal approach for pituitary adenomas: is one nostril enough? Acta Neurochir (Wien) 2013;155(9):1601–1609

24. Elhadi AM, Hardesty DA, Zaidi HA, et al. Evaluation of surgical freedom for microscopic and endoscopic transsphenoidal approaches to the sella. Neurosurgery 2015;11(1, Suppl 2): 69–78, discussion 78–79

25. Kamphuis GM, de Bruin DM, Fallert J, et al. Storz professional image enhancement system: a new technique to improve endoscopic bladder imaging. J Cancer Sci Ther 2016;8(3): 71–77

26. Hong SM, Cho JG, Chae SW, Lee HM, Woo JS. Coblation vs. electrocautery tonsillectomy: a prospective randomized study comparing clinical outcomes in adolescents and adults. Clin Exp Otorhinolaryngol 2013;6(2):90–93

27. Marcason W. Should albumin and prealbumin be used as indicators for malnutrition? J Acad Nutr Diet 2017;117(7): 1144

11

Surgical Techniques Involved in Stage-Wise Management of Rhino-Orbito-Cerebral Mucormycosis

Chapter 11

Surgical Techniques Involved in Stage-Wise Management of Rhino-Orbito-Cerebral Mucormycosis

Narayanan Janakiram, Shilpee Bhatia Sharma, Lekshmy R. Kurup, and Harshita Singh

Introduction

Sinonasal mucormycosis is a life-threatening fungal infection that usually occurs in immunocompromised patients and requires extensive surgical debridement and systemic antifungal therapy.[1] Despite these measures, prognosis remains bleak. The incidence rate of global mucormycosis varies from 0.005 to 1.7 per million population. Prevalence of mucormycosis in India is 140 per million population, which is approximately 80 times that of other developed countries.[2]

Coexistence of COVID-19 with diabetes and immunosuppressive treatments have unexpectedly increased the incidence and severity of mucormycosis. Fungemia may be responsible for skull base osteomyelitis.[3]

Early diagnosis is crucial to prevent any devastating sequelae and to improve surgical outcome.[4]

Regional involvement of invasive *mucor* and interval between the onset of infection and treatment determines the survival, morbidity, and mortality of the patient.

Effectiveness of treatment depends on the following factors: Early diagnosis, correction of predisposing factors, surgical debridement of affected parts, and systemic antifungal therapy.

Endonasal endoscopic approach has superseded open approaches like Caldwell–Luc surgery, radical maxillectomy, sublabial palatectomy, open craniofacial resection, and maxillary swing. In-depth knowledge of anatomy clubbed with evolution of endoscopes and advanced camera system has enabled complete disease clearance, except in those cases where there was lateral spread and open approaches had to be combined.

Preoperative Preparation

All patients with post-COVID-19 mucormycosis underwent thorough preoperative evaluation including complete blood profile, reverse transcriptase polymerase chain reaction (RT-PCR), and computed tomography (CT) of the chest. Expert opinions were taken from different specialties including cardiologists, nephrologists, physicians, and pulmonologists for all cases. Ophthalmologists, oral and maxillofacial surgeons, and neurosurgeons were involved depending on the particular organ involved for each case. A multidisciplinary approach by a team of skilled specialists was done in all cases.

Magnetic resonance imaging (MRI) of the nose and paranasal sinuses with the orbit and brain (T1-weighted [T1W], T1W with contrast, T2-weighted [T2W], T2 short tau inversion recovery [STIR] sequences, and diffusion-weighted imaging [DWI]) was done in all patients to assess the complete extent of the disease and specifically to rule out subtle soft-tissue involvement of the dural and extradural space.

Also, cone beam computed tomography (CBCT) of the maxilla and 3D CT of the facial bones were done to aid in assessing the palatal disease and in planning reconstruction later.

Clinical examination included a detailed anterior rhinoscopy, otoendoscopy, videolaryngoscopy, intraoral examination, assessment of vision and extra-ocular movements, and a detailed neurological examination.

In those cases, where biopsy was confirmative of mucormycosis, preoperative systemic antifungal therapy was initiated after test dose and adequate hydration.

Patients and attenders were counseled in their native language regarding the need for intravenous amphotericin-B, as surgical and medical therapy plays synergistic role in the outcome. If cosmetic defects were anticipated, the patients were explained in detail about the possible defects with the help of reconstruction diagrams and photographs of previous patients who had undergone a similar procedure.

Preoperative Anesthesia Checkup

All patients were preoperatively assessed by an anesthetist for airway, comorbidities, blood parameters, and treatment history. Premedication was given to all patients prior to surgery for reducing anxiety and facilitating induction. In our center, we prefer to administer benzodiazepine and H2 blocker on the night before surgery as well as in the morning. If the systolic blood pressure of the patient was more than 100 mm Hg, beta-blockers were administered to ease hypotensive anesthesia.

This chapter deals with an array of post-COVID-19 mucormycosis with varied presentations. All cases are assigned a particular stage, according to the Janakiram staging for post-COVID-19 mucormycosis (JSPM) described in the previous chapter. Each case is dealt with in detail with clinical history, physical examination, and further management till follow-up.

Clinical Cases

Stage IA: Anterior Disease (Involvement of the Premaxilla, Maxilla, Osteomeatal Complex, Septum, Ethmoid Sinus, and Frontal Sinus)

Case 1: A 43-year-old nondiabetic patient with a history of COVID-19 infection presented 2 weeks after discharge with left-sided facial pain and swelling. The patient was diagnosed with recent onset of type II diabetes mellitus after initiation of steroid treatment for COVID-19.

Nasal endoscopy showed slough and purulent discharge over the left middle turbinate (MT) and osteomeatal complex (**Fig. 11.1**). On the opposite side, nasal endoscopy showed no abnormality. The orbit and palate were clinically not

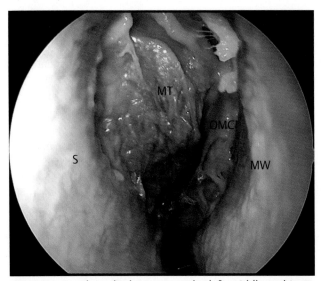

Fig. 11.1 Purulent discharge over the left middle turbinate (MT) with slough in the osteomeatal complex (OMC). (MW, medial wall; S, septum.)

involved. A detailed otorhinolaryngologic, ophthalmologic, and neurological examinations were done. The proinflammatory marker values were monitored and are mentioned in **Table 11.1**.

CT of the paranasal sinuses (CT-PNS) and contrast-enhanced MRI (CE-MRI) of the PNS, orbit, and brain, including T1, T2, T1 fat suppression (FS), T2 FS, T1 FS postcontrast, and DWI were taken to study the extent of the disease and to plan the surgical approaches and excision.

Initial CT-PNS showed mild left ethmoidal sinusitis without any bone erosion evidence. The coronal postcontrast MRI T1 FS images showed nonenhancing soft tissue in the left maxilla, frontal recess, and posterior ethmoid suggestive of fungal soft tissue with a surrounding enhancement of inflammatory tissue (**Fig. 11.2**). In addition, it was noted that the right side sinuses were uninvolved.

All the patients with rhino-orbital-cerebral mucormycosis (ROCM) were planned for endoscopic radical debridement with a sample for KOH and a frozen section to confirm the diagnosis of RCOM. The surgical plan was based on the MRI findings of left-sided maxilla, ethmoid, and frontal sinus involvement. A left endoscopic modified Denker's (EMD) procedure with full-house functional endoscopic sinus surgery (FESS) was performed for aggressive debridement.

After orotracheal intubation, the patient was placed in the reverse Trendelenburg position, and normotensive anesthesia was administered. The nasal cavities were examined, and swabs were taken for gram stain and KOH mount. Povidone-iodine nasal antiseptic washes (0.5%) were given before the onset of surgery. Bilateral nasal cavities were decongested with adrenaline-soaked gauze pieces (1:1,000).

On endoscopic examination, the anterior end of the inferior turbinate had black crusts. The osteomeatal complex had sloughed mucosa over the medial wall of the uncinate process.

Table 11.1 Hematological findings of the patient

	Total count (per µL)	CRP (mg/L)	D-dimer (ng/mL)	LDH (IU/L)	Ferritin (ng/mL)
Preoperative	7,500	160	1,700	320	328
Immediate postoperative	9,000	225	2,200	300	314
At discharge	7,000	45	850	170	88

Abbreviations: CRP, C-reactive protein; LDH, lactate dehydrogenase.

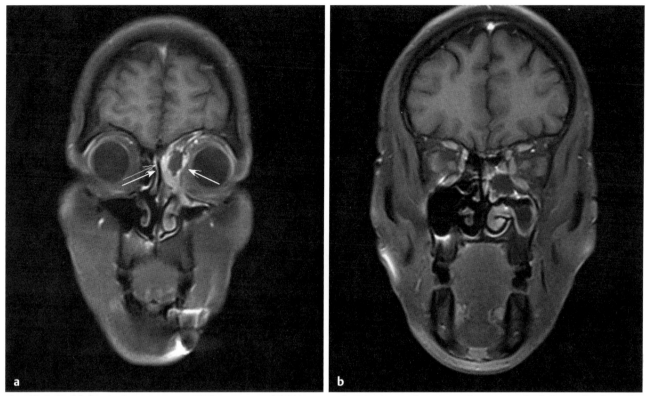

Fig. 11.2 (a, b) Coronal postcontrast T1 fat-saturated (FS) images showing nonenhancing soft tissue in the left maxilla, frontal recess (*white arrows*), and posterior ethmoid suggestive of an invasive fungal disease.

Surgical Steps

Step 1: Left Inferior Turbinectomy

Left inferior turbinate was medialized, in-fractured, and cut along the entire length using sharp turbinectomy scissors, and the specimen was sent separately for KOH mount and histopathology (**Fig. 11.3**). The author has noted that a normal bleeding turbinate signifies patency of the sphenopalatine vascular pedicle and thus decreased probability of thrombosis in the internal maxillary artery. The posterior end of the inferior turbinate was cauterized after turbinectomy.

Step 2: Left Endoscopic Modified Denker's Procedure

Mucosal incisions for Denker's procedure are described below. The superior incision was placed from the anterior attachment of the middle turbinate (MT) to the pyriform aperture (**Fig. 11.4**). The inferior incision was made at the junction of the lateral nasal wall and floor of the nasal cavity (**Fig. 11.5**). Both incisions were joined along the anterior border of the pyriform aperture (**Fig. 11.6**). The subperiosteal plane was identified over the anterolateral wall of the maxillary sinus and elevated laterally till the infraorbital foramen (**Fig. 11.7**). The assistant ensures adequate retraction using the curved tip of the Freer's elevator, which was lodged at the junction of the anterolateral and posterolateral walls of the maxilla (**Fig. 11.8**).

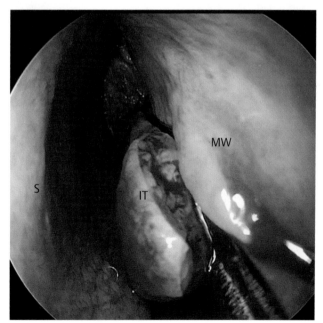

Fig. 11.3 Left inferior turbinectomy. (IT, inferior turbinate; MW, medial wall of the maxilla; S, septum.)

The surgeon shifts to a "four-handed technique" at this stage. Using a Karl Storz S III Neuro drill, an inspection window was created over the anterolateral wall of the maxilla (**Fig. 11.9**).

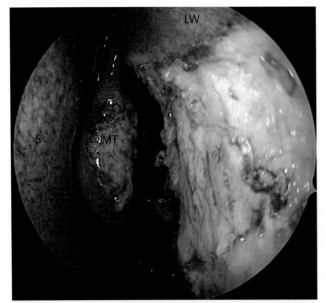

Fig. 11.4 Superior incision for Denker's procedure: Anterior to the middle turbinate (MT) attachment up to the edge of the pyriform aperture. (LW, lateral wall of the nose; S, septum.)

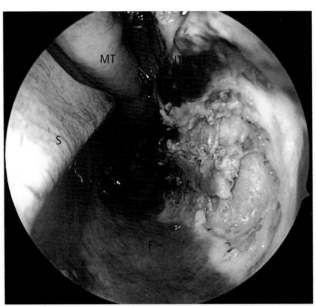

Fig. 11.5 Inferior incision for Denker's procedure at the junction of the lateral wall and floor of the nasal cavity. (F, floor of the nasal cavity; IT CUT, cut end of the inferior turbinate; MT, middle turbinate; S, septum.)

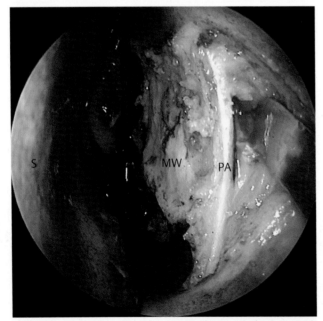

Fig. 11.6 Anterior incision for Denker's procedure along with the bony aperture of the pyriform sinus. (MW, medial wall of maxilla; PA, pyriform aperture; S, septum.)

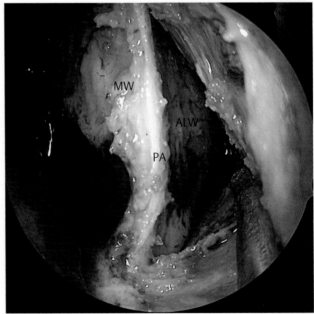

Fig. 11.7 Subperiosteal plane over the anterolateral wall of the maxillary sinus (ALW). (MW, medial wall of the maxilla; PA, pyriform aperture.)

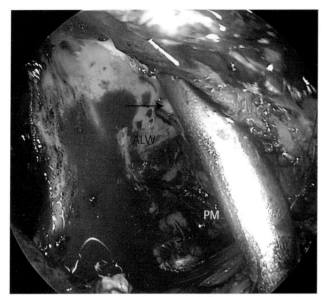

Fig. 11.8 Anterolateral wall of the maxilla (ALW) with contents of the infraorbital foramen (*black arrow*). (PM, premaxilla.)

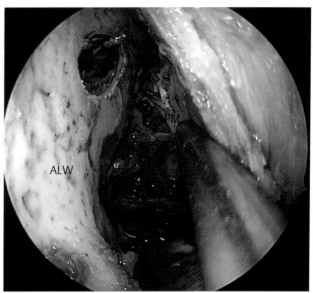

Fig. 11.9 Inspection window (IO) over the anterolateral wall of the maxilla. (ALW, anterolateral wall; PM, premaxilla.)

Superior osteotomy was made inferior to the infraorbital nerve and inferior osteotomy at the floor of the nasal cavity. The low inferior bony cut can cause injury to alveolar roots and a thin alveolar arch; hence, it should be done with caution. After osteotomies, the anterolateral wall of the maxilla was removed and sent for histopathological examination (HPE; **Fig. 11.10**). The nasolacrimal duct (NLD) was transected. In this case, the patient had no gross involvement in the anterolateral wall of the maxillary sinus, frontal process of the maxilla, or the NLD.

Step 3: Left Maxillary Sinus Debridement

On examination, the antral wall mucosa over the medial wall was necrosed (**Fig. 11.11**). The entire antral mucosa was elevated using a curette and removed.

Specimens were sent separately for KOH mount and HPE. Posterior, posterolateral, and alveolar surfaces of the maxilla were carefully examined for disease. The posterior wall of the sinus was intact (**Fig. 11.12**).

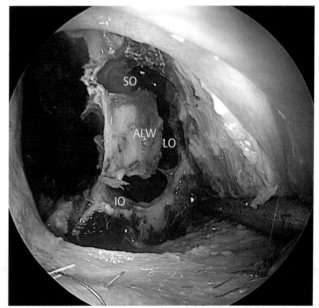

Fig. 11.10 Osteotomies for Denker's procedure. (ALW, anterolateral wall; IO, inferior osteotomy; LO, lateral osteotomy; SO, superior osteotomy.)

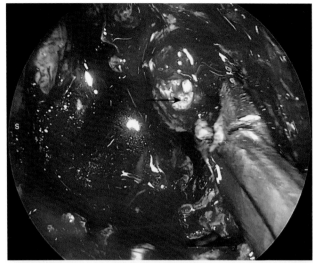

Fig. 11.11 Necrosed maxillary antral mucosa (*black arrow*). (ASM, alveolar surface of maxilla; S, septum.)

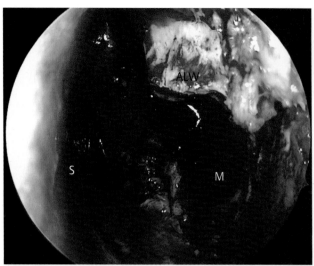

Fig. 11.12 Complete clearance of the left maxilla (M). (ALW, anterolateral wall; S, septum.)

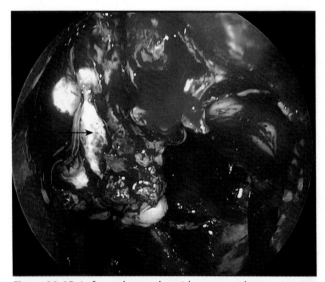

Fig. 11.13 Left sphenoethmoidectomy done. Lamina papyracea (*black arrow*).

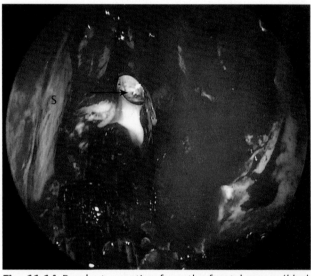

Fig. 11.14 Purulent secretion from the frontal recess (*black arrow*) (S, septum).

Step 4: Left MT Resection

The MT on the left side was necrosed, and partial middle turbinectomy was done.

Step 5: Complete Sphenoethmoidectomy

MRI showed involvement of the left anterior and posterior ethmoids, and the same were filled with fungal debris and were debrided (**Fig. 11.13**). The lamina papyracea was found intact. A wide sphenoidotomy was done, and the sphenoid sinus was found free of disease.

Step 6: Frontal Sinus Debridement

When visualized using a 70-degree endoscope, purulent secretions were seen draining from the frontal recess (**Fig. 11.14**). An on-table decision was made to proceed with the Draf IIb procedure. It was done as the two-handed uninostril approach. The mucosa anterior to the axilla of the MT over the frontonasal process of the maxilla was denuded. The frontonasal process of the maxilla was drilled, nasofrontal beak identified, and frontal recess widened till the septum medially (**Fig. 11.15**). After completion of the Draf IIb procedure, the frontal sinus was cleared off of disease (**Fig. 11.16** and **Video 11.1**).

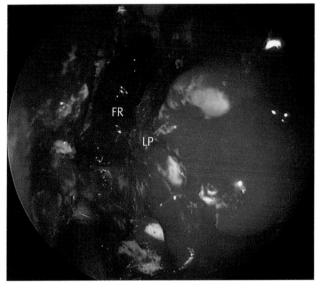

Fig. 11.15 Completed Draf IIB. (FR, frontal recess; LP, lamina papyracea.)

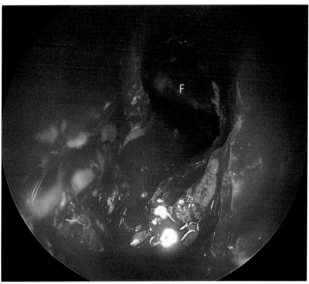

Fig. 11.16 Disease-free frontal sinus (F).

Packing

Diluted amphotericin washes were given, and the nasal cavity was packed.

Postoperative Management

After the surgery, the patient was treated with a cumulative dose of 2.0 g of intravenous liposomal amphotericin-B, which was supplemented with a whole 8-week duration of oral posaconazole. Renal function tests and serum electrolytes were serially monitored, and the patient tolerated the treatment well. The postoperative scan showed complete disease clearance (**Fig. 11.17**). **Figs. 11.18** and **11.19** show healed postoperative cavity.

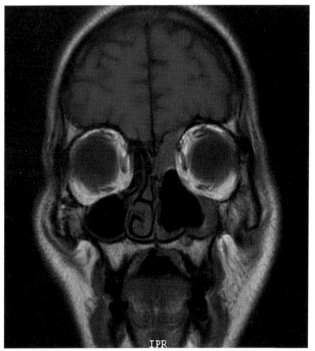

Fig. 11.17 Postoperative T1-weighted (T1W) magnetic resonance imaging (MRI) scan showing complete clearance of disease.

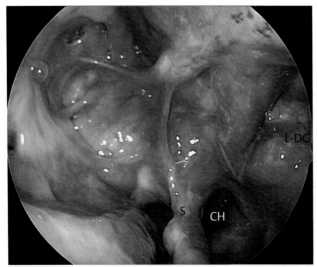

Fig. 11.18 Zero-degree endoscopic view of a well-healed nasal cavity at 2 months postoperatively. (CH, choana; L-DC, healed left Denker's cavity; S, septum.)

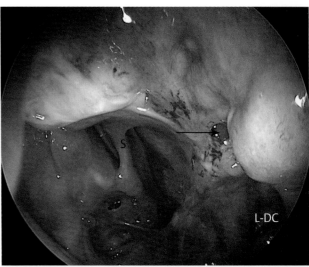

Fig. 11.19 Seventy-degree endoscopic view of the left frontal opening (*broken arrow*). (L-DC, left Denker's cavity; S, superior part of the septum.)

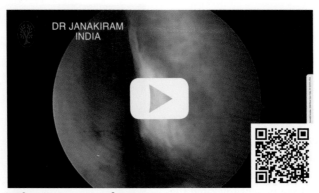

Video 11.1 A case of stage IA.

Stage IB: Anterior Disease (Involvement of the Premaxilla, Maxilla, Ethmoid Sinus, Palate, Infratemporal Fossa, and Pterygopalatine Fossa)

Case 2: A 35-year-old nondiabetic man admitted with COVID-19 pneumonia developed steroid-induced hyperglycemia on the third day of admission. The patient received oral and inhalational steroids, high-flow nasal oxygen, and insulin. After 7 days of steroid use, he complained of headaches, left-sided facial pain, and facial swelling with trismus.

On examination, left-sided diffuse facial swelling was noted with normal overlying skin. In addition, mouth opening was reduced with grade 1 trismus.

Nasal endoscopic examination revealed purulent discharge in the left osteomeatal complex. Ocular and oral cavity examinations showed no abnormality.

On further evaluation, MRI of the brain and PNS with orbit T1W, T1W with contrast, T2W, and T2 STIR sequences were performed. T1W contrast showed nonenhancing soft tissue in the left maxilla, sphenoid, and retroantral area suggestive of fungal debris. In addition, a nonenhancing left pterygoid wedge was suggestive of the sequestrum. The premaxillary and retroantral tissues were edematous compared to the right side (**Fig. 11.20**).

T2W STIR image showed central hypointense areas with air pockets within the hyperintense mucosal thickening of the left sphenoid, retroantral area, and pterygoid wedge. Contralateral sinuses were uninvolved (**Fig. 11.21**).

The patient underwent a detailed evaluation with a complete blood profile and serum inflammatory markers every alternate day (**Table 11.2**). At admission, the mean blood sugar was 276 mg/dL. The patient was continued with insulin, and oral hypoglycemics and strict glycemic control were ensured. A significant reduction was noted in the inflammatory mediators at discharge.

The surgical plan formulated was a left-sided transmaxillary approach via EMD procedure along with clearance of the left pterygoid wedge. In addition, the surgical debridement of the ethmoidal sinus with frontal sinusotomy was planned.

After orotracheal intubation, the patient was placed in a reverse trendelenburg position; the nasal cavity was packed with 1:1,000 adrenaline-soaked patties and adequately decongested. Diluted 0.5% povidone-iodine nasal antiseptic washes were given before the onset of surgery.

Surgical Steps

Transmaxillary Approach

Step 1: Left Endoscopic Modified Denker's Approach
Left EMD procedure was performed to increase accessibility to the pterygoid wedge and infratemporal fossa (ITF).

An incision was placed at the pyriform aperture, and the mucoperiosteal layer over the anterolateral maxillary wall was elevated. Fat stranding of the premaxilla, tissue edema, and relative avascularity were noted (**Fig. 11.22**). The subcutaneous tissue, mucoperiosteal layer, and muscle attachment were debrided. The infraorbital nerve was uninvolved and thus preserved. The anterolateral wall was grayish yellow and thinned out with increased porosity (**Fig. 11.23**). The anterior wall was drilled till the normal bleeding bony edges were noted. Similarly, the floor of the maxillary sinus appeared pale and unhealthy and thus was drilled.

Step 2: Medial Maxillectomy
Only minimal bleeding was noted when resecting the inferior turbinate, which was suggestive of possible sphenopalatine arterial thrombosis. The mucosa covering the medial wall of the maxillary sinus was avascular and covered with slough, and the same was debrided. The bony canal of the NLD was removed, and the duct was transected sharply (**Fig. 11.24**).

Step 3: Left Maxillary and Ethmoid Sinus Debridement
The mucosa over the anterolateral and posterolateral maxillary walls were involved grossly and denuded. The bony walls of the maxilla were inspected, and the posterior wall was found to be avascular and necrotic (**Fig. 11.25**). The anterior and posterior ethmoids were diseased, and a complete sphenoethmoidectomy was performed (**Fig. 11.26**). The lamina papyracea and skull base were found to be intact and healthy.

Table 11.2 Hematological findings of the patient

	Total count (per µL)	CRP (mg/L)	D-dimer (ng/mL)	LDH (IU/L)	Ferritin (ng/mL)
Preoperative	7,800	180	1,875	320	324
Immediate postoperative	10,000	215	1,900	290	284
At discharge	6,500	60	550	150	92

Abbreviations: CRP, C-reactive protein; LDH, lactate dehydrogenase.

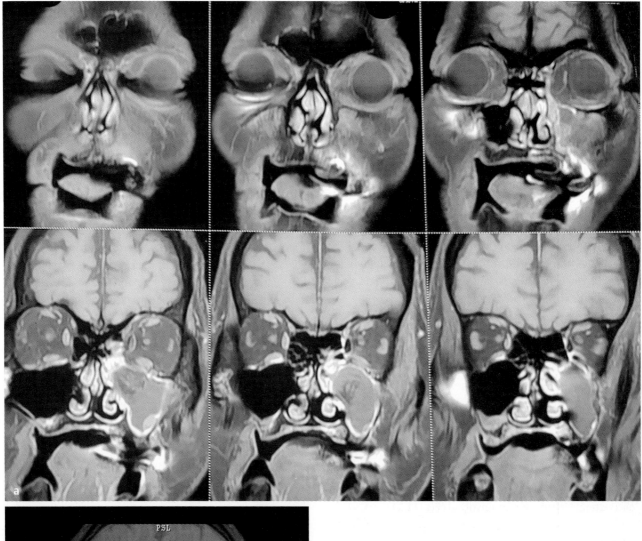

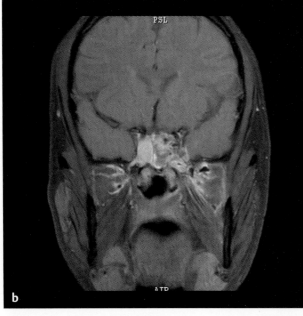

Fig. 11.20 (a, b) T1-weighted (T1W) contrast nonenhancing soft tissue in the left maxilla, sphenoid, and retroantral area suggestive of fungal debris.

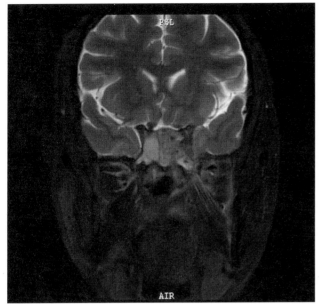

Fig. 11.21 T2-weighted (T2W) short tau inversion recovery (STIR) image showing central hypointense areas with air pockets within the hyperintense mucosal thickening of the left sphenoid, retroantral area, and pterygoid wedge.

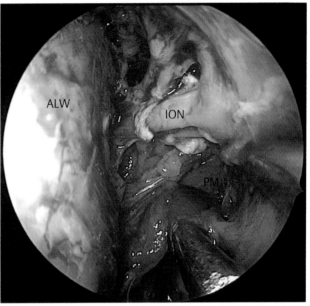

Fig. 11.22 Involvement of the left premaxilla (PM) with fat stranding and relative avascularity. (ALW, anterolateral wall; ION, infraorbital nerve.)

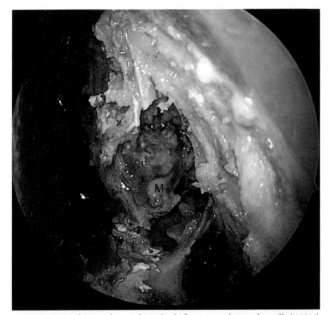

Fig. 11.23 Thinned-out brittle left anterolateral wall (ALW) with gross fungal disease in the left maxilla (M).

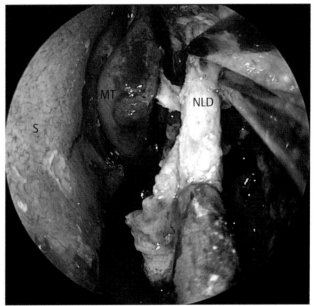

Fig. 11.24 Sharp resection of the left nasolacrimal duct (NLD). (MT, middle turbinate; S, septum.)

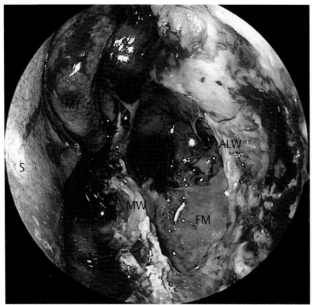

Fig. 11.25 Gross mucosal disease in the left maxilla. (ALW, anterolateral wall; FM, floor of the maxilla; MT, middle turbinate; MW, medial wall; S, septum.)

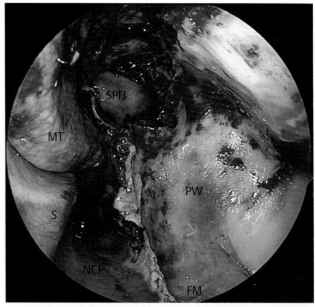

Fig. 11.26 Maxilla denuded of diseased mucosa; left complete sphenoethmoidectomy was done. (FM, floor of the maxilla; MT, middle turbinate; NCF, floor of the nasal cavity; PW, posterior wall of the maxilla; S, septum; SPH, sphenoid sinus.)

Step 4: Dissection and Debridement of the Left Infratemporal Fossa

MRI of the PNS demonstrated significant left-side retroantral fat stranding and sequestrum in the pterygoid wedge and anteroinferior wall of the sphenoid sinus with vidian canal and foramen rotundum involvement.

The left sphenopalatine artery was coblated, and the posterior maxillary sinus wall was drilled. The periosteum over the pterygopalatine fossa (PPF) and ITF was grayish and necrotic (**Fig. 11.27**). The periosteum was incised and dissected using sharp scissors. The adipose tissue and muscles inside the ITF were thinned, necrosed, and the internal maxillary artery was found to be thrombosed (**Fig. 11.28**). The contents of the ITF were debrided till bleeding was noted from the pterygoid and temporalis muscle fibers (**Fig. 11.29**).

The proximal end of the internal maxillary artery was clipped, the distal end with the thrombus was sent for histopathology (**Fig. 11.30**).

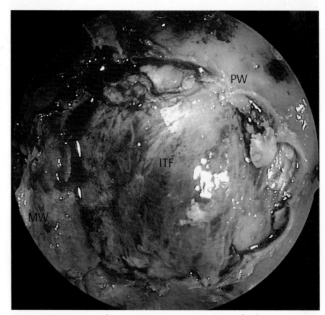

Fig. 11.27 Grayish necrotic periosteum of the pterygopalatine and infratemporal fossa (ITF). (MW, medial wall; PW, posterior wall.)

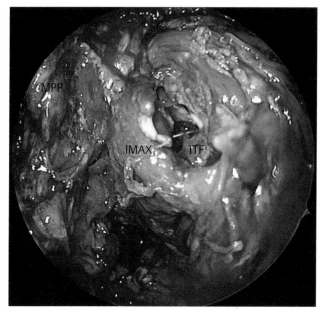

Fig. 11.28 Contents of left infratemporal fossa (ITF) necrosed and internal maxillary artery (IMAX) thrombosed. (MPP, medial pterygoid plate.)

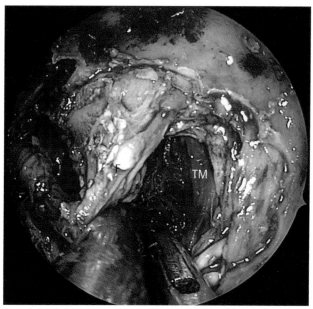

Fig. 11.29 Normal temporalis muscle (TM) seen in deep infratemporal fossa (ITF). Necrosed fat (F) in the ITF.

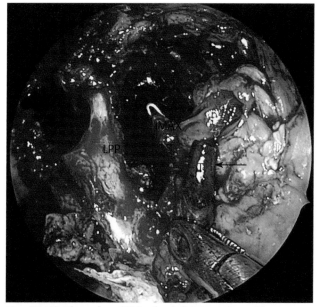

Fig. 11.30 Thrombus (T) in the left internal maxillary artery (*black arrow*). (IMAX, internal maxillary artery; LPP, lateral pterygoid plate.)

Clearance of the Pterygoid Wedge

Step 5: Left Pterygoid Wedge Clearance

The pterygoid wedge, vidian nerve, and both pterygoid plates were demarcated. The pterygoid wedge and vidian nerve were grayish, necrotic, and excised (**Fig. 11.31**). The transpterygoid drilling was performed with binostril four-handed technique. The pterygoid wedge was seen as a low-density friable sequestrum with the vidian and V2 nerves necrosed.

Step 6: Skull Base Debridement

The anterior and inferior walls of the sphenoid sinus were drilled. Pneumatization of the lateral recess was small, and the bone over the greater wing of the sphenoid (GWS) was drilled to ensure the removal of the infective nidus. The drilling of the central skull base is highly recommended, as through the marrow, the fungal hyphae extend to involve the skull base causing avascular necrosis. The superior boundary of the lateral recess is close to the temporal fossa dura. Thus, utmost care should be taken to avoid cerebrospinal fluid (CSF) leaks (**Video 11.2**).

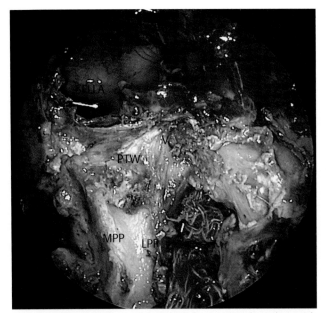

Fig. 11.31 Avascular and brittle left pterygoid wedge with necrosed vidian nerve and V2 (V). (LPP, lateral pterygoid plate; MPP, medial pterygoid plate; PTW, pterygoid wedge.)

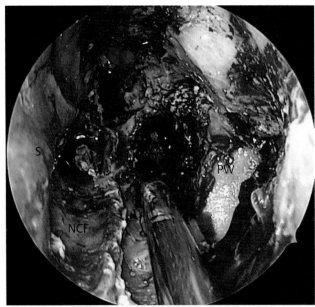

Fig. 11.32 Cavity after clearance (NCF, floor of the nasal cavity; PW, posterior wall; S, septum).

Packing

The nasal cavity after complete disease clearance is shown in **Fig. 11.32**. Nasal washes with amphotericin-B were given, and anterior nasal packing was done. The patient developed a reaction to lyophilized amphotericin-B, and due to the unavailability of liposomal amphotericin, medical management was delayed by 10 days. The patient received a cumulative dose of 2 g of liposomal amphotericin-B with 8 weeks of oral posaconazole.

Postoperative Management

After 1 month, a postoperative scan showed disease resolution (**Fig. 11.33**), and nasal cavity healing after 1 month of surgery is depicted in **Fig. 11.34**.

Three months following surgery, the patient had loosening of the left upper alveolar teeth, and the left palate was eroded in a CBCT showed erosion of left palate. He underwent a left partial palatectomy and primary mucosal suturing. Six months after surgery, the patient was symptom free, and taking feeds by mouth. No palatal dehiscence was noted.

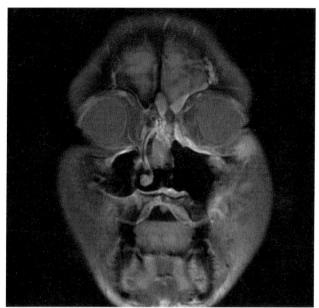

Fig. 11.33 Postoperative scan showing resolution of disease.

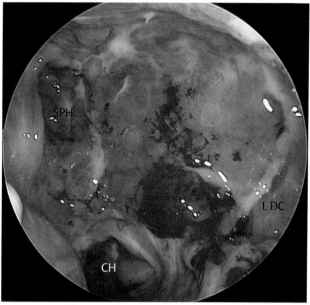

Fig. 11.34 Postoperative healed left nasal cavity. Note the healing of the left Denker's cavity (L-DC). (CH, choana; SPH, sphenoid.)

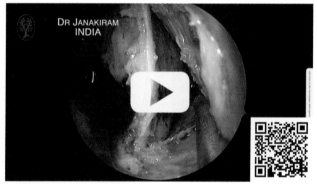

Video 11.2 A case of stage IB.

Stage IIA (Case 1): Rhino-Orbital: Involvement of Bony Orbital Walls (Medial Wall)

Case 3: A 55-year-old woman, known case of post-COVID-19 pneumonia, with steroid-induced hyperglycemia presented with complaints of foul-smelling discharge from the left nasal cavity since 10 days associated with one episode of mild self-limiting nasal bleed. She also noticed left-sided periorbital swelling and drooping of the left eyelid for a duration of 3 days.

On examination of the face, swelling and tenderness were present over the left side of the cheek with left eye ptosis (**Fig. 11.35**).

Nasal endoscopic examination showed black discoloration of the left MT with nasal discharge and crustations (**Fig. 11.36**). Right-sided nasal cavity showed no abnormality.

Ocular examination revealed left preseptal cellulitis, ptosis, and conjunctival congestion with intact vision. The right eye revealed no abnormal findings. In addition, the palatal examination was within normal limits.

Hematological examination details are mentioned in **Table 11.3**.

Coronal CT-PNS without contrast showed left maxillary opacification with left ethmoid sinusitis. MRI of the brain and PNS with the orbit (T1W, T1W with contrast, T2W, T2 STIR sequences) showed T1W hypointensity in the left maxilla with left medial orbital wall erosion and preseptal cellulitis (**Figs. 11.37** and **11.38**). Contralateral sinuses and both palates were uninvolved.

The surgical plan was a left-sided EMD procedure with full-house FESS with medial orbital decompression and left transcutaneous retrobulbar injection of amphotericin-B (TRAMB).

After orotracheal intubation, the patient was placed in the reverse trendelenburg position; the nasal cavity was packed with 1:1,000 adrenaline-soaked patties and decongested adequately. Diluted 0.5% povidone-iodine nasal antiseptic washes were given before the surgery.

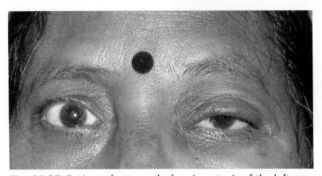

Fig. 11.35 Patient photograph showing ptosis of the left eye.

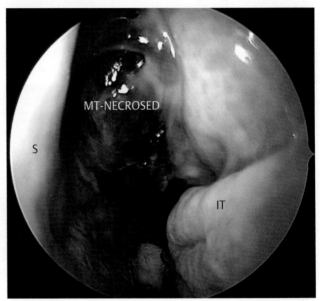

Fig. 11.36 Anterior rhinoscopy showing necrosed black middle turbinate (MT). (IT, left inferior turbinate; S, septum.)

Table 11.3 Hematological findings of the patient

	Total count (per µL)	CRP (mg/L)	D-dimer (ng/mL)	LDH (IU/L)	Ferritin (ng/mL)
Preoperative	6,000	200	1,900	333	344
Immediate postoperative	8,000	187	2,300	320	334
At discharge	6,000	50	350	135	90

Abbreviations: CRP, C-reactive protein; LDH, lactate dehydrogenase.

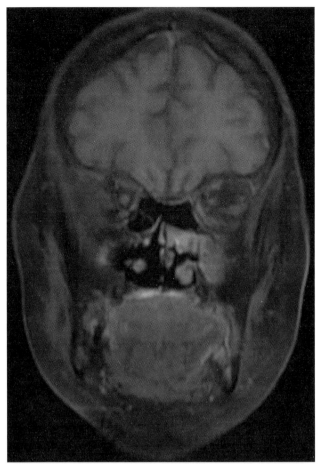

Fig. 11.37 Magnetic resonance imaging (MRI) T1-weighted (T1W) fat-suppressed (FS) coronal image showing hypodensity in the left maxilla.

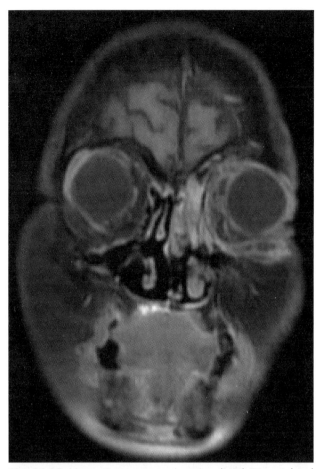

Fig. 11.38 Magnetic resonance imaging (MRI) T1-weighted (T1W) fat-suppressed (FS) coronal image showing left ethmoid disease with erosion of the left lamina papyracea.

Surgical Steps

Step 1: Left Endoscopic Modified Denker's Procedure

Left inferior turbinectomy and EMD procedure was performed for exposure of all the walls of the maxillary sinus and alveolar recess to ensure complete excision of gross disease. The anterolateral bony wall was brittle, cancellous, and necrotic (**Fig. 11.39**). The bony margins of the osteotomies were enlarged till healthy bone was noted. The mucosa of the medial wall of the maxilla was sloughed and thus excised.

Step 2: Contact Endoscopy in the Nasolacrimal Duct

During mucosal excision from the frontal process of the maxilla, the necrosis had extended toward the NLD. As a result, the bone over the NLD was osteomyelitic and porous. Therefore, the bone was drilled, and the NLD was delineated and resected (**Fig. 11.40**). A contact endoscopy over the NLD mucosa showed necrotic mucosa and fungal debris (**Figs. 11.41** and **11.42**). Contact endoscopy is a noninvasive

optical technique that demonstrates real-time visualization of the superficial mucosal layer's cellular architecture and the submucosal plane's vascularization pattern.

Step 3: Left Maxillary Sinus Debridement

The mucosa over all walls of the maxillary sinus was necrotic and was removed entirely. The bony walls were inspected, and the medial aspect of the posterior wall was discolored (**Fig. 11.43**). A medial maxillectomy was performed. Left sphenoethmoidectomy demonstrated sloughed mucosa (**Fig. 11.44**).

Step 4: Left Medial Orbital Decompression

MRI findings suggested the involvement of the left lamina papyracea. Therefore, a left medial orbital decompression was performed. The medial bony wall of the orbit was elevated using a freer elevator, leaving 2-mm bone of superior aspect. The periorbita was inspected and found uninvolved (**Fig. 11.45**).

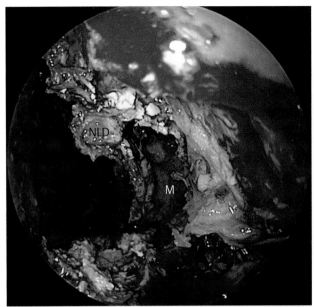

Fig. 11.39 Left endoscopic modified Denker's procedure. The left maxilla shows gross involvement with disease. (M, maxilla; NLD, nasolacrimal duct.)

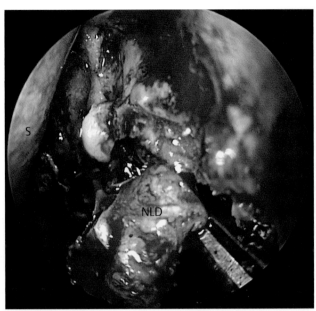

Fig. 11.40 Resection of the involved left nasolacrimal duct (NLD). (S, septum.)

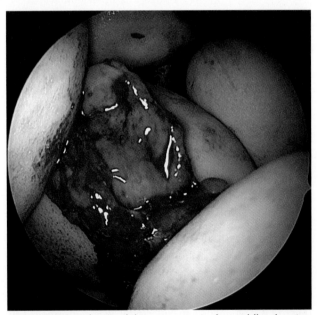

Fig. 11.41 Nasolacrimal duct cut open in the middle, showing fungal debris (F).

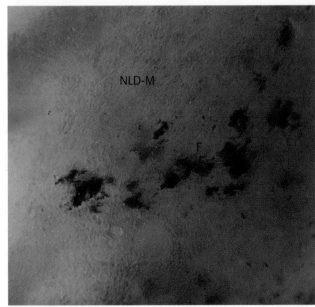

Fig. 11.42 Contact endoscopy showing fungal debris (F) in the nasolacrimal duct mucosa (NLD-M).

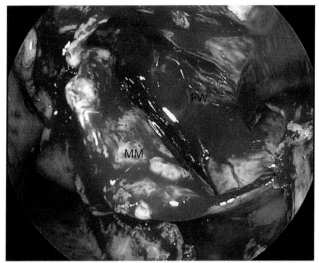

Fig. 11.43 Maxillary sinus mucosa denuded off all the walls, exposing the posterior wall (PW). (MW, maxillary mucosa.)

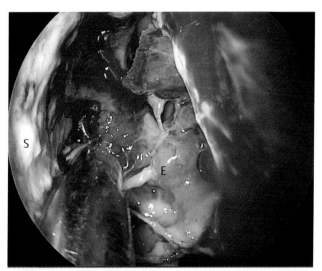

Fig. 11.44 Disease in the left ethmoid sinus (E) debrided. (S, septum.)

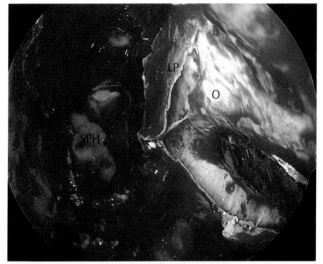

Fig. 11.45 Left medial orbital decompression. (LP, lamina papyracea; O, left orbit; S, septum; SPH, sphenoid sinus.)

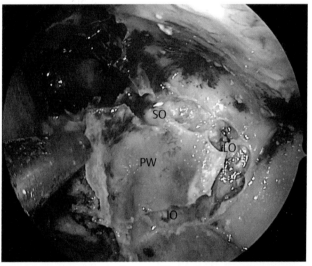

Fig. 11.46 Window in the maxilla posterior wall (PW), with osteotomies. (IO, inferior osteotomy; LO, lateral osteotomy; SO, superior osteotomy.)

Step 5: Inspection of the Left Infratemporal Fossa

Black discoloration was noted in the medial aspect of the posterior wall of the maxillary sinus. However, the MRI scan suggested no retromaxillary disease.

The surgeon created a window in the posterior maxillary wall to inspect recent disease extension to the retroantral space. The posterior maxillary wall was drilled with a 1-cm margin around the discoloration, and the specimen was sent for histopathology. The periosteum of the PPF and ITF was intact and opened using straight scissors (**Figs. 11.46** and **11.47**). Normal adipose tissue with patent descending artery and sphenopalatine artery were observed (**Fig. 11.48**).

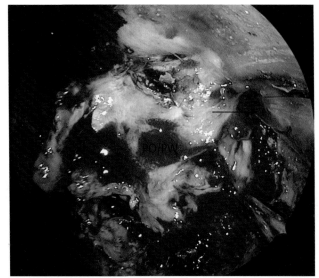

Fig. 11.47 Opening the periosteum of the infratemporal fossa with sharp scissors (*black arrow*). (PO/PW, periosteum of posterior wall.)

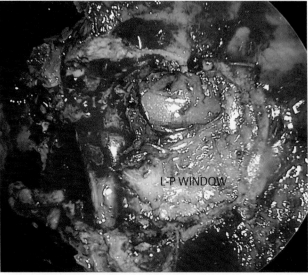

Fig. 11.48 Left infratemporal fossa contents, descending palatine artery, left posterior window (L-PW).

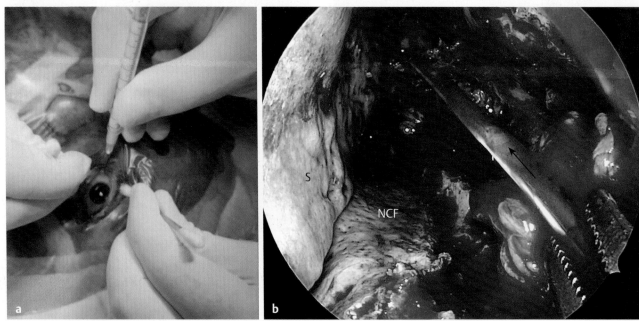

Fig. 11.49 (a) Retrobulbar injection of amphotericin-B. **(b)** Placing infant feeding tube (*black arrow*) in the nasal cavity for amphotericin wash. (NCF, the floor of the nasal cavity; S, septum.)

Step 6: Left Transcutaneous Retrobulbar Amphotericin-B

The standard treatment for the progressive orbital disease is exenteration; however, organ salvage should be attempted. Early intervention in orbital disease can avert a more radical procedure. This patient was treated locally with retrobulbar deoxycholate amphotericin-B (1 mL of 3.5 mg/mL AMB deoxycholate with an antecedent retrobulbar injection of anesthetic comprising 2 mL of 2% lidocaine). The patient remained clinically stable with no further evidence of progression (**Fig. 11.49**). The inpatient medical team continued aggressive antifungal treatment and blood sugar control. For amphotericin irrigations, an infant feeding tube was placed in the left maxillary and ethmoid sinus (**Fig. 11.50** and **Video 11.3**).

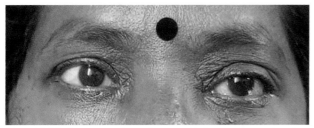

Fig. 11.50 Postoperative picture of the patient showing improved left eye ptosis.

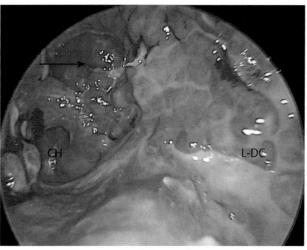

Fig. 11.52 Postoperative left nasal cavity healing (CH, choana; L-DC, healed left Denker's cavity). The *black arrow* shows polypoidal changes in the sphenoid region.

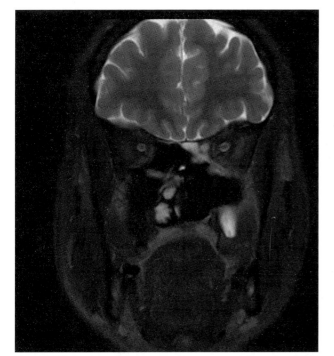

Fig. 11.51 Postoperative magnetic resonance imaging (MRI) coronal image showing complete clearance.

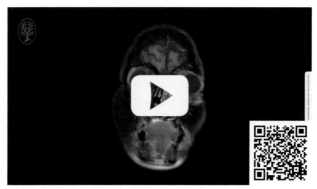

Video 11.3 A case of stage IIA—case 1.

Packing

Hemostasis was achieved, and anterior nasal packing was done with merocel packs.

Postoperative Management

Postoperatively the patient received a cumulative dose of 2 g of conventional amphotericin-B, which was supplemented with a whole 8-week duration of oral posaconazole. Ptosis in the left eye improved after 20 days of surgery. Postoperative MRI (T1W and T2W STIR) done 1 month postsurgery showed no residual disease (**Fig. 11.51**). Postoperative healing of the left nasal cavity after 45 days of surgery is depicted in **Fig. 11.52**. The patient showed complete resolution of orbital symptoms and is now clinicoradiologically disease free.

Stage IIA (Case 2): Rhino-Orbital: Involvement of the Floor of the Orbit

Case 4: A 69-year-old post-COVID-19 patient on treatment for diabetes mellitus, systemic hypertension, and peripheral neuropathy who was discharged 1 month back presented with left-sided headache, facial pain, and paresthesia over the left side of the cheek for 10 days. During hospitalization, he was treated with systemic steroids and oxygen supplementation with persistently high blood sugar levels for 3 days.

On examination, swelling of the left side of the face with decreased sensation around the periorbital area was noted.

Anterior rhinoscopy showed discharge in the left middle meatus. Ocular and oral cavity examination revealed no significant abnormality.

Evaluation at presentation included a detailed otorhinolaryngologic, ophthalmologic, and neurological examinations to assess the extent of the disease. The proinflammatory marker values were recorded every alternate day. Hematological values are mentioned in **Table 11.4**.

He was further evaluated with MRI of the brain and PNS with the orbit (T1W, T1W with contrast, T2W, T2 STIR sequences). Coronal T1W scan showed contrast-enhancing intraorbital, extraconal soft tissue along the floor of the left orbit. In addition, the bilateral maxillary sinus showed peripherally enhancing centrally nonenhancing soft tissue. The left retroantral area revealed subtle perisinus inflammation (**Figs. 11.53** and **11.54**).

The patient underwent a thorough preoperative evaluation with a complete blood profile, serum inflammatory markers, and complete systemic workup. Serum ferritin and D-dimer were normal (ferritin: 100 ng/mL; D-dimer: 450 ng/mL). At admission, mean blood sugar was 340 mg/dL. Strict glycemic control was ensured under the physician's supervision.

Ophthalmological examination showed normal vision with no restriction of extraocular movements. The ophthalmologist advised surgical clearance of sinonasal disease followed by TRAMB. A biopsy from the left middle meatus confirmed the diagnosis.

After a thorough preanesthetic checkup, he was taken up for surgery. The treatment plan was a bilateral EMD procedure, left ITF exploration with orbital decompression, and a full house FESS on both sides. Orotracheal intubation was done, and the patient was placed in the reverse trendelenburg position. The nasal cavity was packed with 1:1,000 adrenaline-soaked patties and adequately decongested. Povidone-iodine nasal antiseptic wash (0.5%) was given before the onset of surgery.

Surgical Steps

Step 1: Left Endoscopic Modified Denker's Procedure
The EMD procedure was done on the left side, and the maxilla was exposed. It was primarily diseased over the posterior wall and roof (floor of the orbit). Diseased mucosa was stripped off the walls, and the bony wall of the floor of the orbit was noted to be discolored and necrosed (**Figs. 11.54** and **11.55**).

Step 2: Debridement of the Floor of the Left Orbit
Using freer's elevator, bone over the roof of the maxilla was elevated carefully to expose the periorbital layer (**Fig. 11.56**). It was thin and brittle. The plane between diseased periorbita and orbital fat was opened by sharp dissection. The involved periorbita was removed and sent for HPE (**Fig. 11.57**). The orbital fat was normal. The infraorbital nerve was involved; therefore, it was resected and sent for HPE separately.

Step 3: Left Infratemporal Fossa Debridement
The posterior wall of the maxilla was drilled to expose the PPF and ITF. Fat stranding was noted, and the same was removed after clipping the internal maxillary artery (**Figs. 11.58** and **11.59**). The muscles were noninflamed, well vascularized, and thus left in situ.

Step 4: Right Endoscopic Modified Denker's Procedure With Full House Fess
The EMD procedure was done on the right side, and fungal debris in the maxillary sinus was cleared (**Fig. 11.60**). The bony walls were normal. A complete FESS was done on the right side, and minimal disease in the right ethmoid sinus was also cleared (**Fig. 11.61**). A transcutaneous retrobulbar injection of deoxycholate amphotericin-B (1 mL of 3.5 mg/mL) with an antecedent local anesthetic injection (2 mL of 2% lignocaine) was given after lateral canthotomy in the left orbit (**Video 11.4**).

Table 11.4 Hematological findings of the patient

	Total count (per µL)	CRP (mg/L)	D-dimer (ng/mL)	LDH (IU/L)	Ferritin (ng/mL)
Preoperative	7,000	200	450	300	100
Immediate postoperative	15,000	336	1,500	325	250
At discharge	5,000	60	450	220	85

Abbreviations: CRP, C-reactive protein; LDH, lactate dehydrogenase.

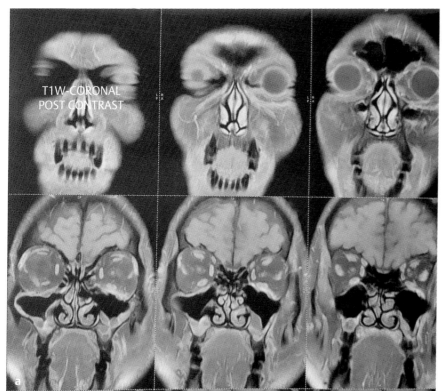

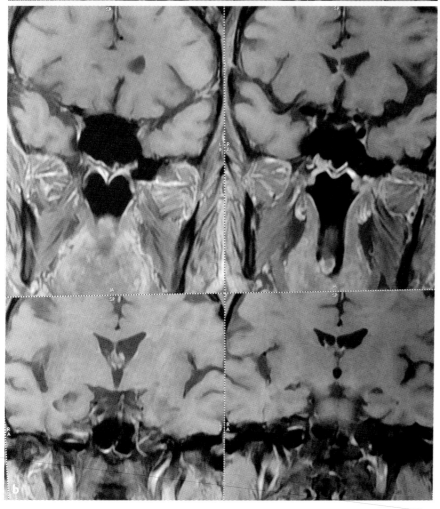

Fig. 11.53 (a, b) Magnetic resonance imaging (MRI) of the paranasal sinus (PNS) coronal T1-weighted (T1W) scan showing contrast-enhancing intraorbital, extraconal soft tissue along the floor of left orbit. Bilateral maxillary sinus showed peripherally enhancing centrally nonenhancing soft tissue. The left retroantral area revealed subtle perisinus inflammation.

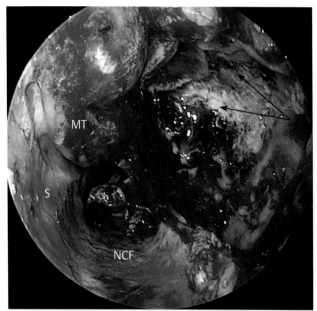

Fig. 11.54 Diseased mucosa of the posterolateral wall and the roof of the maxilla (*black arrows*). (MT, middle turbinate; NCF, nasal cavity floor; S, septum.)

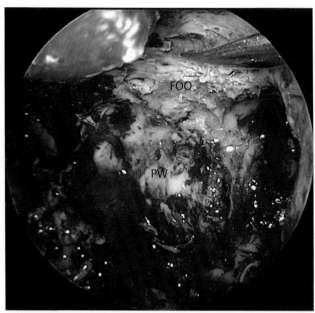

Fig. 11.55 Diseased bone of the floor of the orbit (FOO). (PW, posterior wall.)

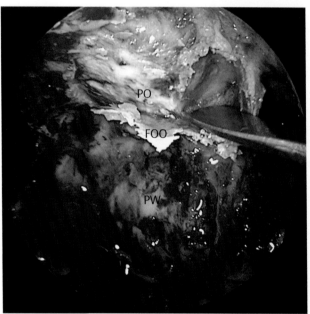

Fig. 11.56 Floor of the orbit being elevated off the periorbita (PO). (FOO, floor of the orbit; PW, posterior wall.)

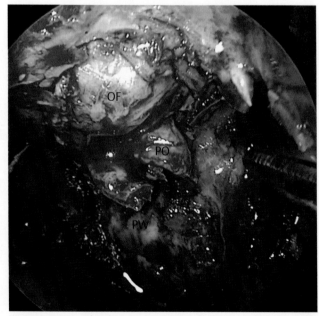

Fig. 11.57 Involved periorbita (PO) dissected off the orbital fat (OF) and removed. (PW, posterior wall.)

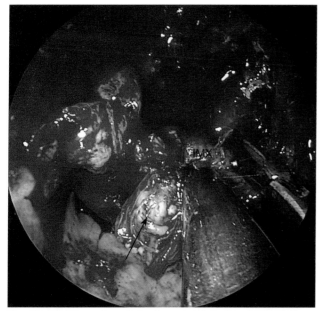

Fig. 11.58 Dissection of the fungal debris (*black arrow*) from the infratemporal fossa (ITF) and clipping of the internal maxillary artery (IMAX).

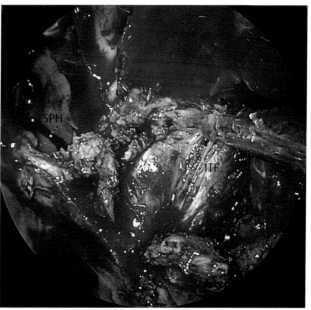

Fig. 11.59 Complete clearance of left infratemporal fossa (ITF). (SPH, sphenoid.)

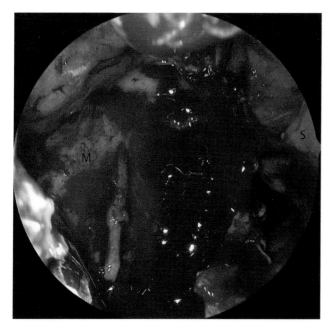

Fig. 11.60 Right side disease clearance after Denker's procedure (M, maxilla; S, septum).

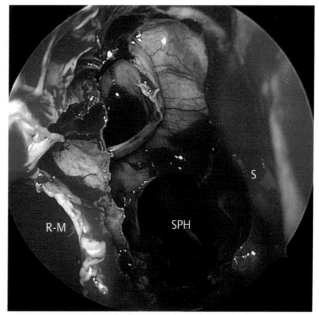

Fig. 11.61 Full house functional endoscopic sinus surgery FESS) done on the right side. (M, right maxilla; SPH, sphenoid.)

Packing

Once hemostasis was achieved, anterior nasal packing was done with merocel packs.

Postoperative Management

The patient was treated with systemic antifungals (liposomal amphotericin-B and oral posaconazole). A cumulative dose of 2.0 g of amphotericin with 8 weeks of oral posaconazole was given to the patient. The patient tolerated the treatment very well.

A postoperative scan done after 3 months showed no residual disease (**Fig. 11.62**). Healing of bilateral Denker's cavity and sphenoid sinus is shown in **Fig. 11.63**.

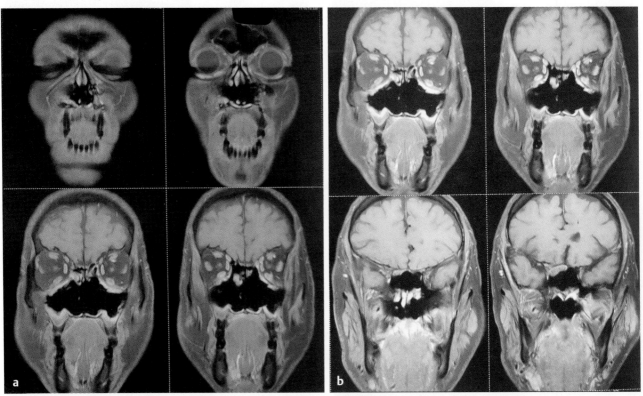

Fig. 11.62 (a, b) Postoperative scan showing complete disease resolution.

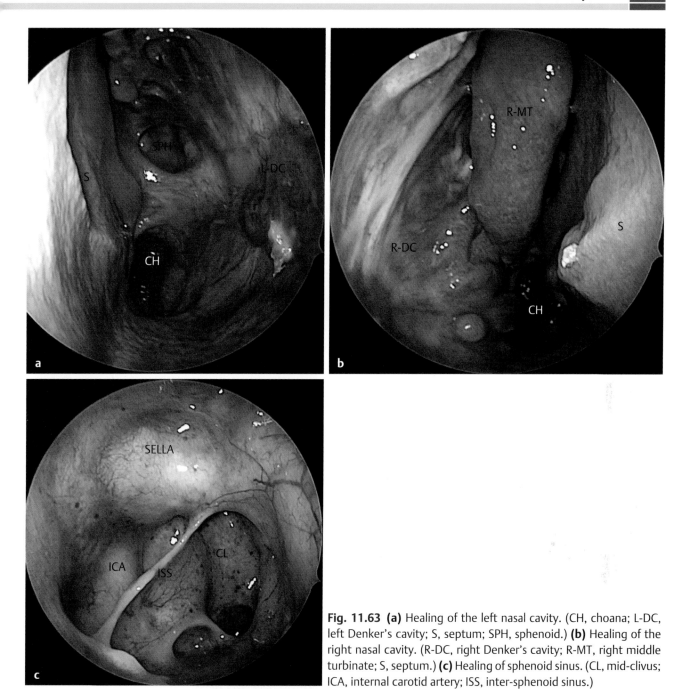

Fig. 11.63 **(a)** Healing of the left nasal cavity. (CH, choana; L-DC, left Denker's cavity; S, septum; SPH, sphenoid.) **(b)** Healing of the right nasal cavity. (R-DC, right Denker's cavity; R-MT, right middle turbinate; S, septum.) **(c)** Healing of sphenoid sinus. (CL, mid-clivus; ICA, internal carotid artery; ISS, inter-sphenoid sinus.)

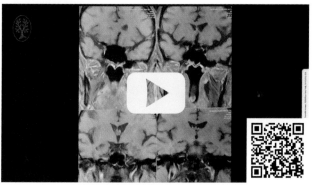

Video 11.4 A case of stage IIA—case 2.

Stage IIB: Rhino-Orbital—Involvement of the Extraocular Muscles with Intact Vision

Case 5: A 63-year-old post-COVID-19 and diabetic man presented with complaints of left-sided headache, periorbital swelling, ptosis, and decreased vision in the left eye for 15 days. On nasal endoscopy, bilateral middle turbinates were covered with slough, purulent discharge, and fungal debris (**Fig. 11.64**). Ocular examination showed total paralysis of all the extraocular muscles with complete ptosis of the left eye, dilated nonreacting pupil, and loss of accommodation suggestive of total ophthalmoplegia. The palate was normal on examination.

Preoperative evaluation included a detailed otorhinolaryngologic, ophthalmologic, and neurological examinations to assess the extent. In addition, the values of the proinflammatory markers were recorded every alternate day. Hematological examination details are mentioned in **Table 11.5**.

MRI of the PNS, orbit, and brain, including T1, T2, T1W fat-suppressed (FS), T2 FS, T1 FS postcontrast, and DWI was taken to study the extent of disease and to plan the surgical approaches.

MRI coronal postcontrast T1WFS showed nonenhancing soft tissue in the middle half of the posterior septum and bilateral anterior and posterior ethmoids. In addition, inflammation and soft-tissue density were noted along the superomedial aspect of the left eye, suggestive of invasive fungal disease (**Fig. 11.65**). The palate and opposite sino-orbital region were marked normal.

Based on the MRI findings, the surgical plan formulated was a left EMD procedure with bilateral full house FESS, left orbital decompression, and limited posterior debridement of the orbit. An explicit consent was taken about the disease status in the left eye and the on-table need for exenteration if the disease proved to be involving the globe.

After orotracheal intubation, the patient was placed in the reverse trendelenburg position. The nasal cavities were examined, and swabs were taken for gram stain and KOH mount. Povidone-iodine nasal antiseptic washes (0.5%) were given before the onset of surgery. Bilateral nasal cavities were decongested with adrenaline-soaked gauze pieces. Sloughed mucosa was noted over bilateral middle turbinates and osteomeatal complexes on endoscopic examination.

Surgical Steps

Step 1: Left Endoscopic Modified Denker's Procedure
Left inferior turbinectomy was done. After the incision over the pyriform aperture, the soft tissue over the left antero-lateral wall was elevated in the subperiosteal plane till the infraorbital foramen. After the osteotomies left maxillary sinus was exposed, only minimal involvement of the posteromedial was noted (**Fig. 11.66**). The mucosa was removed from all the walls and sent for histopathology (**Fig. 11.67**).

Step 2: Resection of the Left Nasolacrimal Duct and Dacryocystorhinostomy
Purulent secretions were noted at the opening of NLD. Hence, the bone over the NLD and the nasolacrimal duct was removed, following which an endoscopic dacryocystorhinostomy was done (**Figs. 11.68** and **11.69**).

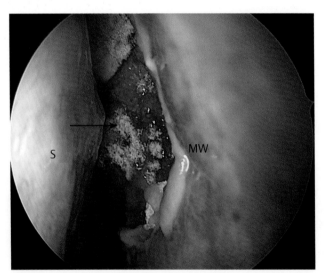

Fig. 11.64 Black eschar–covered left middle turbinate (MT; *black arrow*). (S, septum; MW, medial wall.)

Table 11.5 Hematological findings of the patient

	Total count (per µL)	CRP (mg/L)	D-dimer (ng/mL)	LDH (IU/L)	Ferritin (ng/mL)
Preoperative	6,000	190	1,500	290	356
Immediate postoperative	7,500	210	2,700	320	350
At discharge	7,000	54	550	200	94

Abbreviations: CRP, C-reactive protein; LDH, lactate dehydrogenase.

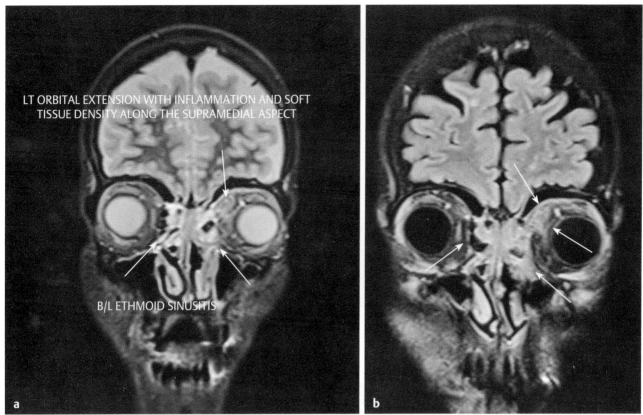

Fig. 11.65 (a, b) Coronal T1 fat-suppressed (FS) image showed nonenhancing soft tissue in the middle half of the posterior septum, bilateral anterior and posterior ethmoids, inflammation, and soft-tissue density along the superomedial aspect of the left eye suggestive of invasive fungal disease (*arrows marked*).

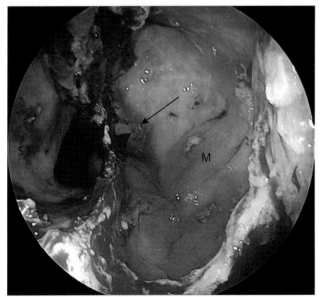

Fig. 11.66 Post-Denker's procedure. The maxilla (M) is exposed and minimal involvement over the posteromedial wall of the maxilla is seen (*black arrow*). (S, septum.)

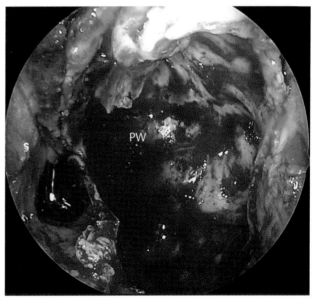

Fig. 11.67 Maxilla (M) mucosa denuded, posterior wall (PW) and septum.

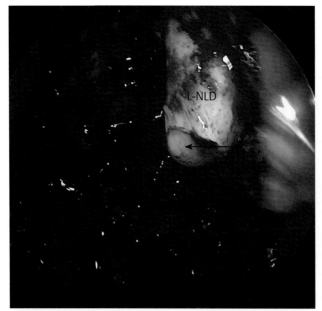

Fig. 11.68 Purulent secretion from the left nasolacrimal duct (L-NLD) expressed (*black arrow*).

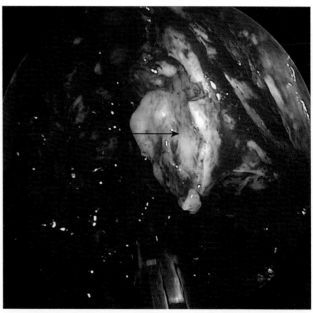

Fig. 11.69 Left dacryocystorhinostomy (*black arrow*).

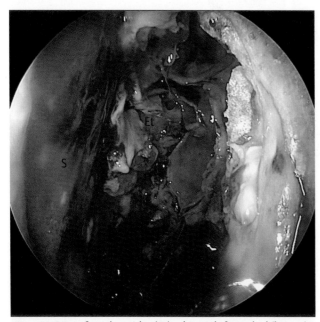

Fig. 11.70 Left ethmoids (Et) showed fungal debris. (S, septum.)

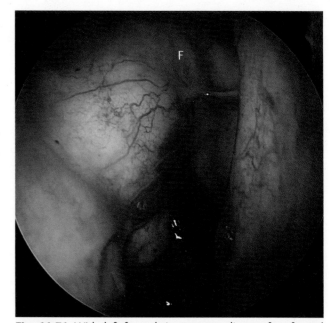

Fig. 11.71 Wide left frontal sinusotomy, disease-free frontal sinus (F).

Step 3: Left Side Full House Fess

As evident in MRI, ethmoid sinus mucosa on the left side was diseased (**Fig. 11.70**), and a complete sphenoethmoidectomy was done along with wide frontal sinusotomy. The frontal sinus was found to be disease free (**Fig. 11.71**). Left diseased MT was resected. All specimens were sent separately for KOH mount and HPE.

Step 4: Medial Orbital Decompression

Following FESS, the left-side lamina papyracea was removed and the periorbita was exposed in its entirety (**Fig. 11.72**). The lamina papyracea was thinned, and black discoloration was noted inferiorly.

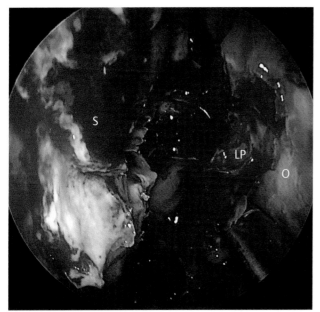

Fig. 11.72 Left side medial orbital decompression. (LP, lamina papyracea; O, orbit; S, serum.)

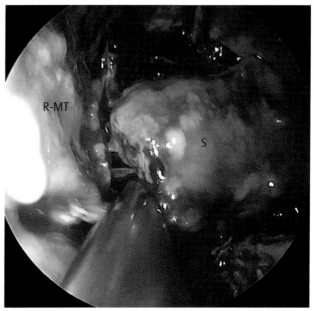

Fig. 11.73 Involved part of the septum (S) is resected. The right middle turbinate (R-MT) is diseased.

Step 5: Extended Posterior Septectomy

The posterior two-thirds of the septal mucosa was found sloughed, and the same was resected with extra mucosal margins (**Figs. 11.73** and **11.74**).

Step 6: Right Full House Fess

The right necrotic MT was partially resected. The maxillary sinus was examined and was found to be disease free (**Fig. 11.75**). However, the ethmoid sinus on the right was diseased; hence, a complete sphenoethmoidectomy was done.

Step 7: Left Limited Orbital Clearance (Globe/Vision Sparing)

A horizontal incision was made over the left periorbita using a no. 15 blade (**Fig. 11.76**). The periorbita was grayish, and the orbital fat was exposed. Fat stranding with thinning of the adipose tissue was noted with fungal debris. After widening the periorbita, the fat was debrided to expose the insertion of muscles and optic nerve. The posterior part of the muscles were avascular and edematous; thus, it was debrided till healthy tissues were seen at the level of the anterior globe (**Figs. 11.77** and **11.78**). However, the anterior contents, globe, and optic nerve were preserved. The disease was not seen extending to the superior orbital fissure (SOF), optic nerve, or orbital apex (OA) (**Video 11.5**).

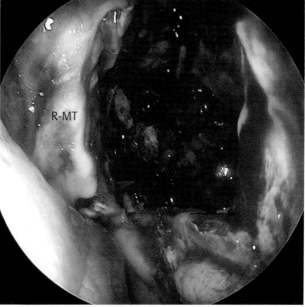

Fig. 11.74 Cut end of the septum is marked (*black arrow*). (R-MT, right middle turbinate.)

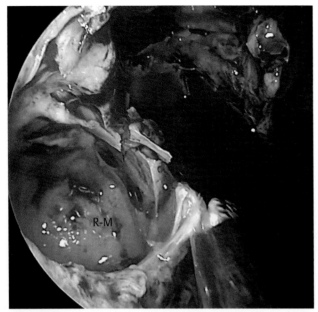

Fig. 11.75 Disease-free right maxilla (R-M) after middle meatal antrostomy.

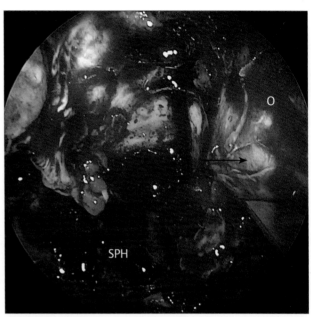

Fig. 11.76 Incision over left periorbita (*black arrow*). (O, orbit; SPH, sphenoid.)

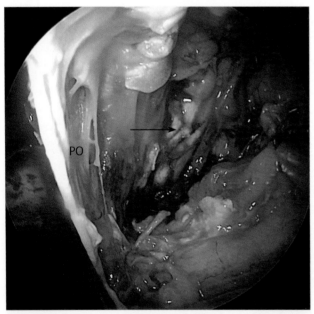

Fig. 11.77 Limited posterior orbital debridement. Periorbita (PO) *black arrow* points to necrotic tissue.

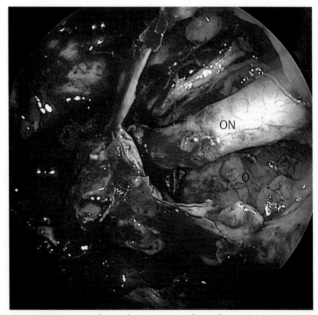

Fig. 11.78 Complete clearance in the orbit (O). (ON, optic nerve.)

Packing

Diluted amphotericin washes were given, and the nasal cavity was packed with merocel in both nostrils. Following surgery, a cumulative dose of 3.0 g of liposomal amphotericin-B was administered along with 8 weeks of posaconazole under strict monitoring of inflammatory markers, renal function tests, serum electrolytes, and blood sugar levels. The patient tolerated the treatment well.

Postoperative Management

A postoperative scan after 1 month showed no residue (**Fig. 11.79**).

The left eye remained ophthalmoplegic in the postoperative period. But the limited posterior orbital debridement saved the patient from the cosmetic deformity of an exenterated socket. Postoperative intranasal mucosalization of the orbital defect is depicted in **Fig. 11.80**. Six months postsurgery, the patient remains clinicoradiologically disease free.

Fig. 11.79 (a, b) Postoperative magnetic resonance imaging (MRI) T1-weighted (T1W) coronal image showing complete clearance of disease.

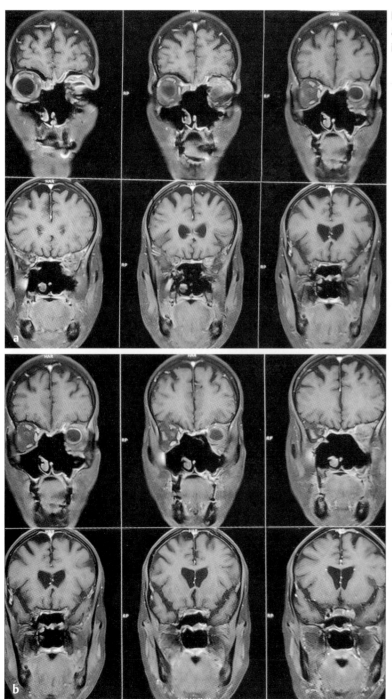

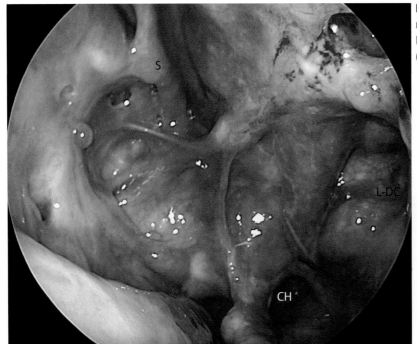

Fig. 11.80 Postoperative healing of bilateral nasal cavities. Healed left Denker's cavity (L-DC), cut end of the septum (S), and choana (CH).

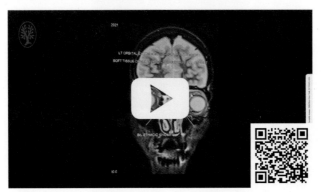

Video 11.5 A case of stage IIB.

Stage IIC: Rhino-Orbital–Involvement of the Superior Orbital Fissure and Orbital Apex

Case 6: A 61-year-old diabetic male with coronary artery disease and post-COVID-19 pneumonia developed right-sided headache, right periorbital pain and drooping of the eyelid after 10 days of discharge. On examination, anterior rhinoscopy revealed no significant findings. Clinically, palate was uninvolved.

Ocular examination showed total paralysis of all the extraocular muscles with complete ptosis of right eye suggestive of total ophthalmoplegia (**Fig. 11.81**). This is termed as "frozen globe," where significant limitation of duction occurs in all directions of gaze (palsy of cranial nerves III, IV, and VI). The visual acuity was 4/60 in both eyes. These findings implied a right-sided superior orbital syndrome (SOF) or an impending orbital apex (OA) syndrome.

Preoperative evaluation included a detailed otorhinolaryngologic, ophthalmologic, and neurological examinations to assess the extent of disease. The proinflammatory marker values were recorded every alternate day. Hematological examination details are mentioned in **Table 11.6**.

MRI of the PNS, orbit, and brain, including T1, T2, T1W fat suppressed (FS), T2 FS, T1 FS postcontrast, and DWI was taken to study the extent of disease and to plan the surgical approaches and excision.

MRI coronal postcontrast T2 FS showed areas of intermediate intensity within bilateral maxillary sinuses, extending to the right ethmoid sinus and medial aspect of the posterior orbit (SOF). Postcontrast T1W image showed isointense shadows over the medial aspect of the SOF suggestive of possible fungal etiology (**Fig. 11.82**). The palate and opposite orbit were marked normal.

The surgical plan based on the MRI findings of the bilateral maxillae, right ethmoid sinus, and SOF included a bilateral EMD procedure with bilateral full house FESS, right transpterygoid approach, and clearance of SOF.

After orotracheal intubation, a central venous pressure (CVP) was inserted into the right subclavian vein. The patient was placed in the reverse Trendelenburg position and normotensive anesthesia was administered. The nasal cavities were examined, and swabs were taken for gram stain and KOH mount. Povidone-iodine nasal antiseptic washes (0.5%) were given before the onset of surgery. Bilateral nasal cavities were decongested with adrenaline-soaked gauze pieces (1:1,000).

Surgical Steps

Step 1: Bilateral Full House Fess
Bilateral middle meatal antrostomy was done and presence of fungal elements in the sinuses was confirmed. A complete sphenoethmoidectomy and bilateral middle turbinectomy were done on both sides (**Figs. 11.83** and **11.84**).

Step 2: Binostril Approach
The mucoperiosteal flaps on either side of the posterior bony septum were removed, and it was disarticulated from the rostrum of the sphenoid (**Fig. 11.85**). Wide sphenoidotomy was performed after "triple osteotomy" and the sphenoid sinus was exposed laterally and till the level of the floor (**Fig. 11.86**). This facilitates four-handed technique. The intersinus septa were carefully drilled keeping internal carotid fully under vision, to prevent any inadvertent fracture or an arterial injury.

Step 3: Right Endoscopic Modified Denker's Procedure
Right EMD procedure was done and disease in the maxillary sinus was cleared. An EMD procedure increases the lateral reach and facilitates the transpterygoid approach (**Fig. 11.87**).

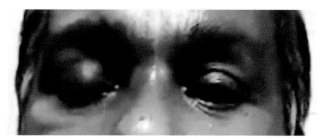

Fig. 11.81 Patient's photograph showing right eye ptosis.

Table 11.6 Hematological findings of the patient

	Total count (per µL)	CRP (mg/L)	D-dimer (ng/mL)	LDH (IU/L)	Ferritin (ng/mL)
Preoperative	6,500	150	1,400	240	265
Immediate postoperative	8,500	200	2,700	310	325
At discharge	5,000	44	500	210	84

Abbreviations: CRP, C-reactive protein; LDH, lactate dehydrogenase.

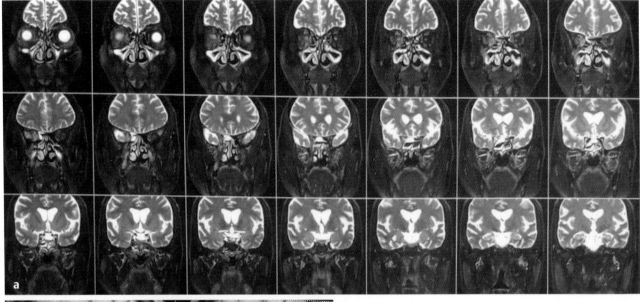

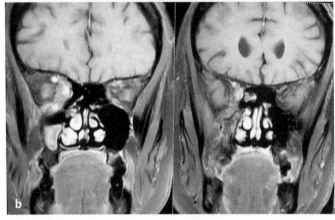

Fig. 11.82 (a) T2-weighted (T2W) fat-suppressed (FS) image showing disease in both maxillary sinuses, right ethmoid sinus and right superior orbital fissure. **(b)** T1-weighted (T1W) contrast image showing isointense shadows over the medial aspect of the superior orbital fissure.

Step 4: Right Transpterygoid Approach

A transpterygoid approach was done for wide exposure of the right cavernous sinus and SOF. The sphenopalatine artery was coblated and the posterior wall of the right maxillary sinus was drilled, and contents of the PPF were removed. The right internal maxillary artery was double clipped, the vidian nerve and V2 branch of trigeminal nerve were identified, and the pterygoid wedge was delineated. Transpterygoid drilling was done while preserving the neurovascular bundles.

Step 5: Clearance of the SOF

Relevant anatomy: The SOF is a three-dimensional communication between the middle cranial fossa and OA; it is bounded superiorly by the lesser wing of the sphenoid, inferiorly by the greater wing of sphenoid (GWS). and medially by the body of the sphenoid. It is situated inferolateral to the canal for the optic nerve. With respect to the transnasal approach, the medial aspect of the SOF is more relevant. In a well-pneumatized sphenoid bone, the optic strut forms the superior boundary, and the maxillary strut forms the inferior boundary of the medial surface of the SOF. Above the optic strut is the optic canal and below the maxillary strut is the foramen rotundum.[5]

The *surgical steps* are as follows:

- After a transpterygoid exposure, the medial surface of the SOF was found to be covered with fungal granulations and necrosis (**Fig. 11.88**). It was carefully scraped off with a blunt elevator (**Fig. 11.89**).
- The posterior end of the lamina papyracea, maxillary strut, and the bone over the SOF were drilled eggshell thin and elevated using a Rosen knife (**Fig. 11.90**). The bone over the cavernous sinus was also drilled and the right cavernous dura was exposed. The clinoidal and cavernous internal carotid arteries were mapped using an endoscopic doppler probe (**Fig. 11.91**).

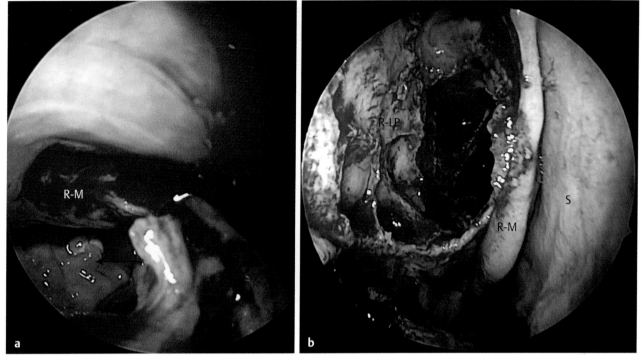

Fig. 11.83 (a) Right middle meatal antrostomy, fungal debris (*black arrow*) in the maxilla (R-M, right maxilla). **(b)** Complete functional endoscopic sinus surgery (FESS) on the right side (R-LP, right lamina papyracea; R-MT, right middle turbinate; S, septum).

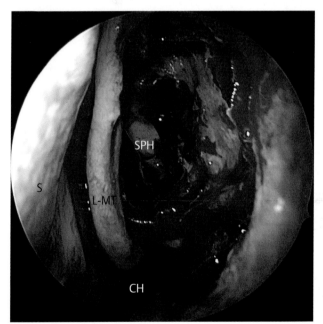

Fig. 11.84 Complete functional endoscopic sinus surgery (FESS) on the left side. (CH, choana; L-MT, left middle turbinate; S, septum; SPH, sphenoid.)

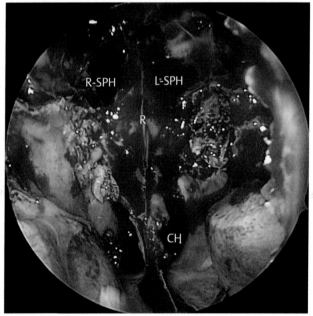

Fig. 11.85 Posterior septectomy and exposure of the anterior wall of the sphenoid sinus. (CH, choana; L-SPH, left sphenoid; R-SPH, right sphenoid.)

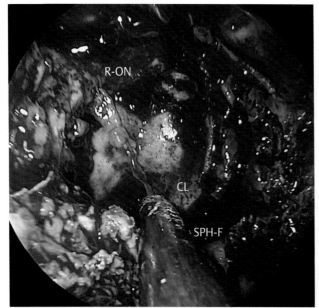

Fig. 11.86 Wide sphenoidotomy. (CL, clivus; R-ON, right optic nerve; SPH-F, floor of the sphenoid.)

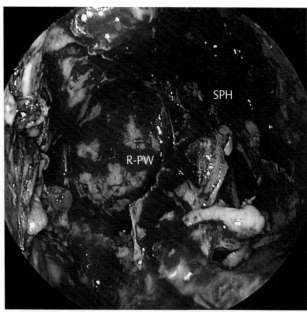

Fig. 11.87 Right endoscopic Denker's cavity. (R-PW, right posterior wall of the maxilla; SPH, sphenoid.)

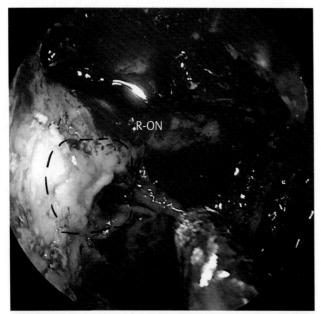

Fig. 11.88 Medial aspect of the right superior orbital fissure (SOF) covered with necrotic debris (*broken square*). (R-ON, right optic nerve.)

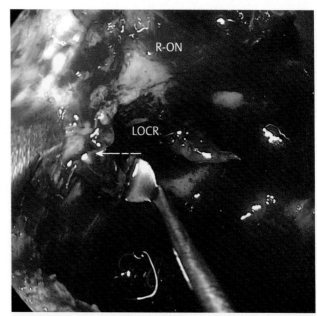

Fig. 11.89 Fungal debris being elevated with a Rosen knife. Note the granulation over the right lateral opticocarotid recess (LOCR). (R-ON, right optic nerve.)

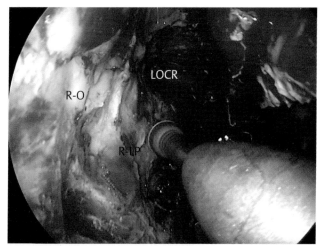

Fig. 11.90 Posterior-most lamina papyracea (R-LP) being drilled. (LOCR, lateral opticocarotid recess; R-O, right orbit.)

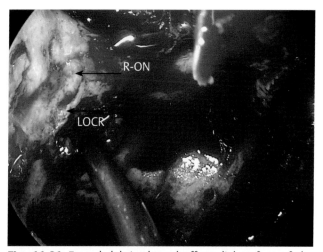

Fig. 11.91 Fungal debris cleared off medial surface of the superior orbital fissure (SOF; *black arrows*). (LOCR, lateral opticocarotid recess; R-ON, right optic nerve.)

- The granulations over the right lateral opticocarotid recess were carefully removed using a blunt-ball probe, taking care to not cause an arterial injury (**Fig. 11.92**).
- The periorbita over the medial aspect of the SOF was incised with a sharp knife (**Fig. 11.93**). The muscles appeared grossly normal and the periorbita alone was found to be infected. It was removed and sent for HPE (**Figs. 11.94** and **11.95**). At the end of the procedure, SOF was completely cleared off the disease.

Step 6: Transcutaneous Retrobulbar Injection of Liposomal Amphotericin-B

The patient was treated locally with retrobulbar deoxycholate amphotericin-B (1 mL of 3.5 mg/mL) with an antecedent retrobulbar injection of anesthetic comprising 2 mL of 2% lidocaine by the oculoplastic surgeon (**Fig. 11.96** and **Video 11.6**).

Packing

Diluted amphotericin washes were given, and nasal cavity was packed with merocel in both nostrils.

Postoperative Management

Following surgery, the patient was treated with systemic antifungal drugs. A cumulative dose of 2.0 g of amphotericin-B was administered along with 8 weeks of posaconazole under

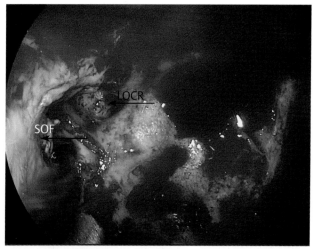

Fig. 11.92 Complete clearance of the lateral opticocarotid recess (LOCR). Right superior orbital fissure (SOF).

strict monitoring of inflammatory markers, renal function tests, serum electrolytes, and blood sugar levels. The patient tolerated the treatment well.

Postoperative scan done 2 months later showed no residue (**Fig. 11.97**).

The left eye remained ophthalmoplegic in the postoperative period, but the periorbital pain subsided very well.

Postoperative healing of the nasal cavity is shown in **Fig. 11.98**.

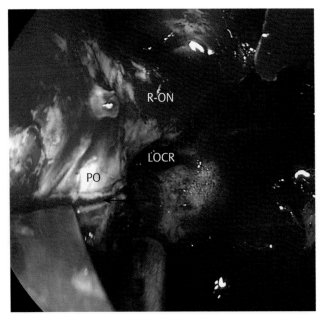

Fig. 11.93 Opening of the periorbita (PO) with a sharp knife. (LOCR, lateral opticocarotid recess; R-ON, right optic nerve.)

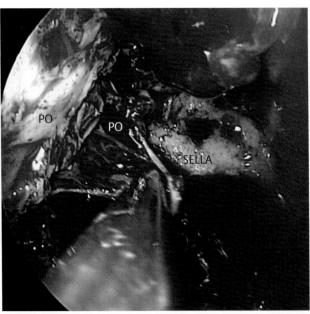

Fig. 11.94 Cut end of the periorbita (PO) being elevated off the muscle layer.

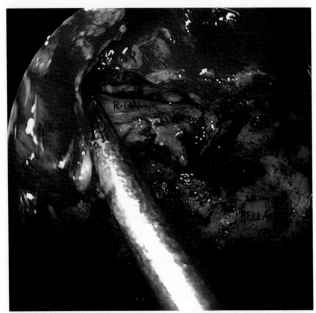

Fig. 11.95 Complete clearance of the right superior orbital fissure (SOF). Note the healthy medial rectus muscle (MRM). (R-ON, right optic nerve.)

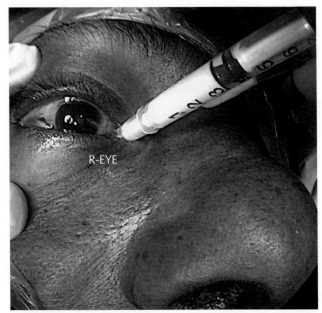

Fig. 11.96 Retrobulbar injection of amphotericin-B in the right eye.

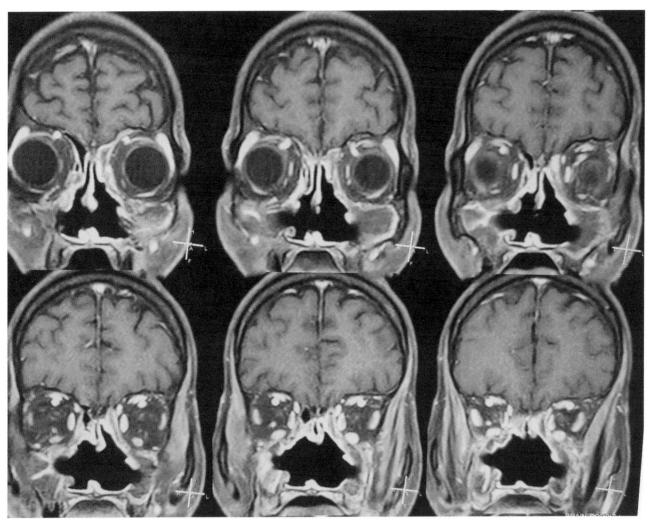

Fig. 11.97 Postoperative magnetic resonance imaging (MRI) paranasal sinus (PNS) showing complete resolution of disease.

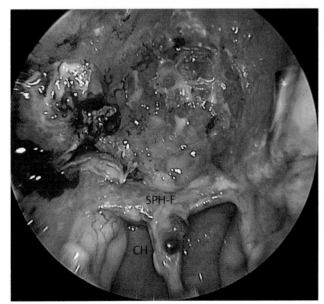

Fig. 11.98 Postoperative healing of both nasal cavities. (CH, choana; SPH-F, sphenoid floor.)

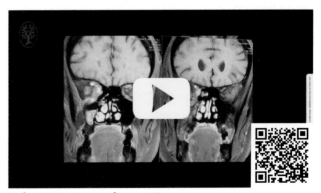

Video 11.6 A case of stage IIC.

Stage IID: Rhino-Orbital—Involvement of the Anterior and Posterior Globe

Case 7: A 46-year-old diabetic male patient was diagnosed with COVID-19-associated mucormycosis 1 month back, when he presented with right facial pain and palatal discoloration. The patient underwent right partial palatectomy and FESS at an outside hospital. Currently, he presented with complaints of epiphora of the right eye, decreased vision, pain while moving the eyeball, and headache with hyperglycemia for 10 days.

On examination, oral cavity showed slough covering the right side of the palate (**Fig. 11.99**). Visual acuity was only perception of light in the right eye with severe chemosis and restricted eye movements (**Fig. 11.100**).

Preoperative evaluation included a detailed otorhinolaryngologic, ophthalmologic, maxillofacial, and neurological examinations to assess the extent of disease. The proinflammatory marker values were recorded every alternate day. Hematological examination details are mentioned in **Table 11.7**.

MRI of the PNS, orbit, and brain, including T1W, T2W, T1WFS, T2WFS, T1WFS postcontrast, and DWI was taken to study the extent of disease and to plan the surgical approaches and excision.

MRI coronal T2WFS showed involvement of bilateral maxillary sinuses and right posterior ethmoids with erosion of the medial and inferior walls of the right orbit with intraorbital abscess formation with inflammation of the extraocular muscles.

Hypodensity infiltrating the area of the right palate and retromaxilla was also seen suggestive of invasive fungal disease (**Fig. 11.101**).

MRI coronal postcontrast T1W image showed nonenhancing right globe with erosion of the medial and inferior orbital walls suggestive of gross invasive fungal disease (**Fig. 11.102**).

The opposite side orbit and palate were normal.

CBCT of the maxilla showed bony defects involving the anterior and lateral walls of the right maxilla, maxillary alveolus, and hard palate. Thinning of the left posterior hard palate was noted in 26 regions (**Fig. 11.103**).

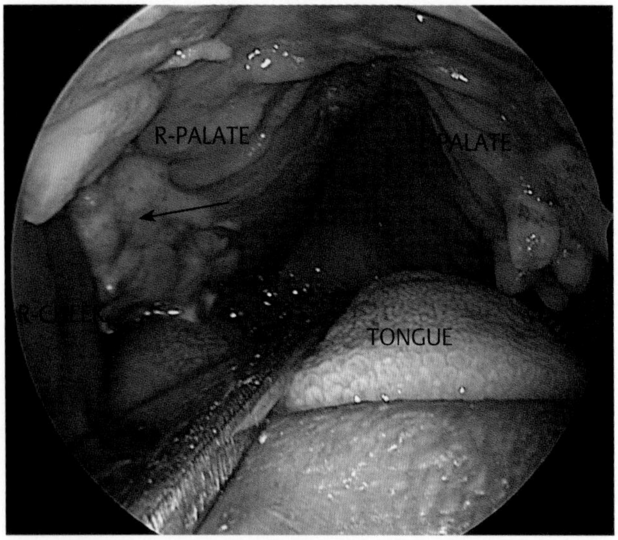

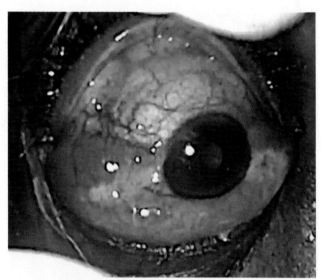

Fig. 11.99 Necrosis of the right palatal mucosa (*black arrow*). (L-PALATE, left palate; R-CHEEK, right cheek; R-PALATE, right palate.)

Fig. 11.100 Preoperative picture of the right eye. Note the chemosis and congestion.

Table 11.7 Hematological findings of the patient

	Total count (per µL)	CRP (mg/L)	D-dimer (ng/mL)	LDH (IU/L)	Ferritin (ng/mL)
Preoperative	7,500	223	1,800	280	376
Immediate postoperative	9,500	230	2,800	345	356
At discharge	4,500	120	580	200	103

Abbreviations: CRP, C-reactive protein; LDH, lactate dehydrogenase.

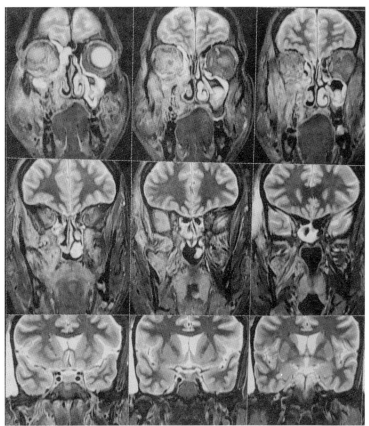

Fig. 11.101 Magnetic resonance imaging (MRI) coronal T2 fat-suppressed (FS) image showing involvement of the bilateral maxillary sinuses and right posterior ethmoids with the erosion of the medial and inferior walls of the right orbit with intraorbital abscess formation. Note the hypodensity infiltrating the area of the right palate and the retromaxilla.

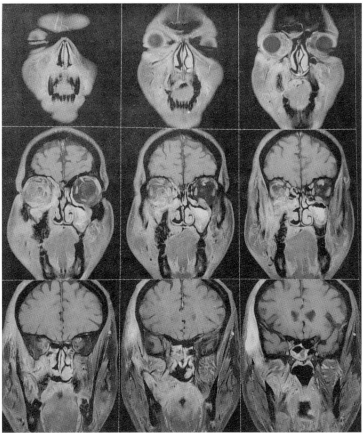

Fig. 11.102 Magnetic resonance imaging (MRI) coronal postcontrast T1-weighted (T1W) image showing nonenhancing right globe with erosion of the medial and inferior orbital walls.

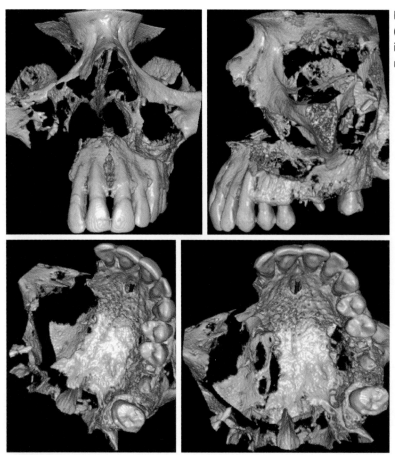

Fig. 11.103 Cone beam computed tomography (CBCT) of the maxilla showing bony defects involving the anterior and lateral walls of the right maxilla, maxillary alveolus, and hard palate.

All patients who presented with a clinical and radiological picture resembling mucormycosis were immediately taken up for radical debridement. Since this patient had gross complete globe involvement, he was taken up for urgent surgical clearance.

The surgical plan based on the MRI findings of bilateral maxilla, ethmoids, palate, and right orbit was bilateral EMD procedure with bilateral full house FESS, right orbital exenteration with clearance of the right SOF and right palatal debridement.

After orotracheal intubation, a central venous line was secured. The patient was placed in the reverse Trendelenburg position and normotensive anesthesia was administered. The nasal cavities were examined, and swabs were taken for gram stain and KOH mount. Povidone-iodine nasal antiseptic washes (0.5%) were given before the onset of surgery. Bilateral nasal cavities were decongested with adrenaline-soaked gauze pieces (1:1,000).

Surgical Steps

Step 1: Left Endoscopic Modified Denker's Procedure

Endoscopic examination of the right nasal cavity revealed post middle meatal antrostomy and ethmoidectomy status.

Left inferior turbinectomy was performed and soft tissue over the left anterolateral wall was elevated in the subperiosteal plane. The left maxillary mucosa was found to be grossly necrosed (**Fig. 11.104**); hence, the mucosa over all the walls was stripped off and sent for HPE. The posterior wall was drilled, and the retroantral area was inspected. Minimal involvement was noted. After clipping of the right internal maxillary artery, the contents of the ITF and PPF were debrided till healthy muscle was seen. Complete sphenoethmoidectomy was done.

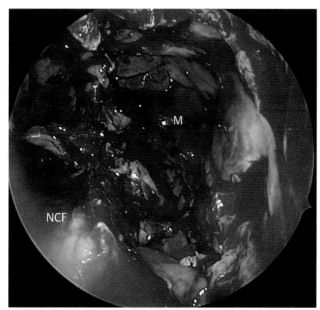

Fig. 11.104 Post left endoscopic modified Denker's procedure. The left maxillary (M) mucosa necrosed. (NCF, nasal cavity floor.)

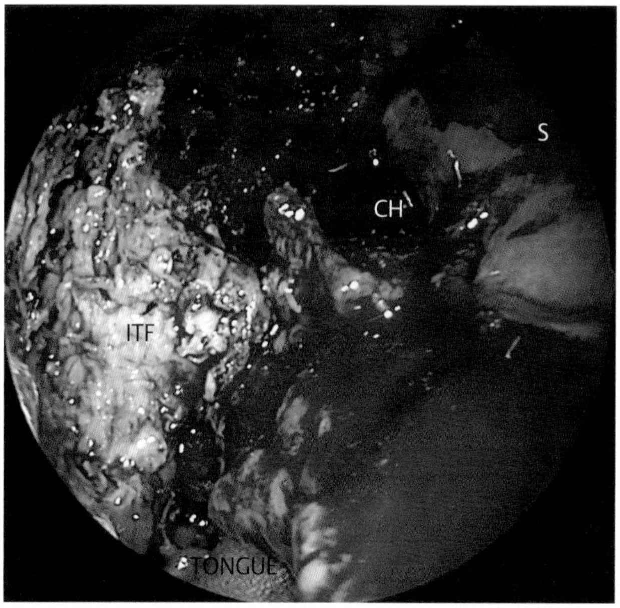

Fig. 11.105 Right infratemporal fossa (ITF) dissection. Note the gross fat stranding and presence of oroantral fistula. (CH, choana.)

Step 2: Dissection of the Right ITF

Right EMD procedure was completed, and the maxilla was inspected. It was filled with slough and necrosed mucosa continuing with the previous palatectomy. The same was debrided completely and the presence of oroantral fistula was noted (**Fig. 11.105**).

The right posterior wall was drilled and the contents of the right ITF were inspected. Fat stranding was noted. The internal maxillary was ligated, and contents of the ITF were debrided till healthy muscle was noted. Complete sphenoethmoidectomy and endoscopic palatal debridement were done on the right side.

Step 3: Right Orbital Decompression and Division of the Optic Nerve

The right orbit was decompressed by removal of the medial and inferior walls. The inferior wall was found to be diseased (**Fig. 11.106**). Using the Karl Storz S III Neuro drill, the OA and medial wall of the optic canal were drilled (**Fig. 11.107**). The optic nerve was found to be sloughed and was divided.

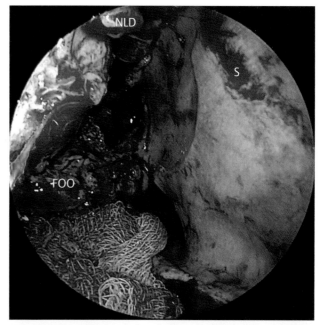

Fig. 11.106 Right medial and inferior orbital walls removed. Note the necrosed inferior wall (*black arrow*). (FOO, floor of the orbit; NLD, nasolacrimal duct.)

Step 4: Right Orbital Exenteration (Lid Sparing)

The NLD on the right side was filled with necrosed material. The same was dissected and divided with sharp scissors (**Fig. 11.108**).

A lid-sparing orbital exenteration was done on the right side. The steps are as follows:

- Medial and lateral canthotomy with a sharp no. 15 surgical blade (**Figs. 11.109** and **11.110**).
- Incision between the orbicularis muscle and the orbital septum to the inferior orbital rim.
- Periosteum at the inferior rim was incised with cautery.
- The same incision was extended in the same plane at 360 degrees.
- A freer's elevator was used to elevate the periosteum all around.
- The zygomaticofacial and zygomaticotemporal bundles were cauterized.
- The posterior orbit was separated using curved scissors (**Fig. 11.111**).
- The orbital contents were removed, and the orbit was packed for hemostasis.

Step 5: Clearance of the Right Superior Orbital Fissure

After the exenteration of the orbit, the surgeon delineated the SOF. The SOF is the communication between the orbital cavity and the middle cranial fossa and is bounded by the greater wing, lesser wing, and body of the sphenoid.[6]

The medial border of it is limited by the optic strut superiorly and the maxillary strut inferiorly.

The disease in the SOF was removed using coblation, in flush with the greater and lesser wings (**Figs. 11.112** and **11.113**).

The orbit was packed and suturing of the lids was done primarily (**Video 11.7**).

Packing

Once hemostasis was achieved, the anterior nasal packing was done. Postoperative picture of the patient 2 weeks after surgery is shown in **Fig. 11.114**.

He was treated with systemic antifungals (liposomal amphotericin-B and oral posaconazole) postoperatively. A cumulative dose of 3.5 g of amphotericin was given for the patient while monitoring the renal parameters and serum electrolytes. The patient tolerated the treatment very well.

Postoperative Management

Postoperative scan taken 1 month later showed complete resolution of the disease (**Fig. 11.115**). Oral rehabilitation was done by an obturator in the postoperative period and strict glycemic control was advised.

Postoperative healing of the exenterated right eye and bilateral nasal cavities are shown in **Figs. 11.116–11.118**.

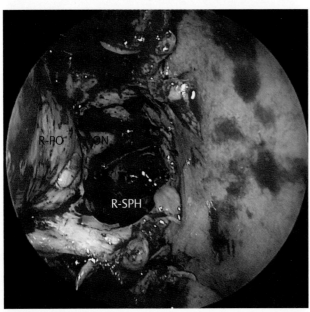

Fig. 11.107 Right side periorbita (R-PO) and optic nerve (ON) exposed in its entirety. (R-SPH, right sphenoid.)

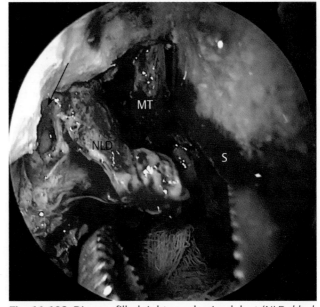

Fig. 11.108 Disease-filled right nasolacrimal duct (NLD; *black arrow*). (MT, middle turbinate; S, septum.)

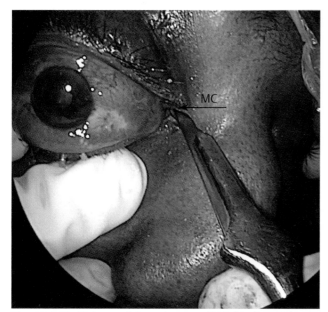

Fig. 11.109 Right medial canthotomy (MC; *black arrow*).

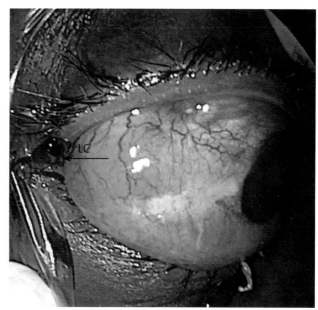

Fig. 11.110 Right lateral canthotomy (LC; *black arrow*).

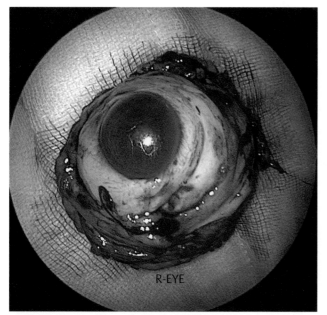

Fig. 11.111 Exenterated right orbital contents.

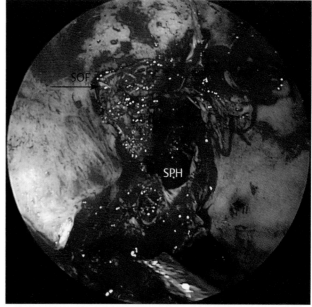

Fig. 11.112 Diseased right superior orbital fissure (SOF; *black arrow*). (SPH, sphenoid sinus.)

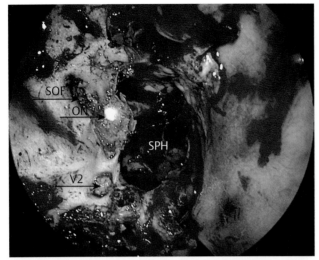

Fig. 11.113 Complete clearance of the right superior orbital fissure (SOF). (ON, optic nerve; SPH, sphenoid sinus; V2, second branch of the trigeminal nerve.)

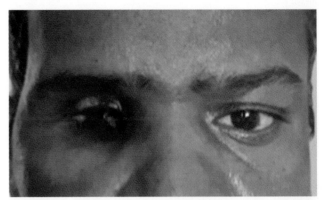

Fig. 11.114 Postoperative photograph of a patient showing healing of the right eyelids.

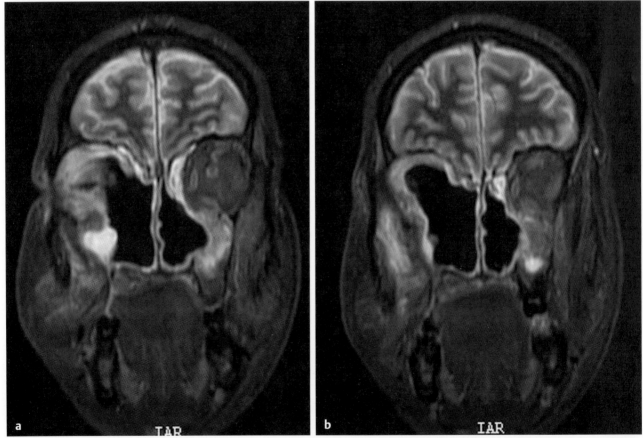

Fig. 11.115 (a, b) Postoperative magnetic resonance imaging (MRI) of the paranasal sinus (PNS) showing complete resolution of disease.

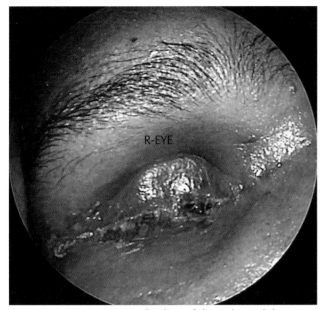

Fig. 11.116 Postoperative healing of the right eyelids.

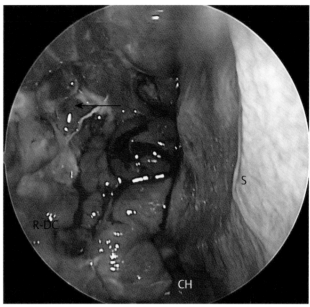

Fig. 11.117 Postoperative healing of the right nasal cavity. Note the polypoidal changes along the exenterated area. (CH, choana; R-DC, right Denker's cavity; S, septum.)

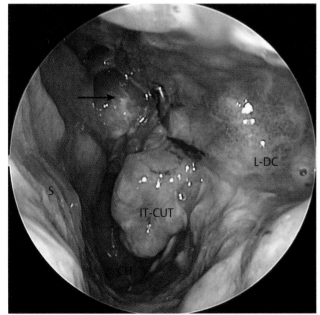

Fig. 11.118 Healing of the left nasal cavity; left Denker's cavity (L-DC). Polypoidal changes along the anterior wall of the sphenoid (*black arrow*). (CH, choana; IT-CUT, cut end of the inferior turbinate; S, septum.)

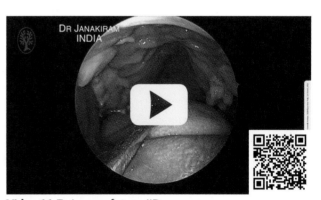

Video 11.7 A case of stage IID.

Stage IIIA: Involvement of the Area Medial to the Internal Carotid Arteries— Planum, Tuberculum, Sella, Clivus, Pterygoid Wedge Sphenoid Sinus, Floor and Keel of Sphenoid, and Rostrum

Case 8: A 36-year-old nondiabetic patient with a history of COVID-19 infection in May 2021 presented 1 month after discharge with complaints of left-sided headache and diplopia. The patient was diagnosed with recent-onset type II diabetes mellitus after initiation of steroid treatment for COVID-19.

Nasal endoscopy showed no abnormality. Orbital examination revealed right lateral rectus palsy (restricted abduction) with no refractory error (**Fig. 11.119**). The palate was clinically not involved.

Evaluation at presentation included a detailed otorhinolaryngologic, ophthalmologic, and neurological examinations to assess the extent of the disease. The pro-inflammatory marker values were recorded every alternate day. Hematological values are mentioned in **Table 11.8**.

CT-PNS showed involvement of the bilateral ethmoids, erosion of the left GWS, and clivus. The bilateral maxillae were free.

MRI of the PNS, orbit, and brain, including T1W, T2W, T2WFS, T1WFS postcontrast, and DWI was taken to study the extent of disease and to plan the surgical approaches and excision.

The coronal postcontrast T1 FS images showed non-enhancing soft tissue in the bilateral ethmoid sinuses, osteomyelitis of the left GWS, and clivus, with surrounding enhancement, suggestive of inflammatory tissue

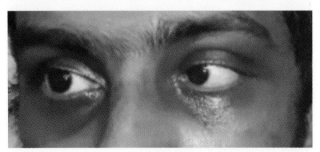

Fig. 11.119 Patient photograph showing right lateral rectus palsy.

(**Fig. 11.120a, b**). The left cavernous sinus showed inflammatory changes. It was noted that the bilateral maxillary sinuses, orbit, and palate were uninvolved.

Considering the patient had orbital involvement, he was immediately taken up for total excision. The surgical plan was based on the MRI findings of the ethmoid, sphenoid, and clivus with cavernous involvement. A left modified EMD procedure with bilateral full house FESS, trans-sellar, transclival, and medial transpetrous approach was performed for aggressive debridement.

After orotracheal intubation, the CVP line was secured. The patient was placed in the reverse Trendelenburg position and hypotensive anesthesia was administered. The nasal cavities were examined, and swabs were taken for gram stain and KOH mount. Povidone-iodine nasal antiseptic washes (0.5%) were given before the onset of surgery. Bilateral nasal cavities were decongested with adrenaline-soaked gauze pieces (1:1,000).

Surgical Steps

Step 1: Left Endoscopic Modified Denker's Procedure

An EMD procedure was performed. The left maxillary sinus mucosa found thickened and necrotic over the anterolateral and posterior walls were removed. The anterolateral wall was drilled further laterally to provide the noninfected margin to the EMD procedure (**Figs. 11.121** and **11.122**). The premaxillary tissues were found to be uninvolved by the disease. Bilateral middle turbinectomy with complete sphenoethmoidectomy was done (**Fig. 11.123**).

Step 2: Left Pterygopalatine Fossa Dissection and Pterygoid Wedge Drilling

The bone over the posterior wall of the left maxilla was drilled (**Fig. 11.124**), the fat in the pterygopalatine fossa was not grossly involved. It was coablated and diseased pterygoid wedge was drilled, keeping the V2 branch of the trigeminal nerve laterally and the vidian nerve medially as landmarks. The posterolateral boundary of drilling was the anterior surface of the lateral pterygoid muscle. Osteomyelitic bone chips were removed, and drilling was done up to the lateral wall of the sphenoid. The vidian nerve was found to be involved and resected.

Table 11.8 Hematological findings of the patient

	Total count (per µL)	CRP (mg/L)	D-dimer (ng/mL)	LDH (IU/L)	Ferritin (ng/mL)
Preoperative	5,000	220	1,900	340	330
Immediate postoperative	8,500	225	3,000	300	320
At discharge	7,000	20	500	180	80

Abbreviations: CRP, C-reactive protein; LDH, lactate dehydrogenase.

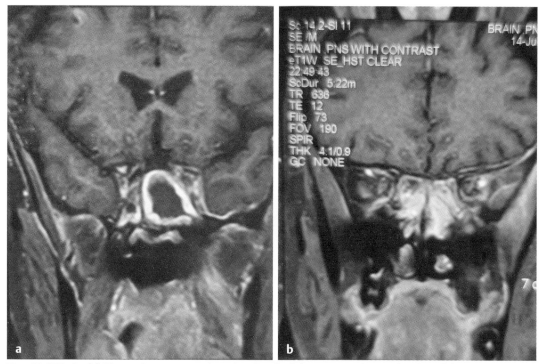

Fig. 11.120 (a, b) Magnetic resonance imaging (MRI) of the paranasal sinus (PNS) with brain coronal T1-weighted (T1W) postcontrast showing nonenhancing soft tissue in the bilateral ethmoids with osteomyelitis of the left greater wing of the sphenoid and clivus.

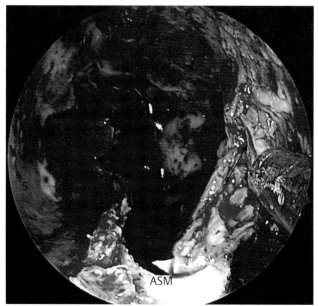

Fig. 11.121 Left endoscopic modified Denker's procedure. The *black arrow* shows the extra-anterolateral wall that was removed to provide noninfected margin. (ASM, alveolar surface of maxilla; S, septum.)

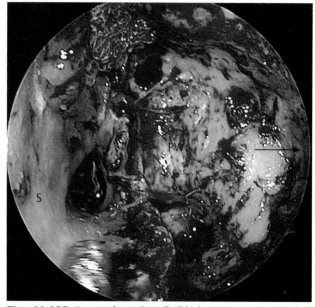

Fig. 11.122 Posterolateral wall (*black arrow*) is seen after extended Denker's procedure. (PW, posterior wall; S, septum.)

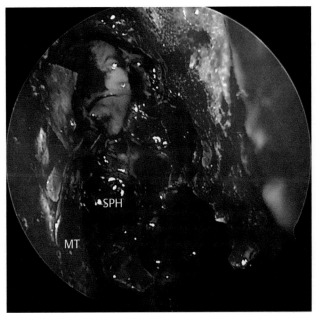

Fig. 11.123 Left complete sphenoethmoidectomy. Sphenoid sinus (SPH) and remnant middle turbinate (MT).

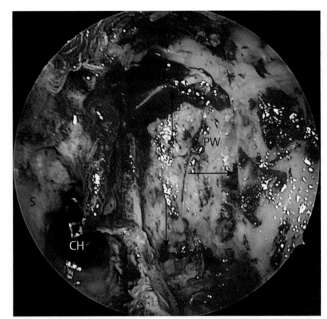

Fig. 11.124 Posterior window osteotomies (*black arrows*) over the posterior wall (PW) of the maxilla. (CH, choana; S, septum.)

Step 3: Wide Sphenoidotomy

The posterior septum was transected and disarticulated from the rostrum of the sphenoid. The septum was uninvolved (**Fig. 11.125**). The rostrum and ventral surface of the sphenoid were denuded of all mucosae, which resulted in the classical "owl's-eye appearance" (**Fig. 11.126**).

The anatomical landmarks on the posterior wall of the sphenoid are identified. The planum sphenoidale was delineated. Planar osteotomy and bilateral "shoulder osteotomy" were done at the level of pterygosphenoid synchondrosis and the bony cut connected inferiorly at the level of the floor of the sphenoid (**Fig. 11.127**).

The sphenoid sinus was widened superiorly up to the planum, laterally up to lateral wall of the sphenoid and medial pterygoid plate, and inferiorly two suction tips below the sellar floor. The sphenoid cavity was smoothened by drilling off all septations using a diamond burr. Wide sphenoidotomy was done for the exposure of the clivus and left GWS.

Over the posterior wall of the sphenoid, the surgeon must identify the sellar bulge, lateral and medial opticocarotid recesses, optic canal, bilateral paraclival carotid prominences, and clival recess.

Step 4: Trans-Sphenoidal Transclival Drilling

The sphenoid mucosa over the floor was found to be necrosed. The same was removed and sent separately for KOH mount and HPE (**Fig. 11.128**). The bone of the lateral

wall of the sphenoid, GWS, and mid-clivus had yellowish discoloration with high porosity. The striking difference could be made between whitish dense healthy bone overlying the sella and yellow porous brittle bone in the lower part of the mid-clivus (**Fig. 11.129**).

The floor of the sphenoid sinus was osteomyelitic and was drilled completely, thus obtaining better access to the mid-clival recess. The outer cortical and inner cancellous bone of the clivus was found to be avascular and necrotic. Bilateral paraclival internal carotid arteries were mapped using the carotid doppler and the mid-third of the clivus drilled until thin bone was left over the clival dura. The authors had noted that the diseased clival bone does not bleed as opposed to the normal clival bone (**Figs. 11.130** and **11.131**).

The surgeon must delineate the drilled pterygoid wedge and follow the infratemporal surface of the GWS posteromedially, inferior to the V2 branch of the trigeminal nerve, to drill the necrosed GWS (**Figs. 11.132** and **11.133**).

Step 5: Medial Transpetrous Approach

Medial transpetrous approach is a type of paramedian endoscopic endonasal approach where access is made posterior to the paraclival internal carotid artery (ICA).

Keeping the vidian nerve as landmark, bone over the bilateral paraclival ICA was drilled till a thin shell of bone was left. Bilateral petroclival windows were found osteomyelitic and the same was drilled and removed (**Figs. 11.134–11.136**).

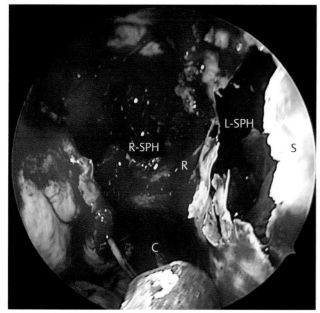

Fig. 11.125 Posterior septectomy. (C, choana; L-SPH, left sphenoid; R, rostrum; R-SPH, right sphenoid; S, septum.)

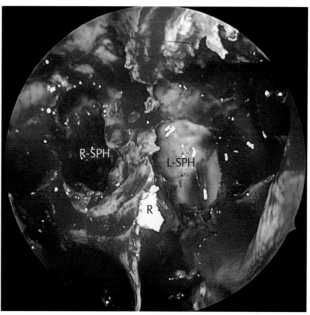

Fig. 11.126 "Owl's eye" appearance. (L-SPH, left sphenoid; R, rostrum; R-SPH, right sphenoid.)

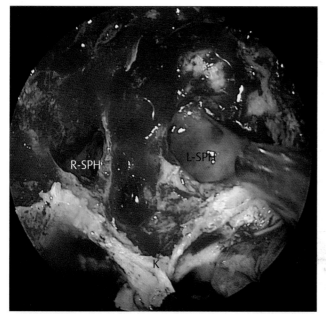

Fig. 11.127 Wide sphenoidotomy following triple osteotomy. (K, keel; L-SPH, left sphenoid; R-SPH, right sphenoid.)

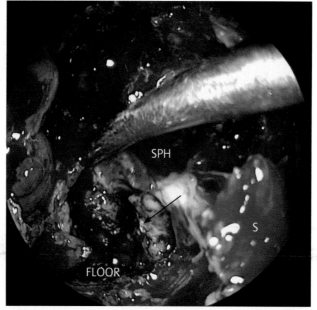

Fig. 11.128 Elevation of the floor of the sphenoid mucosa, showing sloughed mucosa (*black arrow*). (SPH, sphenoid sinus.)

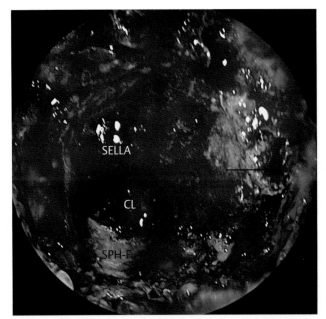

Fig. 11.129 Posterior wall of the sphenoid sinus. Avascular bone of the lower end of the clival recess is visible. Clivus (CL), floor of the sphenoid (SPH-F), and the V2 branch of the trigeminal nerve (*black arrow*).

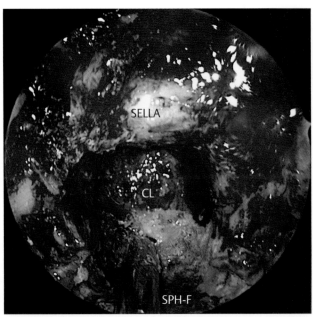

Fig. 11.130 Outer cortical and inner cancellous bone of the clivus (CL) diseased. The floor of the sphenoid (SPH-F) and sella are marked.

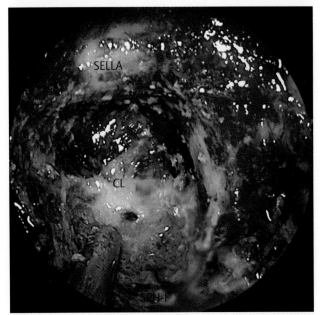

Fig. 11.131 No bleeding is noted from the avascular bone of the clival recess. The clivus (CL), floor of the sphenoid (SPH-F), and sella are marked.

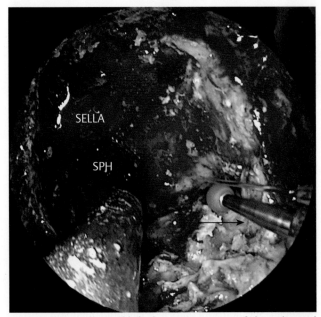

Fig. 11.132 Drilling of left the greater wing of the sphenoid (GWS; *black arrow*). Sella and sphenoid sinus (SPH) are marked.

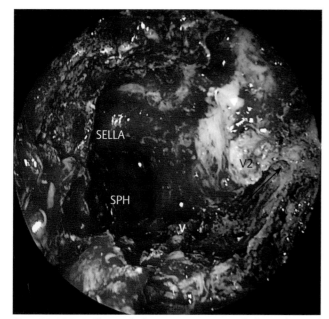

Fig. 11.133 Drilling of the greater wing of the sphenoid (GWS) inferior to the V2 branch of the trigeminal nerve (V2). Sella and sphenoid sinus (SPH) are marked.

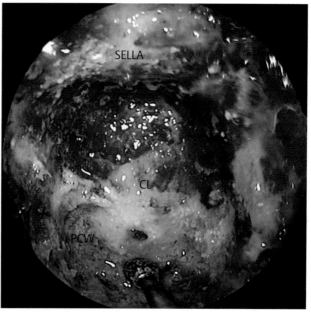

Fig. 11.134 Drilling of the mid-clivus (mid-CL); necrosis of the bilateral petroclival window (PCW) is noted.

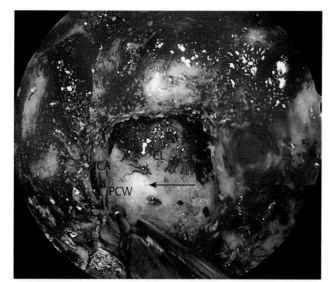

Fig. 11.135 Bone over the right petroclival window (PCW) is drilled and thinned out. The clival dura is visible on the right side (*black arrow*). (CL, clivus; ICA, internal carotid artery.)

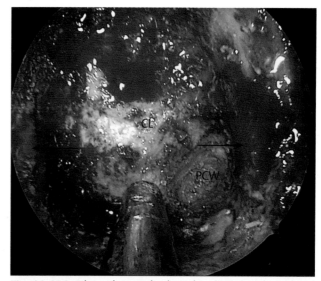

Fig. 11.136 Bilateral petroclival window (PCW) is cleared and both internal carotid arteries are marked (*black arrows*).

Thick granulation tissue was noted in the dehiscence of the inner clival bone with intact dura. It was excised using rosen's elevator and sent for histopathology (**Figs. 11.137** and **11.138**). Cavity after debridement is depicted in **Fig. 11.139 (Video 11.8)**.

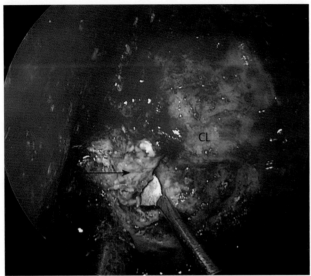

Fig. 11.137 Thick granulation tissue (*black arrow*), in the dehiscence of the inner clival bone. (CL, clivus.)

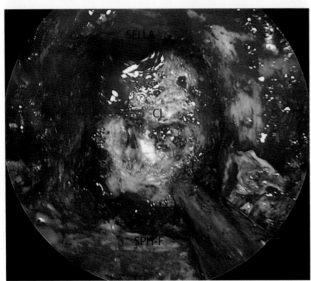

Fig. 11.138 Complete clearance of the granulation tissue; the clival dura is intact. The clivus (CL), sella, and the floor of the sphenoid sinus (SPH-F) are marked.

Packing

Diluted amphotericin washes were given, and nasal cavity was packed with merocel 8 cm in both nostrils.

Postoperative Management

Postoperative scan showed complete disease clearance (**Fig. 11.140**). The lateral rectus palsy recovered after 1 week of intravenous amphotericin treatment. Although no gross changes were noted in MRI of the brain in the sixth nerve, proximity of the nerve and continuous inflammatory spread of the disease explain the sixth nerve involvement.

The postoperative picture showed recovered lateral rectus function (**Fig. 11.141**). Healing of the nasal cavity 2 months following surgery is depicted in **Fig. 11.142**.

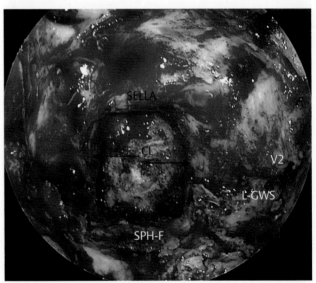

Fig. 11.139 Cavity after complete clearance. The clivus (CL), sella, floor of the sphenoid sinus (SPH-F), left greater wing of the sphenoid (L-GWS), and bilateral paraclival internal carotid arteries are marked (*black arrows*).

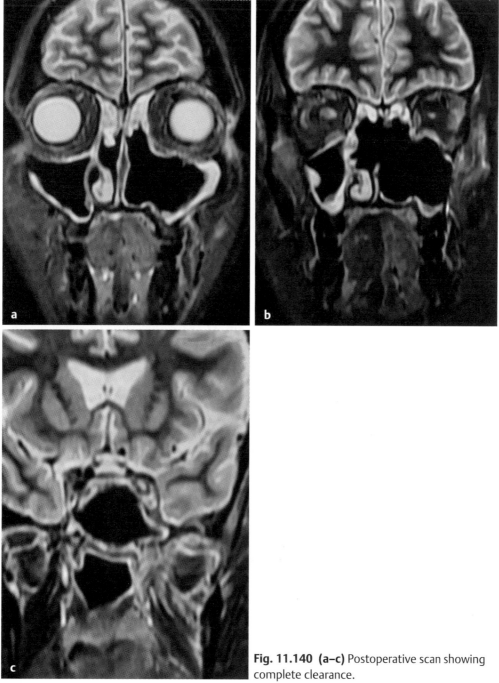

Fig. 11.140 (a–c) Postoperative scan showing complete clearance.

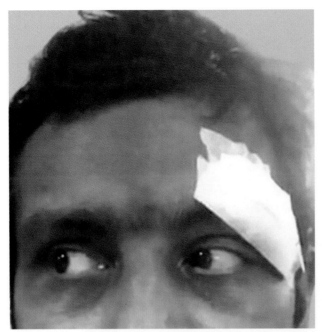

Fig. 11.141 Postoperative resolution of the right lateral rectus palsy.

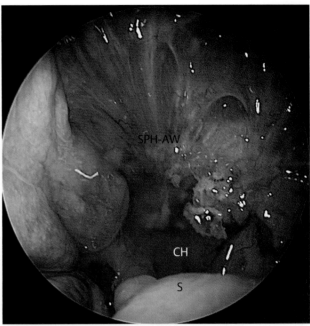

Fig. 11.142 Postoperative healing of the nasal cavity. Note the healed anterior wall of the sphenoid (SPH-AW). (CH, choana; S, septum.)

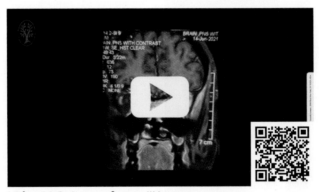

Video 11.8 A case of stage IIIA.

Stage IIIB (Case 1): Involvement of the Paramedian Anterior Compartment— Medial and Lateral Pterygoid Plates, V2 Branch of the Trigeminal Nerve, and Quadrangular Space

Case 9: A 32-year-old nondiabetic patient with a history of COVID-19 infection in June 2021 presented 15 days after discharge with complaints of severe headache, not responding to medications. The patient was diagnosed with recent-onset type II diabetes mellitus after initiation of steroid treatment for COVID-19.

Nasal endoscopy revealed purulent secretions with sloughed mucosa in the right middle meatus (**Fig. 11.143**). Orbital examination showed no abnormality. The palate was clinically not involved.

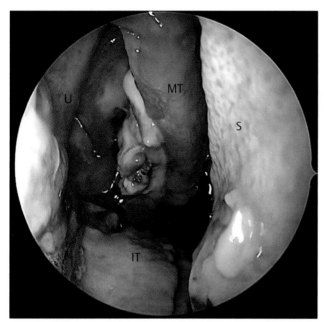

Fig. 11.143 Fungal debris seen lateral to the right middle turbinate (MT). (IT, inferior turbinate; S, septum; U, uncinate.)

Evaluation at presentation included a detailed otorhinolaryngologic, ophthalmologic, and neurological examinations to assess the extent of disease. The proinflammatory marker values were recorded every alternate day. Hematological values are mentioned in **Table 11.9**.

CT-PNS showed erosion of the bilateral GWS and the clivus with soft-tissue density. Bilateral maxillary sinuses were free.

MRI of the PNS, orbit, and brain, including T1W, T2W, T2WFS, T1WFS postcontrast, and DWI was taken to study the extent of disease and to plan the surgical approaches and excision.

The coronal T2W STIR images showed nonenhancing soft tissue in the bilateral ethmoid sinuses, osteomyelitis of the bilateral GWS, and clivus, with surrounding soft-tissue edema (**Fig. 11.144**). The sequestra of the cortical bone appear as low signal on T1, T2, and STIR and do not enhance. The sequestra of the cancellous bone also do not enhance but are relatively hyperintense to cortical sequestra on T1, T2, and STIR. Both ethmoid sinus and retromaxillae showed hypodensities suggestive of fungal disease. Bilateral maxillary sinuses, orbit, and palate were uninvolved.

The patient was taken up for surgical clearance after a thorough preoperative checkup. The surgical plan was based on the MRI findings of ethmoid, sphenoid, clivus, and bilateral GWS involvement. Bilateral EMD procedure with bilateral full house FESS, transclival, and drilling of the infratemporal aspect of the GWS was performed for aggressive debridement.

After orotracheal intubation, a central venous line was secured. The patient was placed in the reverse Trendelenburg position and hypotensive anesthesia was administered. The nasal cavities were examined, and swabs were taken for gram stain and KOH mount. Povidone-iodine nasal antiseptic washes (0.5%) were given before the onset of surgery. Bilateral nasal cavities were decongested with adrenaline-soaked gauze pieces (1:1,000).

Table 11.9   Hematological findings of the patient

	Total count (per μL)	CRP (mg/L)	D-dimer (ng/mL)	LDH (IU/L)	Ferritin (ng/mL)
Preoperative	7,500	243	2,225	300	310
Immediate postoperative	10,000	234	3,000	345	310
At discharge	5,000	45	410	200	75

Abbreviations: CRP, C-reactive protein; LDH, lactate dehydrogenase.

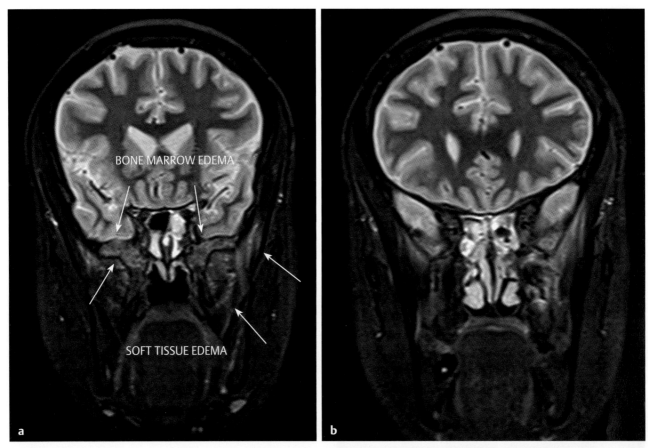

Fig. 11.144 (a, b) Preoperative magnetic resonance imaging (MRI) of the paranasal sinus (PNS) T2-weighted (T2W) short tau inversion recovery (STIR) coronal images showing osteomyelitis of the bilateral greater wing of the sphenoid and clivus along with fungal hypodensity in the bilateral ethmoid sinus and bilateral retroantral area.

Surgical Steps

Step 1: Bilateral Fess with Posterior Septectomy
Bilateral complete sphenoethmoidectomy was done with posterior septectomy for the binostril approach (**Fig. 11.145**). Bilateral ethmoidal mucosa was sloughed.

Step 2: Transellar and Trans Mid-Clival Drilling
Triple osteotomy was performed, and the anterior wall of the sphenoid was found to be thinned and necrotic. The rostrum, keel, and inferior wall of the sphenoid were thinned out and hence excised. The sella and mid-clivus were exposed. The outer cortex of the mid-clival bone was discolored and appeared more granular and sclerotic. During drilling, it was noted that the outer cortex could not be differentiated from the bone marrow of the mid-clivus. The marrow spaces of the mid-clivus were avascular and highly porous. This signifies obliteration of the vascular marrow spaces by thrombosis and how it becomes a nidus for fungus and bacterial biofilms.

Biopsy was taken for histopathological study from the outer diseased cortical bone of the clivus, and it was drilled completely to give disease clearance (**Figs. 11.146–11.149**). The drilling was continued till the inner cortical bone, which was also thinned out. In areas where the inner cortical bone was grossly involved, the dura was noted to be friable but not dehiscent. The inner cortical bone drilling was performed carefully, and the dura was kept intact.

Step 3: Left Infratemporal Fossa Dissection and Transpterygoid Approach
After a left EMD procedure, the posterior wall of the left maxilla was drilled. Gross fat stranding was noted in the PPF and ITF (**Fig. 11.150**). The internal maxillary artery was identified and ligated, and the contents of the fossa were debrided till healthy muscle was seen.

The pterygoid wedge was granular, thinned, and decalcified. During drilling, the bone appeared brittle and avascular. The pterygoid sequestrum was noted from the V2 branch of the trigeminal nerve laterally to the vidian nerve medially. The vidian foramen and its neurovascular bundle were found to be discolored and necrotic. The foramina were drilled and the vidian canal was followed till the precarotid area.

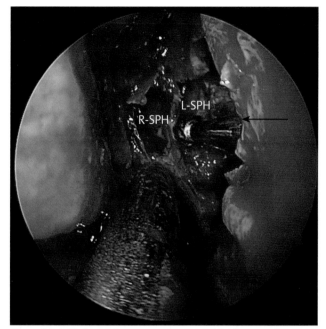

Fig. 11.145 Posterior septectomy (*black arrow*). Both sphenoid sinuses exposed, and the right sphenoid (R-SPH) and left sphenoid (L-SPH) are marked.

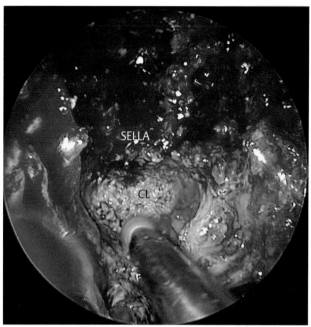

Fig. 11.146 Gross disease in the clivus (CL). The sella is marked.

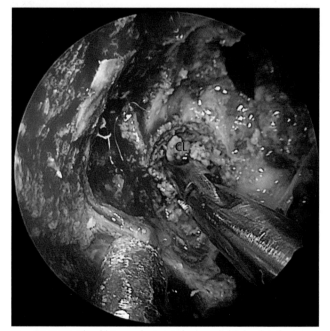

Fig. 11.147 Clival biopsy being taken with blakesley forceps.

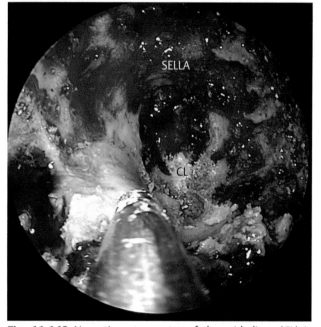

Fig. 11.148 Necrotic outer cortex of the mid-clivus (CL) is drilled. The sella is marked.

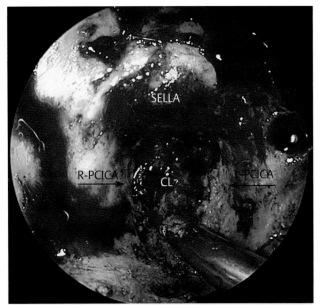

Fig. 11.149 Mid-clivus (CL) cleared off disease. Right para-clival internal carotid artery (R-PCICA) and left paraclival internal carotid artery (L-PCICA).

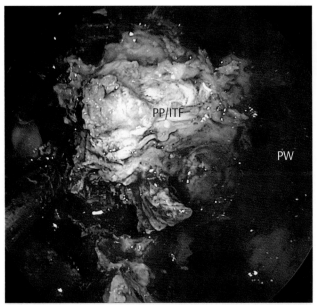

Fig. 11.150 Gross fat stranding of the left infratemporal fossa (ITF) and pterygopalatine (PP) fossa. Posterior wall of the maxilla (PW).

Step 4: Drilling of the Left Greater Wing of the Sphenoid

Following the drilling of the left pterygoid wedge, with V2 as the landmark, the infratemporal surface of the GWS was exposed after coblation of muscular attachments. The GWS was granular and brittle in gross appearance (**Fig. 11.151**). Since the disease was extending laterally till V3, the left quadrangular space was delineated. The quadrangular space is bounded laterally by V2, superiorly by the sixth cranial nerve, and inferomedially by the ICA. It is referred to as the "front door to Meckel's cave."[7] Laterally, the soft tissue till the foramen ovale was coblated and sent for histopathology. The V3 nerve was identified and was found to be intact (**Fig. 11.152**).

Step 5: Right Endoscopic Modified Denker's and Dissection of the Right Infratemporal Fossa

An EMD procedure was done on the right side for increasing surgical maneuverability. The posterior wall of the right maxilla was drilled, and the pterygopalatine and ITF were exposed. Comparable to the left side, gross fat stranding was also observed on the right side, and the same was coblated and excised after clipping of the internal maxillary artery.

Step 6: Endoscopic Endonasal Transpterygoid Approach: Right Side

This approach provides excellent visualization of the foramen rotundum, vidian nerve, foramen ovale, and V3 branch of the

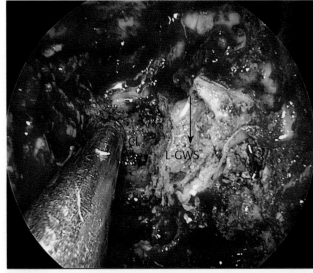

Fig. 11.151 Osteonecrosis of the left greater wing of the sphenoid (L-GWS, *black arrow*); mid-clivus (CL).

trigeminal nerve. The right pterygoid wedge was osteomyelitic and was drilled out completely. The vidian nerve was resected since it was sloughed (**Fig. 11.153**). The necrosed infratemporal surface of the GWS was drilled posteromedially till the V3 branch of the trigeminal nerve was identified. The whole cavity after clearance is shown in **Figs. 11.154** and **11.155 (Video 11.9)**.

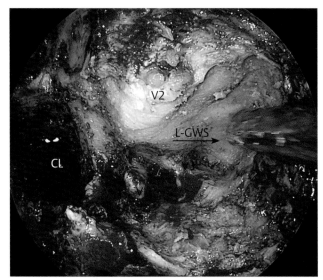

Fig. 11.152 Left greater wing of the sphenoid (L-GWS) cleared off disease, vidian (V), second division of the trigeminal nerve (V2), third division of the trigeminal nerve (V3), and the clivus (CL) are seen.

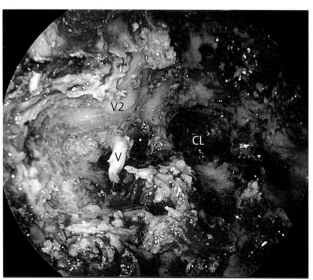

Fig. 11.153 Necrosed right greater wing of the sphenoid. note the sloughed vidian nerve (V). Second branch of the trigeminal nerve (V2) and mid-clivus (CL).

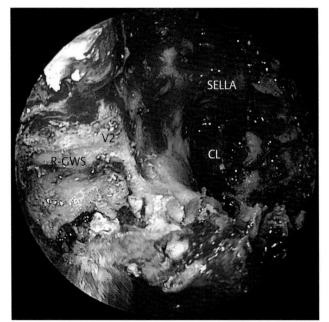

Fig. 11.154 Right greater wing of the sphenoid (R-GWS) cleared off disease. Second branch of the trigeminal nerve (V2) and mid-clivus (CL).

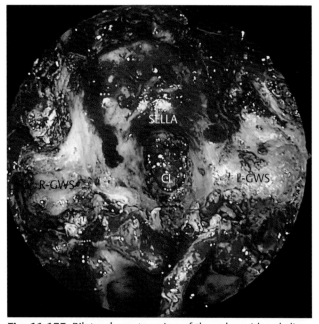

Fig. 11.155 Bilateral greater wing of the sphenoid and clivus completely cleared off disease. The left greater wing of the sphenoid (L-GWS), the right greater wing of the sphenoid (R-GWS), and the clivus (CL) are marked.

Packing

Diluted amphotericin washes were given, and nasal cavity was packed with merocel 8 cm in both nostrils.

Postoperative Management

Postoperatively the patient was treated with systemic antifungals (conventional amphotericin-B and oral posaconazole). He received a total dose of 2 g of amphotericin-B with total 8 weeks' duration of 400 mg of posaconazole.

A postoperative scan was done and it showed complete disease clearance (**Fig. 11.156**).

The surgeon has described the postoperative MRI of the PNS at the level of the pterygoid wedge of the patients with the bilateral GWS involvement appear as a "*holy cross sign.*" The vertical limb of the cross extends from the floor of the nasal cavity to the planum superiorly. The horizontal limb of the cross extends between the bone over the bilateral temporal fossa (**Fig. 11.157**).

The undersurface of the greater wing of sphenoid, which forms the base of the middle cranial fossa, when undergoes necrosis, due to invasive fungal disease, there is a major chance of dural breach and thus subsequent brain abscess is its sequalae.

In a patient when the scan is suggestive of disease process in the GWS, if the surgeon can achieve a bony clearance in the primary setting itself, this major intracranial complication may be avoided. The authors would like to stress the importance of complete clearance of the diseased bone in

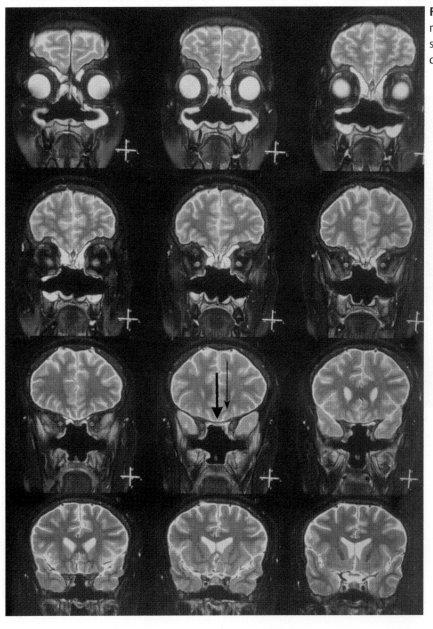

Fig. 11.156 Postoperative magnetic resonance imaging (MRI) of the paranasal sinus (PNS) shows complete resolution of disease.

the primary surgery itself. This is the importance of the *holy cross sign* in postoperative imaging when the unilateral or greater wing of sphenoid is involved.

Postoperative healing of the nasal cavity at the second and third months is depicted in **Figs. 11.158** and **11.159**, respectively.

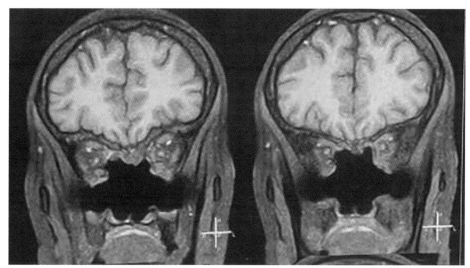

Fig. 11.157 Depiction of "holy cross sign" on magnetic resonance imaging (MRI).

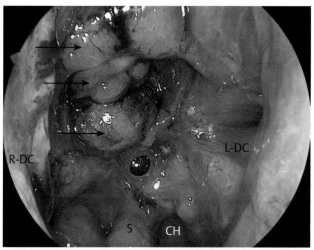

Fig. 11.158 Healing of the nasal cavity at the second month after surgery. (CH, choana; L-DC, left Denker's cavity; S, resected septum; R-DC, right Denker's cavity.) Note the polypoidal changes during the normal healing process (*black arrows*).

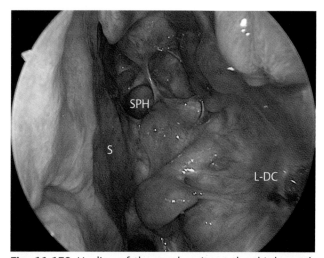

Fig. 11.159 Healing of the nasal cavity at the third month after surgery. (L-DC, left Denker's cavity; S, septum; SPH, sphenoid.)

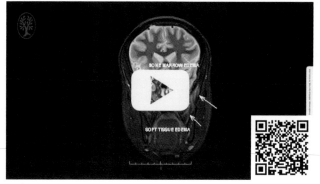

Video 11.9 A case of stage IIIB—case 1.

Stage IIIB (Case 2): Involvement of the Paramedian Middle Compartment—the Cavernous Sinus

Case 10: A 36-year-old nondiabetic man diagnosed with COVID-19-associated rhino-orbital mucormycosis 2 months back had undergone right endoscopic sinus surgery with right orbital decompression surgery elsewhere. The patient noted loss of vision in the right eye after 1 month and underwent right orbital exenteration in the same hospital. Currently, he presented with severe headache that was not responding to treatment. The patient had received a total of 15 g of intravenous amphotericin-B till the time of presentation. He was referred to the authors' center for further assessment and management.

Nasal endoscopy revealed status post maxillary antrostomy and ethmoidectomy on the right side with polypoidal changes. Orbital examination showed right exenterated socket with wound gaping and normal visual acuity in the left eye (**Figs. 11.160** and **11.161**). The palate was clinically not involved.

Evaluation at presentation included a detailed otorhinolaryngologic, ophthalmic, and neurological examinations to assess the extent of disease. The proinflammatory marker values were recorded every alternate day. Hematological values are mentioned in **Table 11.10**.

MRI of the PNS, orbit, and brain including T1W, T2W, T2WFS, T1WFS postcontrast, and DWI was taken to study the extent of disease and to plan the surgical approaches and excision.

The coronal T1WFS images showed heterogeneously enhancing mucosal thickening with hypointensities within the right maxillary and ethmoid sinus. STIR hyperintensity was noted in the body of the sphenoid causing erosions of the posterior and lateral walls of the sphenoid sinus on the right side.

Heterogeneously enhancing soft-tissue density was seen in the right orbital apex (OA), PPF, retroantral fat pad, and infratemporal region, with erosion of the right pterygoid

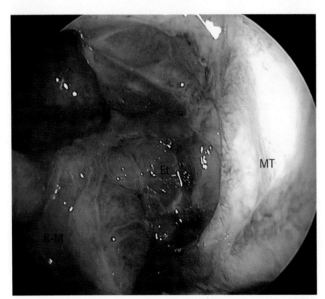

Fig. 11.160 Anterior rhinoscopy showing status post maxillary antrostomy and ethmoidectomy on the right side with polypoidal changes. (Et, ethmoids; MT, middle turbinate; R-M, right maxilla.)

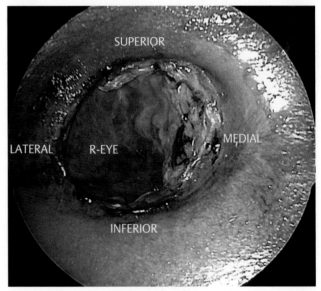

Fig. 11.161 Right exenterated socket.

Table 11.10 Hematological findings of the patient

	Total count (per μL)	CRP (mg/L)	D-dimer (ng/mL)	LDH (IU/L)	Ferritin (ng/mL)
Preoperative	5,000	250	2,500	300	285
Immediate postoperative	12,000	245	3,100	325	300
At discharge	4,000	60	500	240	95

Abbreviations: CRP, C-reactive protein; LDH, lactate dehydrogenase.

wedge and GWS. Thickening and enhancement of the dural sheath of the right cavernous sinus with preserved flow void of the ICA was noted (**Fig. 11.162**).

After thorough preoperative workup, the patient was taken up for total excision. The surgical plan was based on the MRI findings of the right maxilla, sphenoid, GWS, and OA

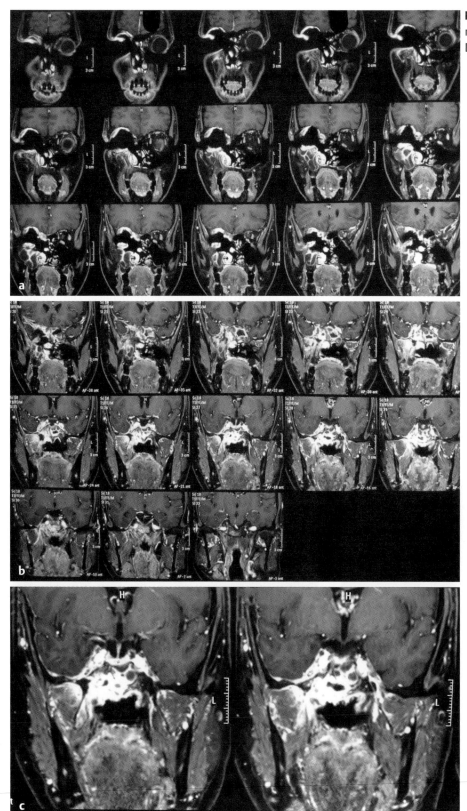

Fig. 11.162 (a–c) Preoperative magnetic resonance (MR) images. Description in the text.

involvement. A right EMD procedure with full house FESS, transclival and transpterygoid approach to the infratemporal aspect of the GWS, clearance of the OA, and decompression of the cavernous sinus was planned for aggressive debridement.

After orotracheal intubation, a central venous line was secured. The patient was placed in the reverse Trendelenburg position and hypotensive anesthesia was administered. The nasal cavities were examined, and swabs were taken for gram stain and KOH mount. Povidone-iodine nasal antiseptic washes (0.5%) were given before the onset of surgery. Bilateral nasal cavities were decongested with adrenaline-soaked gauze pieces (1:1,000).

Surgical Steps

Step 1: Right Endoscopic Modified Denker's Procedure with ITF Dissection

A EMD procedure was done on the right side, and on inspection of the maxillary sinus no gross disease was seen (**Fig. 11.163**). The posterior wall of the maxilla was drilled to access the pterygopalatine and the ITF. Gross fat stranding with tissue necrosis was noted and the same was dissected till healthy bleeding tissue was noted. The pterygoid wedge and medial pterygoid plate were found to be eroded and devascularized.

Step 2: Transclival Drilling

Posterior septectomy and triple osteotomy were done. The rostrum of the sphenoid was removed. Fungal debris inside

the right side of the sphenoid sinus was removed and sent for HPE. The sella, floor of the sphenoid, and mid-clivus were exposed. The outer cortical bone of the mid-clivus was found to be avascular and diseased, with porous marrow cavities (**Figs. 11.164** and **11.165**). The mucosa inside the sphenoid sinuses was elevated and removed; the floor was osteomyelitic and it was drilled in flush with the lower clivus, and transclival drilling was done till thin bone was left over the clival dura. At the end of clival disease clearance, bleeding from the marrow was noted (**Figs. 11.166** and **11.167**).

The clivus is divided into the upper, middle, and lower parts. The upper clivus is the part above the crossing of the trigeminal and abducens nerves from the posterior to the middle cranial fossa. This includes the dorsum sellae and the posterior clinoid processes. The mid-clivus is between the exits of the trigeminal nerve and the glossopharyngeal nerves. The lower clivus is the part from the glossopharyngeal nerve to the foramen magnum.

Step 3: Right Transpterygoid Approach

Following the right ITF dissection, the vidian nerve and V2 branch of the trigeminal nerve are defined. The pterygoid wedge was found eroded by the disease, and the same was drilled keeping the above landmarks in the line of vision. The vidian nerve and V2 were involved, and their respective canals were drilled till the precarotid area. The GWS on the right side was also found involved. It appeared brittle and osteonecrotic (**Fig. 11.168**). The infratemporal surface of the greater wing was drilled till healthy bone was seen (**Fig. 11.169**).

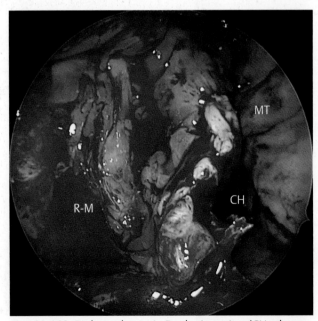

Fig. 11.163 Right endoscopic Denker's cavity. (CH, choana; MT, middle turbinate; R-M, right maxilla.)

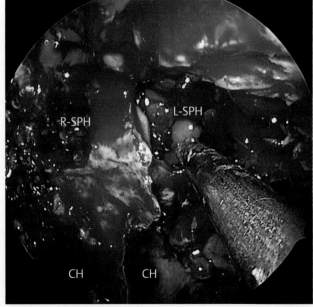

Fig. 11.164 "Owl's eye appearance." (CH, choana; L-SPH, left sphenoid; R-SPH, right sphenoid.)

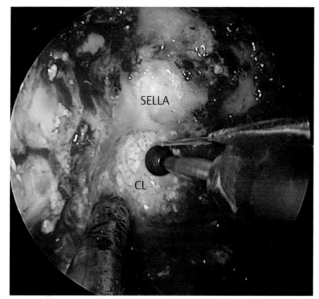

Fig. 11.165 Diseased and avascular bone of the mid-clivus. (CL, clivus.)

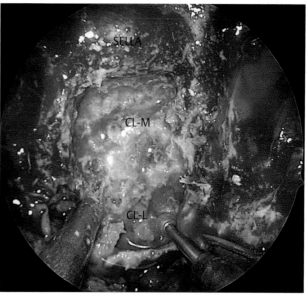

Fig. 11.166 Drilling of unhealthy bone over the mid-clivus (CL-M) and lower clivus (CL-L).

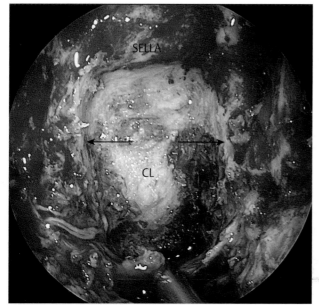

Fig. 11.167 Complete disease clearance from the mid-clivus (CL-M) and lower clivus (CL-L). Bilateral paraclival carotid arteries are marked (*black arrows*).

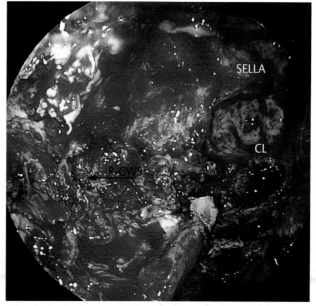

Fig. 11.168 Osteonecrosis of the right greater wing of sphenoid (R-GWS). (CL, clivus.)

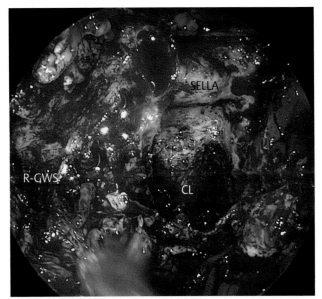

Fig. 11.169 Complete clearance of the right greater wing of the sphenoid (R-GWS). (CL, clivus.)

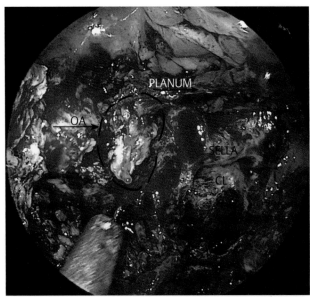

Fig. 11.170 Necrosis of tissues at the level of the orbital apex (OA) on the right side (*broken square*). (CL, clivus.)

Step 4: Clearance of the Right Superior Orbital Fissure

The planum was defined and drilled, and was followed toward the right lesser wing of the sphenoid. The area of the OA was defined, and the contents were found to be infected and sloughed (**Fig. 11.170**). The necrosed tissue was debrided with care (**Fig. 11.171**).

Step 5: Decompression and Clearance of the Right Cavernous Sinus

The authors describe this step as "decompression" of the cavernous sinus (aptly referred to as lateral sellar compartment) and not "radical removal" of disease. This is to avoid the risk of increasing the neural damage and thus improving the neuropathies.

The transpterygoid approach exposes the inferolateral portion of the cavernous sinus. To approach the cavernous sinus, the surgeon needs to define the SOF and the maxillary strut. The SOF is lateral to the cavernous sinus and the maxillary strut forms the inferior border of the medial aspect of the SOF. The maxillary strut is a constant bony landmark useful for indicating the SOF and the front door to the cavernous sinus.

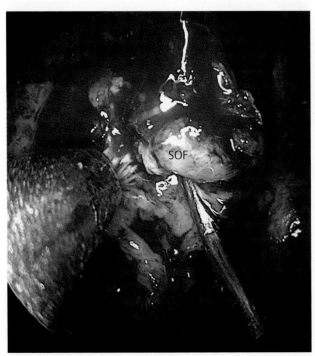

Fig. 11.171 Clearance of infected tissue from the right superior orbital fissure (SOF) using a ball probe.

The bone to be drilled to approach the cavernous sinus is a quadrilateral structure located between the opticocarotid recess and the paraclival carotid artery prominence medially and the OA and trigeminal nerve prominence laterally (**Fig. 11.172**).

The vidian canal is a useful landmark on the floor of the sphenoid sinus and it indicates the junction of the horizontal petrous and the vertical paraclival part of the ICA.

The diseased OA is depicted in **Fig. 11.173**.

Dural incision of the cavernous sinus depends on which segment of the sinus is affected. In this case, the anterolateral compartment was invaded by the disease. After confirming the position of the ICA using carotid doppler, the surgeon made an incision over the dura over the medial aspect just anterior to the cavernous sinus, thus decompressing the sinus (**Fig. 11.174**). The flow in the intracavernous part of the carotid was normal at the end of dissection.

Complete hemostasis was achieved, and the cavity was inspected for any residue (**Fig. 11.175** and **Video 11.10**).

Packing

Diluted amphotericin washes were given, and nasal cavity was packed with merocel 8 cm in both nostrils.

Postoperative Management

Postoperatively the patient was found to have mildly elevated serum creatinine levels, and the nephrologist's opinion was sought for the same. Amphotericin-B and posaconazole were withheld for 10 days and after the renal parameters were normalized, these were restarted on low dose. After the current surgery, the patient was administered a total of 3 g of amphotericin-B, strictly under renal monitoring. The patient tolerated the same well.

Postoperative scan showed complete disease clearance (**Fig. 11.176**).

Postoperative healing of the nasal cavity and right exenterated eye at 1 month after surgery is shown in **Figs. 11.177** and **11.178**, respectively.

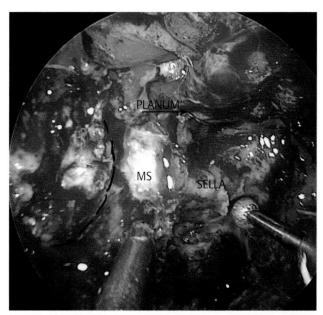

Fig. 11.172 Medial aspect of the superior orbital fissure (SOF) is marked in *broken curve*. (MS, maxillary strut.)

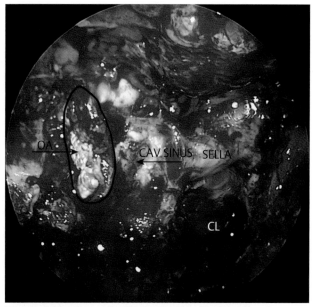

Fig. 11.173 Diseased orbital apex (OA; *black oval*) and cavernous sinus (CAV SINUS) are marked. (CL, clivus.)

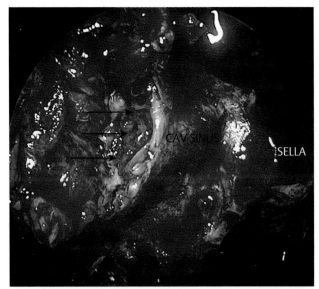

Fig. 11.174 Decompression of the right cavernous sinus (CAV SINUS; *black arrows*) with orbital apex clearance.

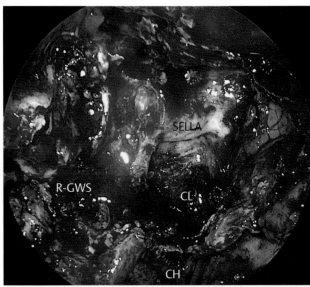

Fig. 11.175 Cavity after complete clearance. (CH, choana; CL, clivus; R-GWS, right greater wing of the sphenoids.)

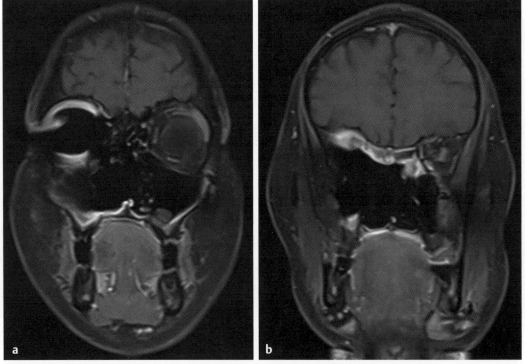

Fig. 11.176 (a, b) Postoperative magnetic resonance imaging (MRI) of the paranasal sinus (PNS) showing complete resolution of disease.

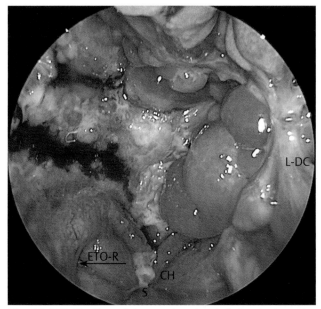

Fig. 11.177 Healing of the nasal cavity. Left Denker's cavity (L-DC), right eustachian orifice (ETO-R), choana (CH), and cut end of the posterior septum (S).

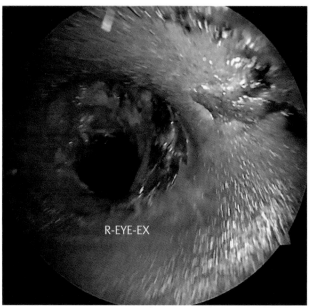

Fig. 11.178 Exenterated right socket.

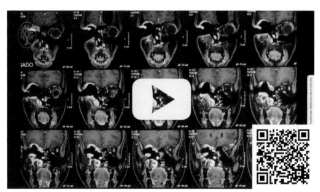

Video 11.10 A case of stage IIIB—case 2.

Stage IIIB (Case 3): Involvement of the Paramedian Posterior Compartment—Medial Petrous Apex

Case 11: This is a 36-year-old newly found diabetic patient (post-COVID-19), operated on in the authors' center previously. He had undergone left EMD procedure with bilateral full house FESS, trans-sellar-trans-clival clearance, and medial transpetrous approach for clearance of the petroclival window. The patient was lost to follow-up for 7 months. Currently he presented back to the authors with intractable headache for 20 days. The patient was apparently symptom free till then.

Nasal endoscopy showed a well-healed anterior face of the sphenoid. The posterior septectomy status is noted. Orbital examination revealed resolved right lateral rectus palsy. The palate was clinically not involved.

Evaluation at presentation included a detailed otorhinolaryngologic, ophthalmic, and neurological examinations to assess the extent of disease. The proinflammatory marker values were recorded every alternate day. Hematological values are mentioned in **Table 11.11**.

MRI of the PNS, orbit, and brain including T1W, T2W, T2WFS, T1WFS postcontrast, and DWI was taken to study the extent of disease and to plan the surgical approaches and excision.

The coronal T2W STIR images showed hyperintense signal with diffusion restriction in the clivus and sphenoid with areas of heterogenous enhancement with contrast suggestive of subacute osteomyelitis. Soft-tissue extension was noted involving the petrous and cavernous segments of the bilateral internal carotid arteries and trigeminal nerves. It was noted that the bilateral maxillary sinuses, orbit, and palate were uninvolved (**Fig. 11.179**).

Considering the impending clival dural breach, he was immediately taken up for total excision. The surgical plan was based on the MRI findings of the clivus with medial petrous apex involvement. A revision of the previously done transsellar, transclival, and a medial trans-sphenoidal approach to petrous apex was planned for aggressive debridement.

After orotracheal intubation, a CVP line was secured. The patient was placed in the reverse Trendelenburg position, and hypotensive anesthesia was administered. The nasal cavities were examined, and swabs were taken for gram stain and KOH mount. The vibrissae were trimmed, and povidone-iodine nasal antiseptic washes (0.5%) were given before the onset of surgery. The bilateral nasal cavities were decongested with adrenaline-soaked gauze pieces (1:1,000).

Surgical Steps

Step 1: Revision of the Trans-Sellar and Transclival Approach

The healed mucosa covering the anterior face of the sphenoid was coblated to identify the anatomical landmarks. The sellar bulge and the region of the clival dura along with the floor of the sphenoid sinus were identified (**Fig. 11.180**). The diseased mucosa covering the sella was coblated, and the anterior wall of the sella drilled (**Fig. 11.181**). Unhealthy granulation tissue covering the upper clivus was removed.

Step 2: Medial Petrous Apex Approach

A "four-handed technique" is mandatory for this approach as it involves manipulation of the ICA and there is a risk of vascular injury.

The three endonasal approaches to the medial petrous apex are (1) the medial trans-sphenoidal approach, (2) the medial approach with lateralization of the ICA, and (3) the transpterygoid infrapetrous approach.[8] A contralateral transmaxillary corridor is used for better visualization of the carotid to avoid injury.[9]

Here the surgeon utilized the medial trans-sphenoidal approach. The remnant of the floor of the sphenoid was found to be porous and diseased. The same was demarcated (**Fig. 11.182**). Using a curved elevator, the bony floor was elevated off the mucosa. The entire osteomyelitic chunk of the lower clivus and the medial petroclival complex on the right side were removed in one piece (**Fig. 11.183**).

The purulent secretion from the right medial petrous apex was drained and saline wash was given. Similarly using a curved curette, the lytic bone from the left medial petrous apex was also removed in a single piece (**Fig. 11.184**). The mid and lower clival dura was covered with unhealthy granulations. It was carefully curetted off with a curved blunt elevator. Complete dural clearance is depicted in **Fig. 11.185**.

Table 11.11 Hematological findings of the patient

	Total count (per µL)	CRP (mg/L)	D-dimer (ng/mL)	LDH (IU/L)	Ferritin (ng/mL)
Preoperative	7,500	200	2,500	300	310
Immediate postoperative	9,000	195	3,500	280	340
At discharge	5,000	50	400	175	100

Abbreviations: CRP, C-reactive protein; LDH, lactate dehydrogenase.

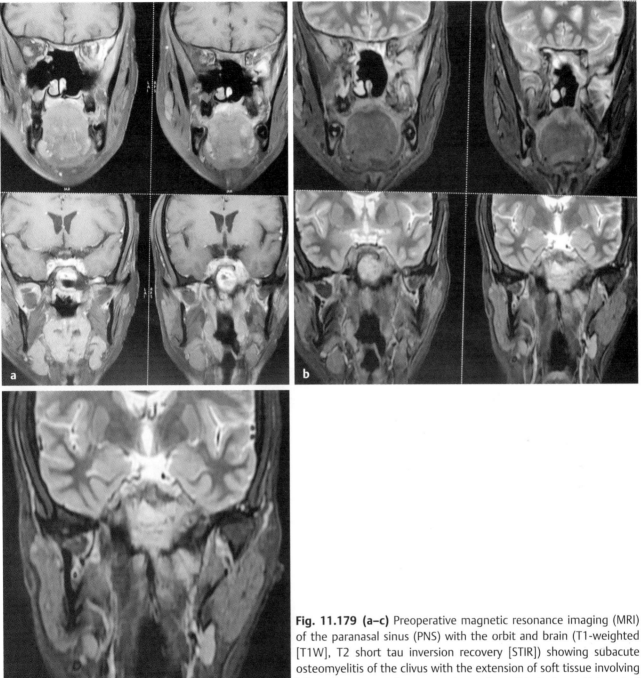

Fig. 11.179 (a–c) Preoperative magnetic resonance imaging (MRI) of the paranasal sinus (PNS) with the orbit and brain (T1-weighted [T1W], T2 short tau inversion recovery [STIR]) showing subacute osteomyelitis of the clivus with the extension of soft tissue involving bilateral petrous and cavernous internal carotid arteries and trigeminal nerves.

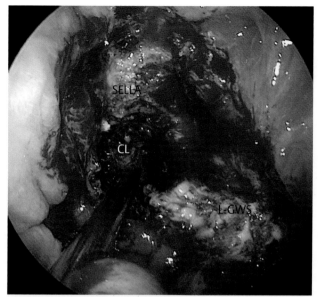

Fig. 11.180 Sellar bulge and clivus (CL) identified inside the sphenoid (L-GWS, left greater wing of the sphenoid).

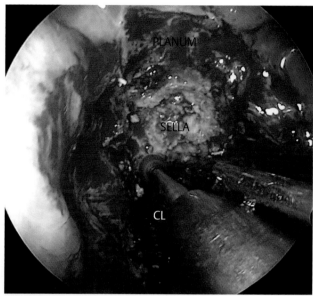

Fig. 11.181 Drilling of the anterior wall of the sella. The planum and clivus (CL) are marked.

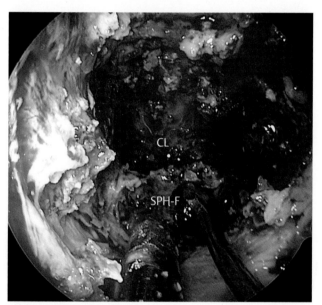

Fig. 11.182 Diseased floor of the sphenoid (SPH-F) being delineated. (CL, clivus.)

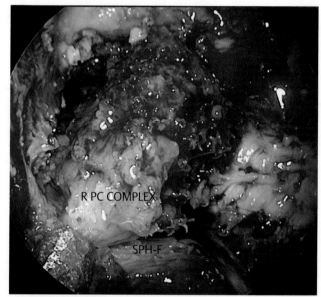

Fig. 11.183 Right petroclival complex (R PC COMPLEX) along with the lower clivus removed in one piece. (SPH-F, floor of the sphenoid.)

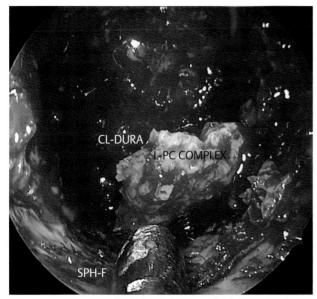

Fig. 11.184 Removal of the left petroclival complex (L PC COMPLEX). (CL-DURA, clival dura.)

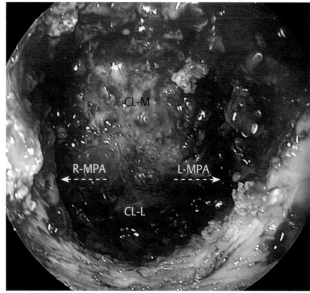

Fig. 11.185 Complete mid-clival and lower clival clearance. Mid-clival dura (CL-M), lower clival dura (CL-L), right medial petrous apex (R MPA), and left medial petrous apex (L MPA).

Step 3: Clearance of the Left Greater Wing of the Sphenoid

Keeping the paraclival carotid as a landmark, the infratemporal surface of the left greater wing was traced. The minimal disease in the region of the left GWS was drilled off completely (**Fig. 11.186** and **Video 11.11**).

Packing

Diluted amphotericin washes were given, and the nasal cavity was packed with merocel 8 cm in both nostrils.

Postoperative Management

Postoperatively the patient was started on intravenous amphotericin-B and oral posaconazole. He received a cumulative dose of 3.5 g as per the expert's advice from the nephrologist. He tolerated the treatment well.

Postoperative MRI of the PNS showed complete resolution of the disease (**Fig. 11.187**).

Postoperative nasal endoscopic picture is shown in **Fig. 11.188**.

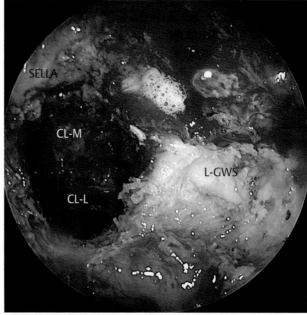

Fig. 11.186 Clearance of the left greater wing of the sphenoid (L-GWS). (CL-L, lower clival dura; CL-M, mid-clival dura.)

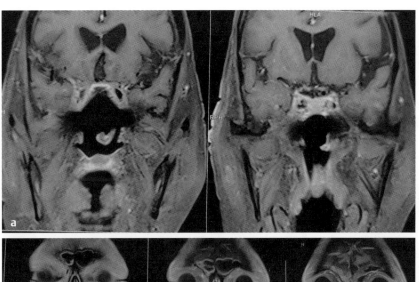

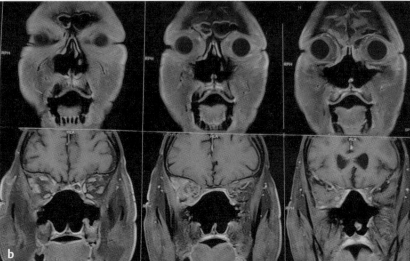

Fig. 11.187 (a, b) Postoperative magnetic resonance imaging (MRI) of the paranasal sinus (PNS) with the orbit and brain shows resolution of disease.

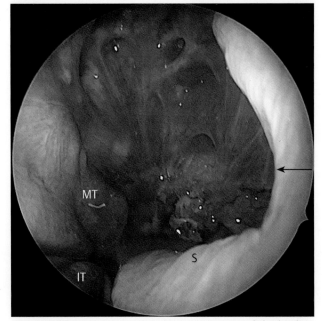

Fig. 11.188 Postoperative endoscopic picture of the healing nasal cavity. Posterior septectomy (*black arrow*). (IT, inferior turbinate; MT, middle turbinate; S, septum.)

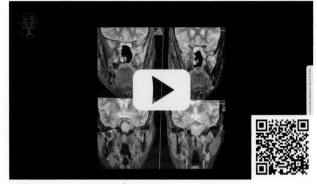

Video 11.11 A case of stage IIIB—case 3.

Stage IIIC: Involvement of the Lateral Posterior Compartment—V3, Greater Wing of the Sphenoid, Base of the Temporal Lobe, Lateral Orbital Wall, and Superior Orbital Wall

Case 12: A 66-year-old post-COVID-19 pneumonia patient who was a known case of type II diabetes mellitus with hypertensive coronary artery disease with the stent in situ presented 1 month after discharge with complaints of severe headache, paresthesia on the left side of the face, and restricted opening of the mouth. At the onset of complaints, 20 days back, the patient had undergone left side molar and premolar teeth extraction, which failed to heal and developed into an oroantral fistula. Following this, he underwent bilateral FESS elsewhere and a biopsy from the maxilla was positive for mucormycosis. He presented at the authors' center for further evaluation since he had no symptomatic relief.

Anterior rhinoscopy showed post-FESS status on the right side; the sphenoid ostium was visualized (**Fig. 11.189**). The left nasal cavity showed polypoidal changes in the middle meatus (**Fig. 11.190**). An oroantral fistula was noted on the left side. Orbital examination showed no abnormality.

Evaluation at presentation included a detailed otorhinolaryngologic, maxillofacial, ophthalmologic, and neurological examinations to assess the extent of disease. The proinflammatory marker values were recorded every alternate day. The hematological values are mentioned in **Table 11.12**.

CT-PNS showed erosion of the left hard palate, pterygoid wedge, GWS, and left temporal fossa region. The bilateral maxilla and left sphenoid showed soft-tissue density (**Fig. 11.191**).

MRI of the PNS, orbit, and brain including T1W, T2W, T2WFS, T1WFS postcontrast, and DWI was taken to study the extent of disease and to plan the surgical approaches and excision.

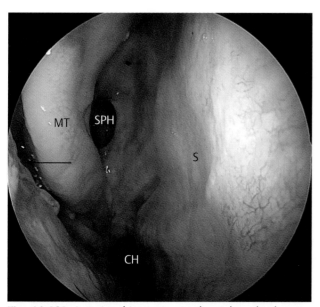

Fig. 11.189 Anterior rhinoscopy on the right side showing post-functional endoscopic sinus surgery (FESS) status. (CH, choana; MT, middle turbinate; S, septum; SPH, sphenoid sinus.)

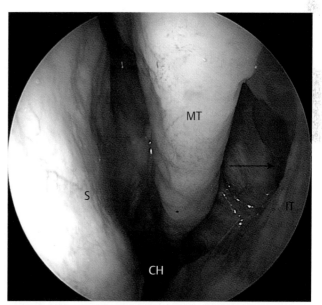

Fig. 11.190 Anterior rhinoscopy on the left side showing polypoidal changes in the middle meatus. (CH, choana; IT, inferior turbinate; MT, middle turbinate; S, septum.)

Table 11.12 Hematological findings of the patient

	Total count (per µL)	CRP (mg/L)	D-dimer (ng/mL)	LDH (IU/L)	Ferritin (ng/mL)
Preoperative	8,000	323	2,250	290	320
Immediate postoperative	10,500	320	3,500	345	300
At discharge	5,500	53	500	210	90

Abbreviations: CRP, C-reactive protein; LDH, lactate dehydrogenase.

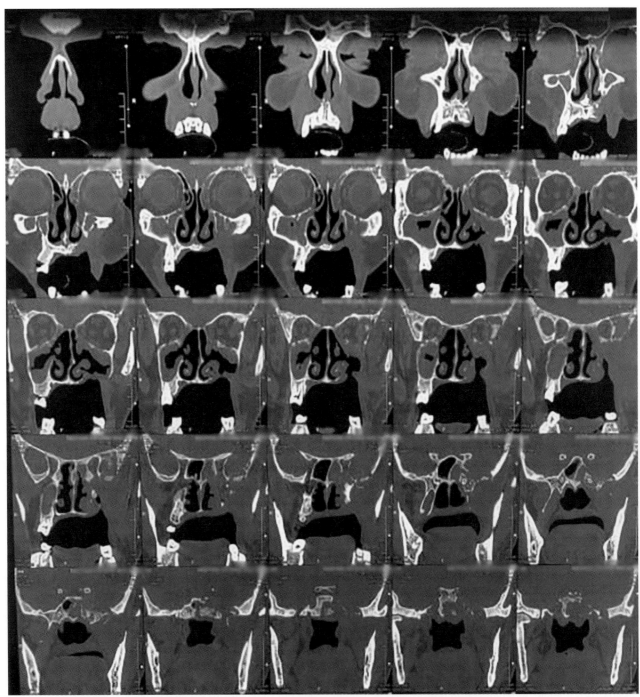

Fig. 11.191 Computed tomography of the paranasal sinus (CT-PNS) showing erosion of the left hard palate, pterygoid wedge, greater wing of the sphenoid, and left temporal fossa region. The bilateral maxilla and left sphenoid showing soft-tissue density.

The MR images showed T1 hypodense nonenhancing mucosal thickening in the left sphenoid sinus with osteonecrosis of the left pterygoid wedge and GWS suggestive of invasive fungal etiology. Also seen was erosion of the base of the left temporal bone with the extension of soft tissue into the left medial temporal lobe abutting Meckel's cave (**Fig. 11.192**). Soft-tissue inflammation of the left temporal fossa was also noted.

On further evaluation, 3D-CT facial bones showed bony erosions involving the left hard palate, floor of the sphenoid on the left side, medial pterygoid plate, lateral wall of the orbit, and temporal fossa region (**Fig. 11.193**).

After thorough preoperative cardiac and anesthetic workup, the patient was taken up for total excision. The surgical plan was based on the MRI findings of the sphenoid, palate, left GWS, and left temporal fossa involvement.

The temporal fossa cannot be approached endoscopically; hence, a combined transnasal, transpterygoid, transoral, and external incision via the bicoronal flap approach to the temporal fossa was planned for aggressive debridement.

After orotracheal intubation, the central venous line was secured. The patient was placed in the reverse Trendelenburg position, and hypotensive anesthesia was administered. The nasal cavities were examined, and swabs were taken for gram stain and KOH mount. Povidone-iodine nasal antiseptic washes (0.5%) were given before the onset of surgery. Bilateral nasal cavities were decongested with adrenaline-soaked gauze pieces (1:1,000).

Surgical Steps

Step 1: Left Endoscopic Modified Denker's Procedure

An EMD procedure (Sturman–Canfield approach) was done to inspect the left maxillary sinus. The maxillary sinus mucosa was edematous and yellowish, and it was denuded off and sent for pathological examination. All the walls of the maxilla appeared healthy except the posterior wall. It was covered with unhealthy granulation and fibrosis with neovascularization around the sequestered bone, a finding that has been consistent in all revision cases (at the authors' center), indicating underlying bony disease (**Fig. 11.194**). A full house FESS was done on the left side; the anterior face of the sphenoid was found to be necrotic.

Step 2: Wide Sphenoidotomy

A posterior septectomy and triple osteotomy were done. The anterior wall and rostrum of the sphenoid were removed. The left side of the sphenoid sinus was filled with fungal debris. The same was debrided and sent for pathological examination. Once the mucosa over the floor of the sphenoid

was removed, the left vidian canal was visualized and the vidian nerve was completely necrosed. The floor of the sphenoid and the left pterygoid wedge were grossly osteomyelitic (**Figs. 11.195–11.198**).

Step 3: Left Infratemporal Fossa Dissection

The bone of the medial aspect of the posterior wall of the left maxilla was removed, and gross fat stranding of the pterygopalatine and infratemporal contents was seen (**Fig. 11.199**). The same was coablated and removed. The internal maxillary artery was thrombosed and clipped. The medial pterygoid plate and the pterygoid wedge on the left appeared avascular and necrotic.

A comparison of the clinical picture on the left side with a radiological picture is depicted in **Figs. 11.200** and **11.201**. Using a curved instrument, the necrotic bone, which consisted of the pterygoid wedge, pterygoid plates, and the left GWS, was removed in one piece, and it was found to be disconnected from healthy bone (**Fig. 11.202**).

In advanced cases with late presentation, the infected skull base bone presents as sequestrum surrounded by inflammatory tissue granulations and it is found separate from the healthy bone.

Step 4: Left Infrapetrous Approach

The infrapetrous approach requires a lateral extension of the middle third transclival approach. In this approach, it is very important to define all the parts of the ICA. The vidian nerve can be followed posteriorly as a landmark for the laceral segment of the internal carotid artery.

After the necrotic pterygoid and GWS were removed, the undersurface of the base of the middle cranial fossa was found to be covered with unhealthy granulations. It was excised completely after mapping the paraclival and horizontal petrous ICA. In this case, since the vidian nerve was necrosed, the remnant of the same was considered a landmark for the laceral carotid. The part of V3 branch of the trigeminal nerve before it enters the ITF was defined, and dissection proceeded lateral to it, under the base of the middle cranial fossa dura (**Fig. 11.203**). The slough and debris were cleared and the abscess was identified. It was drained and the dura was found to be intact. Amphotericin and antibiotic washes were given.

Step 5: Transclival Drilling

The mid-clivus was covered with granulation tissue. Using a powered drill, the outer cortical bone which was found to be avascular was drilled to a thin layer. Bone covering the anterior face of the sella appeared unhealthy; hence, the same was drilled off until healthy sellar dura was seen (**Fig. 11.204**).

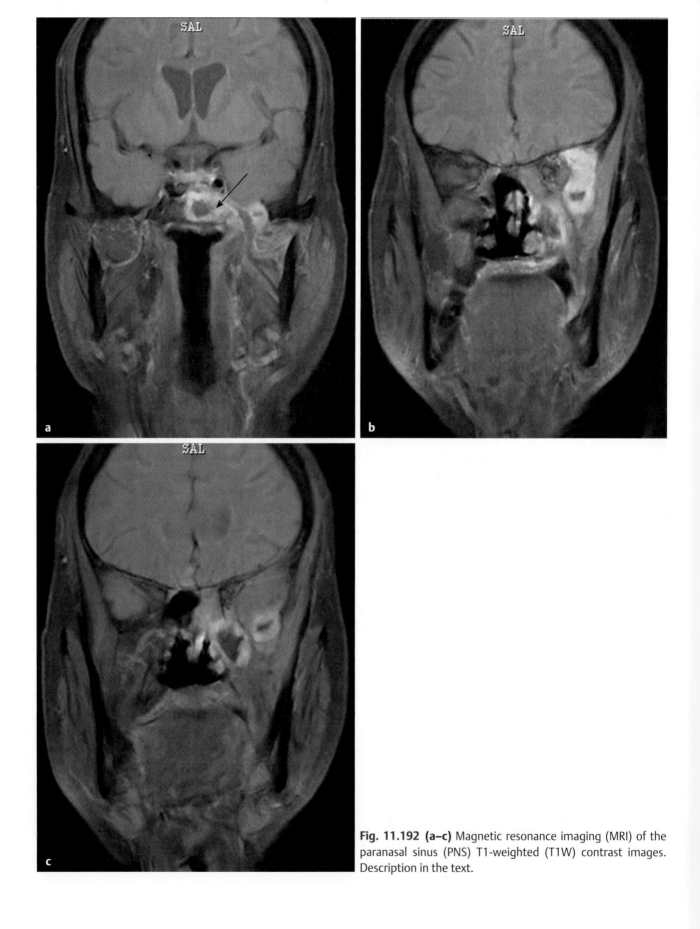

Fig. 11.192 (a–c) Magnetic resonance imaging (MRI) of the paranasal sinus (PNS) T1-weighted (T1W) contrast images. Description in the text.

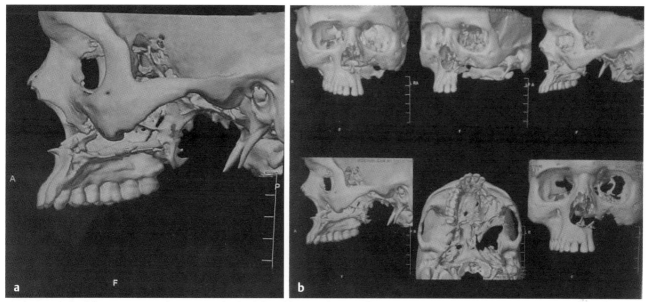

Fig. 11.193 (a, b) 3D computed tomography (CT) facial bones showing bony erosions involving the left hard palate, floor of the sphenoid on the left side, medial pterygoid plate, lateral wall of the orbit, and temporal fossa region.

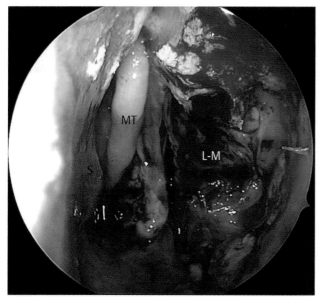

Fig. 11.194 Left endoscopic Denker's cavity. (L-M, left maxilla; MT, middle turbinate; S, septum.)

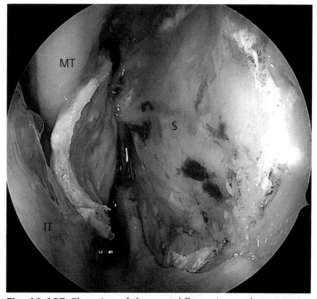

Fig. 11.195 Elevation of the septal flap prior to the posterior septectomy. (IT, inferior turbinate; MT, middle turbinate; S, septum.)

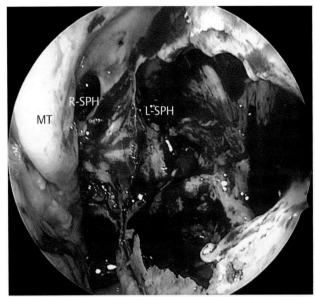

Fig. 11.196 "Owl's eye appearance." (L-SPH, left sphenoid; M, middle turbinate; R-SPH, right sphenoid.)

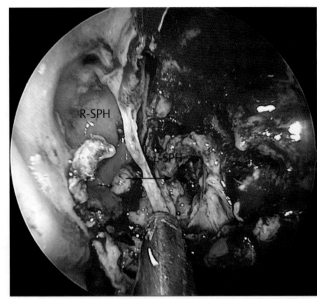

Fig. 11.197 Diseased mucosa of the left sphenoid (*black arrow*). (L-SPH, left sphenoid; R-SPH, right sphenoid.)

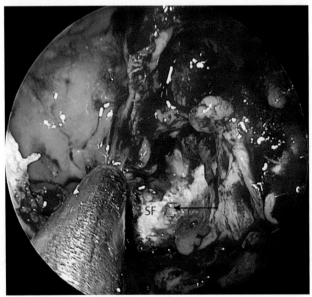

Fig. 11.198 Necrosed floor of the sphenoid (SF). The *black arrow* points to the vidian canal.

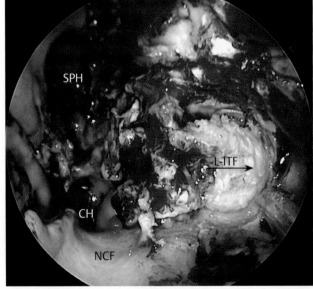

Fig. 11.199 Gross fat stranding of the contents of left infratemporal fossa (L-ITF). (CH, choana; NCF, floor of the nasal cavity; SPH, sphenoid sinus.)

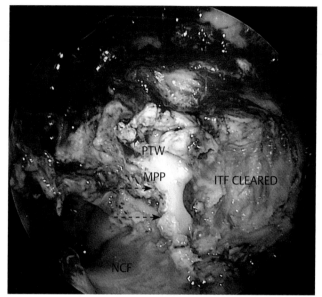

Fig. 11.200 Osteonecrosis of pterygoid wedge (PTW) and medial pterygoid plate (MPP). The left infratemporal fossa (ITF) is cleared. (NCF, floor of the nasal cavity.)

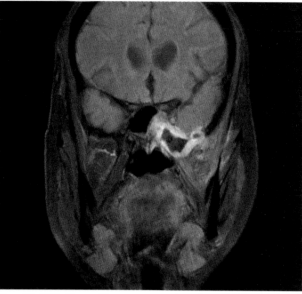

Fig. 11.201 Magnetic resonance imaging (MRI) paranasal sinus (PNS) T1-weighted (T1W) contrast, for comparison with **Fig. 11.200**, showing similar findings.

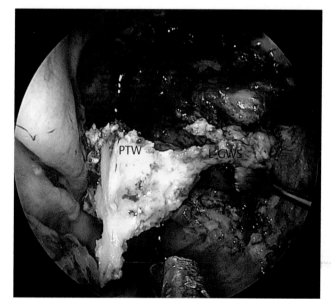

Fig. 11.202 Pterygoid wedge (PTW), pterygoid plates, and the left greater wing of the sphenoid (L-GWS) being removed in one single piece.

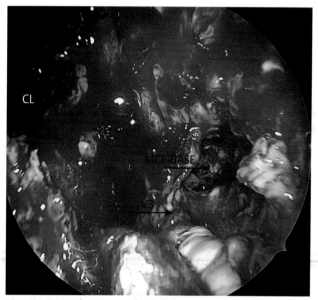

Fig. 11.203 Abscess in the left base of the middle cranial fossa (MCF-BASE) drained; the third branch of the trigeminal nerve (V3) is marked.

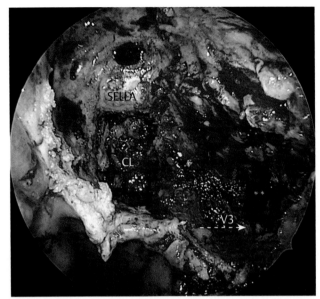

Fig. 11.204 Cavity after complete clearance. (CL, clivus; V3, third branch of trigeminal nerve; **, abscess cavity.)

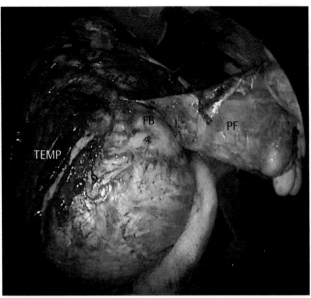

Fig. 11.205 Pericranial flap (PF) raised. (FB, frontal bone; TEMP, temporalis muscle.)

Step 6: Bicoronal Approach (Bi-Temporal Approach)

As per 3D-CT finding the left temporal fossa, lateral orbital wall and zygoma were eroded (refer to **Fig. 11.193a**). Anatomically, the temporal fossa is bounded by the temporal lines superiorly and terminates below the level of the zygomatic arch. This area cannot be approached endoscopically. Hence, as previously planned, a bi-coronal approach was commenced.

Preoperatively, the patient's head was shaved and washed thoroughly with antiseptic soap. A curvilinear incision was made through the skin, subcutaneous tissue, and galea aponeurotica extending from one superior temporal line to the other. Underneath the flap, the subgaleal plane of loose areolar tissue is seen. The flap is elevated below this plane. A preauricular extension of the incision is made up to the level of the helix of the pinna. Anteriorly the flap is elevated till a point 3 cm superior to the supraorbital rims bilaterally. This flap is based on the supratrochlear and supraorbital pedicles. Anteroinferiorly the flap is elevated till the zygomatic arch. The temporal branch of the facial nerve was preserved. Once the flap was reflected anteriorly, the supraorbital rim was palpated, and a straight incision was made over the pericranium medial to the vascular bundle. Laterally a similar but curvilinear incision was made lateral to the pedicle; both incisions were connected posteriorly and a subperiosteal dissection of the flap was done (**Fig. 11.205**).

The temporalis muscle was cut off from its anteroposterior attachment on the temporal line and reflected anteriorly to access the temporal fossa. The part of the temporalis muscle inside the deep temporal fossa was edematous and necrosed (**Fig. 11.206**).

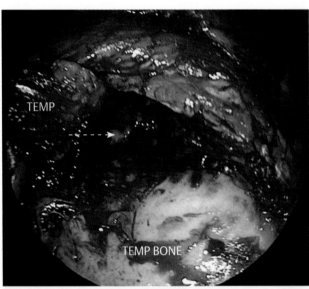

Fig. 11.206 Edematous and necrosed temporalis muscle in the temporal fossa (*broken white arrow*). (TEMP, temporalis muscle; TEMP BONE, temporal bone.)

The necrosed muscle was debrided, and the temporal fossa and lateral orbital wall were exposed. The bone was osteomyelitic. The same was drilled until the healthy counterpart was visualized (**Figs. 11.207** and **11.208**). The temporal fossa was communicated with the ITF as seen endoscopically (**Fig. 11.209**).

The temporalis muscle was cut and reflected anteriorly to fill the temporal fossa defect along with the pericranial flap (**Figs. 11.210** and **11.211** and **Video 11.12**).

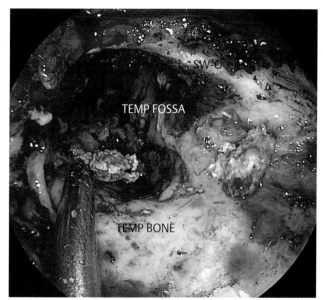

Fig. 11.207 Osteomyelitic bone within the temporal fossa; part of the lateral orbital wall. (TEMP BONE, temporal bone; TEMP FOSSA, temporal fossa.)

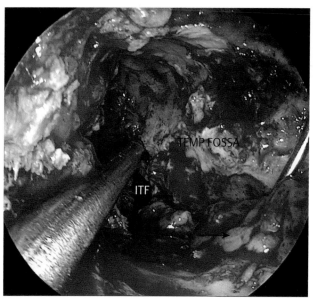

Fig. 11.208 Necrosed contents of the temporal fossa being removed using curved curette. (ITF, infratemporal fossa; TEMP FOSSA, temporal fossa.)

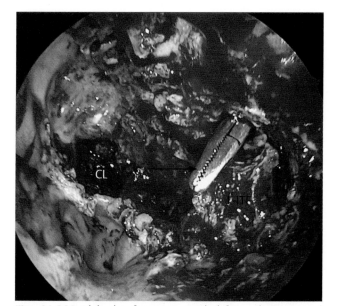

Fig. 11.209 Blakesley forceps tunneled from the temporal fossa to the infratemporal fossa (L-ITF). (CL, clivus.)

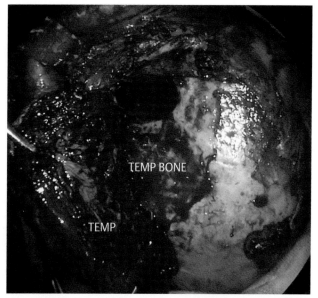

Fig. 11.210 Temporalis muscle cut to reflect anteriorly to cover the temporal fossa. (TEMP, temporalis muscle; TEMP BONE, temporal bone.)

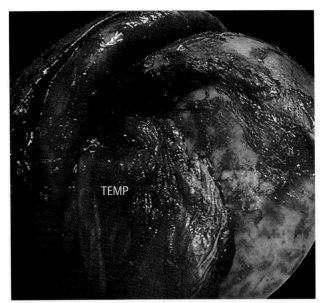

Fig. 11.211 Rotation of the temporalis muscle (TEMP) into the temporal fossa (*black arrow*) to fill the bony defect.

Packing

Diluted amphotericin washes were given, and nasal cavity was packed with merocel 8 cm in both nostrils.

Postoperative Management

Postoperatively the patient was treated with a cumulative dose of 4.0 g of liposomal amphotericin-B along with oral posaconazole for 8 weeks.

Postoperative scan showed complete disease clearance with inflammatory edema of the temporalis muscle (**Fig. 11.212**).

Healing of the nasal cavity at the 2-month postoperative period is depicted in **Fig. 11.213**.

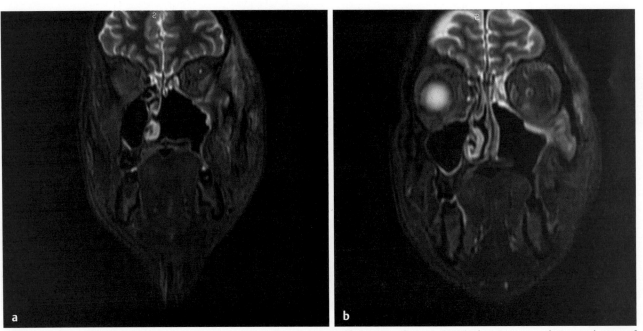

Fig. 11.212 (a, b) Postoperative magnetic resonance imaging (MRI) paranasal sinus (PNS) showing complete resolution of disease.

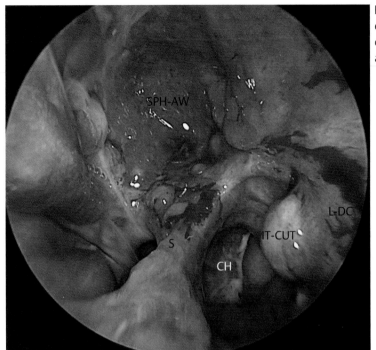

Fig. 11.213 Postoperative healing of nasal cavity. Left endoscopic Denker's cavity (L-DC) healed. (IT-CUT, cut end of the inferior turbinate; S, septum; SPH-AW, anterior wall of the sphenoid.)

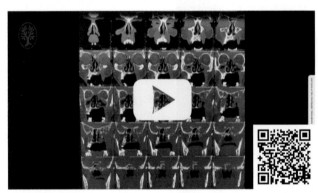

Video 11.12 A case of stage IIIC.

Stage IVA: Involvement of the Frontal Bone without Abscess

Case 13: A 36-year-old patient with no known comorbidities developed left-sided headache with periorbital swelling 3 weeks after treatment for COVID-19 infection. The patient had undergone left middle meatal antrostomy and tissue sampling. Histopathology was positive for fungus.

He was referred to our center for further management. Nasal endoscopy showed the left middle meatus filled with purulent discharge and synechiae between the septum and the left inferior turbinate (**Fig. 11.214**). Orbital examination revealed normal vision and extraocular movements. The palate was clinically normal.

Evaluation at presentation included a detailed otorhinolaryngologic, ophthalmologic, and maxillofacial examinations to assess the extent of disease. The proinflammatory marker values were recorded every alternate day. The hematological values are mentioned in **Table 11.13**.

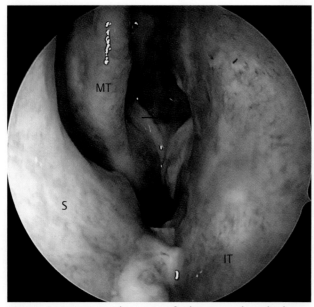

Fig. 11.214 Anterior rhinoscopy findings: purulent discharge in the left middle meatus (*black arrow*). Note the synechiae between the inferior turbinate (IT) and the septum (S). (MT, middle turbinate.)

MRI of the PNS, orbit, and brain including T1W, T2W, T2WFS, T1WFS post contrast, and DWI was taken to study the extent of disease and to plan the surgical approaches and excision.

The coronal postcontrast T2WFS images showed nonenhancing soft tissue in the bilateral maxillary and ethmoid sinuses, osteomyelitis of the superolateral wall of the left orbit with extradural T2 hyperintense fluid density inside the left frontal sinus (**Fig. 11.215**).

The patient was taken up for surgical debridement under general anesthesia. Left-sided EMD procedure with bilateral full house FESS, modified endoscopic Lothrop procedure, and external Lynch–Howarth procedure was planned. External approach was planned in addition to endoscopic procedure because supero-lateral wall of left orbit cannot be accessed by endoscopy alone.

After orotracheal intubation, a CVP line was secured. The patient was placed in the reverse Trendelenburg position, and hypotensive anesthesia was administered. The nasal cavities were examined, and swabs were taken for gram stain and KOH mount. Povidone-iodine nasal antiseptic washes (0.5%) were given before the onset of surgery. Bilateral nasal cavities were decongested with adrenaline-soaked gauze pieces (1:1,000).

Surgical Steps

Step 1: Left Endoscopic Modified Denker's Procedure
An EMD was performed (**Fig. 11.216**). The mucosa of the maxillary sinus grossly appeared normal. The same was removed and sent for HPE. Left middle turbinectomy with complete sphenoethmoidectomy was done. The ethmoid and sphenoid sinuses were uninvolved.

Step 2: Endoscopic Modified Lothrop Procedure (Draf III)
As per the MRI findings, the left frontal sinus walls were grossly involved. Hence, an endoscopic modified Lothrop procedure was commenced as planned previously. This involved removal of the superior part of the nasal septum, inferior portion of the interfrontal septum, and the floor of the frontal sinus till the lamina laterally on either side (**Fig. 11.217**).

Table 11.13 Hematological findings of the patient

	Total count (per μL)	CRP (mg/L)	D-dimer (ng/mL)	LDH (IU/L)	Ferritin (ng/mL)
Preoperative	7,500	235	1,700	250	255
Immediate postoperative	10,000	225	2,200	250	300
At discharge	5,000	35	300	160	75

Abbreviations: CRP, C-reactive protein; LDH, lactate dehydrogenase.

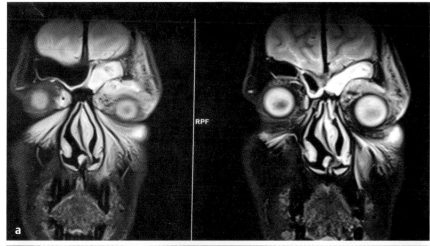
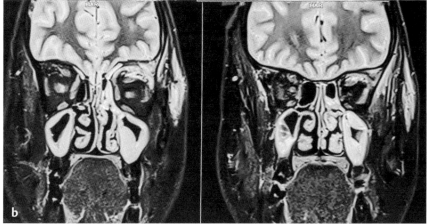

Fig. 11.215 (a, b) Magnetic resonance imaging (MRI) paranasal sinus (PNS) coronal image (T2 fat-suppressed [FS]) showing enhancing soft tissue in the bilateral maxillary and ethmoid sinuses, osteomyelitis of the superolateral wall of the left orbit with extradural T2-hyperintense fluid density inside the left frontal sinus.

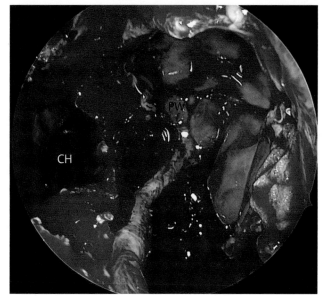

Fig. 11.216 Left Denker's cavity; normal maxillary mucosa. (CH, choana; PW, posterior wall of the maxilla.)

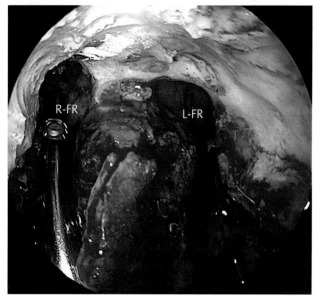

Fig. 11.217 Completed Draf III procedure; bilateral frontal recess widened. (L-FR, left frontal recess; R-FR, right frontal recess.)

Upon exteriorizing the left frontal, it was found to be filled with fungal debris, which was extending laterally beyond the scope of an endoscopic approach (**Fig. 11.218**). Hence, the surgeon proceeded with an external Lynch–Howarth procedure as previously planned.

Step 3: Lynch–Howarth Procedure—Left Side

Incision was made at the inferior margin of the medial aspect of the eyebrow and was extended down toward the medial canthus. It was carried up to the level of the periosteum. The angular vessels were cauterized, and the supratrochlear and supraorbital bundles were preserved. The orbicularis oculi muscle was incised and the mucoperiosteum was elevated to visualize the anterior table of the frontal sinus and the same was drilled (**Fig. 11.219**). The mucosa inside the sinus was diseased, and the same was denuded and sent for pathological examination (**Fig. 11.220**). The lateral-most aspect of the posterior table was seen to be necrotic after removal of the mucosa (**Fig. 11.221**).

Step 4: Removal of the Superolateral Wall of the Orbit

The superior wall (roof) of the left orbit was thinned out due to disease and was removed. Following this, the orbit was pushed inferomedially. The lateral wall of the orbit was exposed and was seen to be completely osteomyelitic (**Fig. 11.222**). The mucosa covering the lateral orbital wall was elevated by sharp dissection and the involved part of the bone was removed using a mallet and a gouge (**Fig. 11.223**). The bone close to the frontal dura was removed using diamond drill (**Fig. 11.224**). The entire necrotic bone was drilled off. Laterally the temporalis muscle was exposed after clearance (**Fig. 11.225**).

Minimal disease was left behind posterior to the temporalis muscle, which was also drilled and removed (**Figs. 11.226** and **11.227**). Cavity after complete clearance is depicted in **Fig. 11.228**. Amphotericin wash was given in the cavity and wound was sutured primarily (**Video 11.13**).

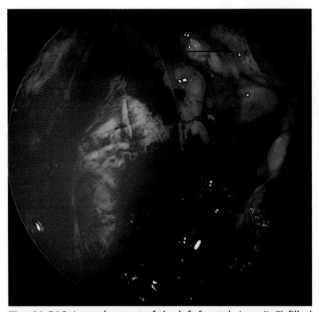

Fig. 11.218 Lateral aspect of the left frontal sinus (L-F) filled with fungal debris (*black arrow*).

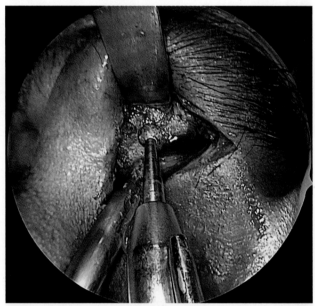

Fig. 11.219 Incision for the Lynch–Howarth procedure.

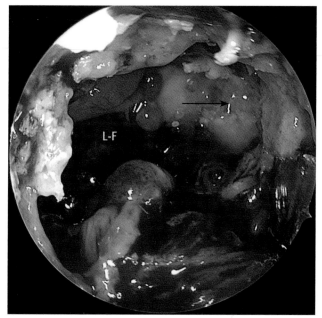

Fig. 11.220 Diseased frontal (L-F) sinus mucosa (*black arrow*).

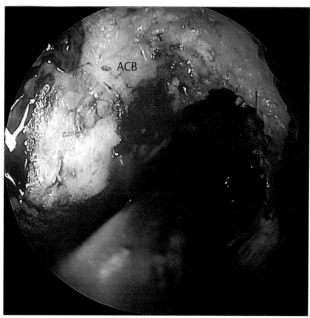

Fig. 11.221 Lateral part of the posterior and anterior table of frontal sinus osteomyelitic (*black arrow*). (ACB, anterior cranial base.)

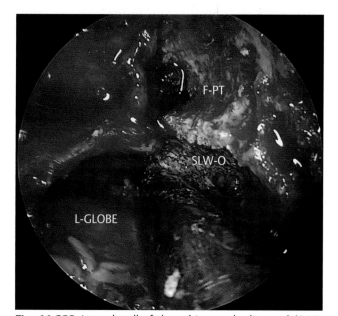

Fig. 11.222 Lateral wall of the orbit grossly diseased (F-PT, posterior table of frontal sinus; L-GLOBE, left globe; SLW-O, superolateral wall of the orbit).

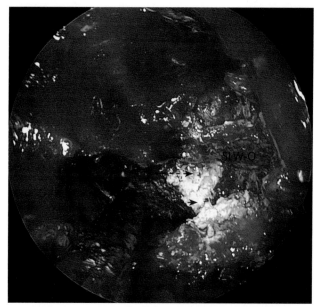

Fig. 11.223 Lateral wall of the orbit being removed with a mallet and a gouge. Note the avascular infected bone (*broken black arrows*). (SLW-O, superolateral wall of the orbit.)

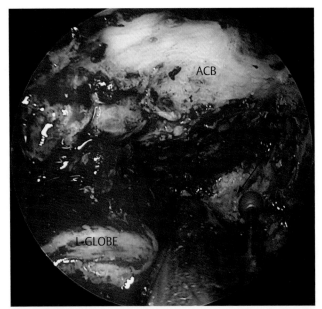

Fig. 11.224 Inferior aspect of the posterior table of the frontal sinus drilled with a diamond burr. (ACB, anterior cranial base; L-GLOBE, left globe.)

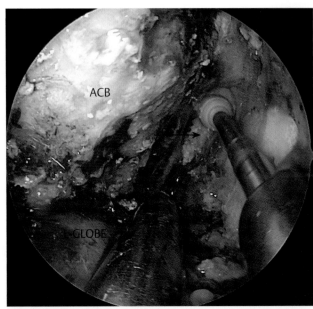

Fig. 11.225 Lateral-most corner of the posterior table of the frontal sinus being cleared (*black arrow*). (ACB, anterior cranial base; L-GLOBE, left globe.)

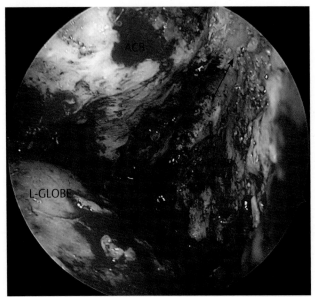

Fig. 11.226 Minimal disease left behind the posterior to temporalis muscle (*black arrow*). (ACB, anterior cranial base; L-GLOBE, left globe; TEMP, temporalis muscle.)

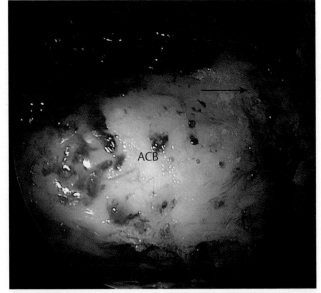

Fig. 11.227 Drilled posterolateral aspect of the posterior table of the frontal sinus (*black arrow*). (ACB, anterior cranial base.)

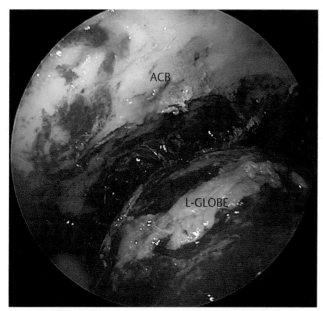

Fig. 11.228 Cavity after complete clearance. (ACB, anterior cranial base; L-GLOBE, left globe.)

Packing

Nasal cavity was packed with merocel 8 cm in both nostrils.

Postoperative Management

Postoperatively the patient's periorbital swelling improved. He was treated with a cumulative dose of 4.0 g of liposomal amphotericin-B along with posaconazole.

Surveillance

Postoperative scan taken 1 month later showed complete disease clearance (**Fig. 11.229**).

Postoperative healing of the nasal cavity is depicted in **Fig. 11.230**.

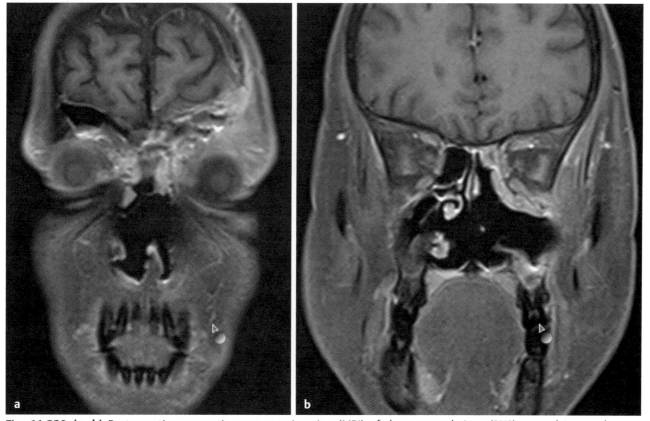

Fig. 11.229 (a, b) Postoperative magnetic resonance imaging (MRI) of the paranasal sinus (PNS) coronal image showing complete clearance.

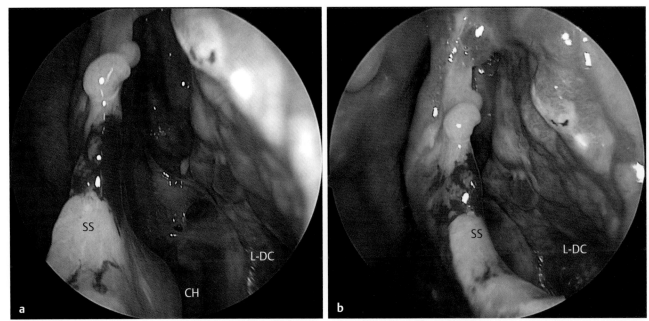

Fig. 11.230 (a, b) Postoperative healing of the nasal cavity. (CH, choana; L-DC, healed left Denker's cavity; SS, superior septectomy edges.)

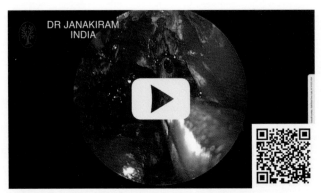

Video 11.13 A case of stage IVA.

Stage IVB (Case 1): Involvement of the Frontal Bone with Abscess

Case 14: A 62-year-old diabetic post-COVID-19 patient developed right-sided yellowish nasal discharge with right-sided severe headache, facial pain, blurring of vision, epiphora, and loosening of teeth on the right upper alveolus 1 month after treatment for COVID-19 infection. The patient was a known case of systemic hypertension. The patient had undergone bilateral endoscopic full house FESS and histopathology was negative for fungus.

Nasal endoscopy showed bilateral wide middle meatus antrostomy and ethmoidal cavity with purulent discharge. Orbital examination revealed right minimal proptosis with inferior displacement of the globe with intact vision and extraocular movements. Palatal discoloration was noted on the right side with numbness in the right malar region.

Evaluation at presentation included a detailed otorhinolaryngologic, ophthalmic, and maxillofacial examinations to assess the extent of disease. The proinflammatory marker values were recorded every alternate day. The hematological values are mentioned in **Table 11.14**.

CT-PNS showed mucosal thickening of the bilateral maxilla and ethmoids, and erosion of the right superior and lateral orbital walls with right palatal erosion.

MRI of the PNS, orbit, and brain including T1W, T2W, T2WFS, T1WFS postcontrast, and DWI was taken to study the extent of disease and to plan the surgical approaches and excision.

The coronal postcontrast T1 images showed nonenhancing soft tissue in bilateral maxillary and ethmoid sinuses, and osteomyelitis of the superolateral wall of the right orbit with extradural abscess (**Fig. 11.231**). The right palate showed features of osteomyelitis.

Cone beam computed tomography (CBCT) scan was taken with field of view of 10 × 10 and reconstructions were made in axial, coronal, and sagittal planes. It revealed an extensive mixed-density lesion involving the entire alveolar process of the right maxilla with a moth-eaten appearance. In addition, a bilateral breach of the maxillary sinus and the floor of the nasal cavity by the lesion with soft-tissue intensity of

both sinuses suggestive of mucosal thickening and resultant blocked ostium was found.

Considering the patient had frontal extradural abscess, he was immediately taken up for surgical debridement and abscess drainage. A bilateral EMD procedure with bilateral full house FESS, right orbital transposition, modified endoscopic Lothrop procedure, and external Lynch–Howarth procedure was planned.

After orotracheal intubation, a CVP line was secured. The patient was placed in the reverse Trendelenburg position and hypotensive anesthesia was administered. The nasal cavities were examined, and swabs were taken for gram stain and KOH mount. Povidone-iodine nasal antiseptic washes (0.5%) were given before the onset of surgery. Bilateral nasal cavities were decongested with adrenaline-soaked gauze pieces (1:1,000).

Surgical Steps

Step 1: Right Endoscopic Modified Denker's Procedure with Palatal Clearance

An EMD was performed on the right side (**Fig. 11.232**). The NLD was uncapped (**Fig. 11.233**). The necrotic mucosa of the maxillary sinus was removed and sent for HPE. The alveolar surface of the maxilla was found to be osteomyelitic, and it was drilled endoscopically till fresh bleeding margins were noted (**Figs. 11.234** and **11.235**). Right middle turbinectomy with complete sphenoethmoidectomy was done. The ethmoid sinus was found to be filled with fungal debris and sloughed mucosa with intact lamina papyracea.

Step 2: Right Orbital Decompression

The thinned lamina papyracea on the right side was delineated and removed to expose the involved periorbita (**Fig. 11.236**).

Step 3: Right Pterygoplaltine Fossa Dissection with Drilling of the Pterygoid Wedge

The right posterior wall of the maxilla was removed, the internal maxillary artery was double clipped, and the PPF contents were coblated and excised for histopathology (**Fig. 11.237**). The yellowish avascular pterygoid wedge was drilled and the necrosed vidian nerve was cut (**Fig. 11.238**).

Table 11.14 Hematological findings of the patient

	Total count (per μL)	CRP (mg/L)	D-dimer (ng/mL)	LDH (IU/L)	Ferritin (ng/mL)
Preoperative	6,000	200	1,500	240	285
Immediate postoperative	8,000	215	2,500	300	328
At discharge	7,000	50	350	180	85

Abbreviations: CRP, C-reactive protein; LDH, lactate dehydrogenase.

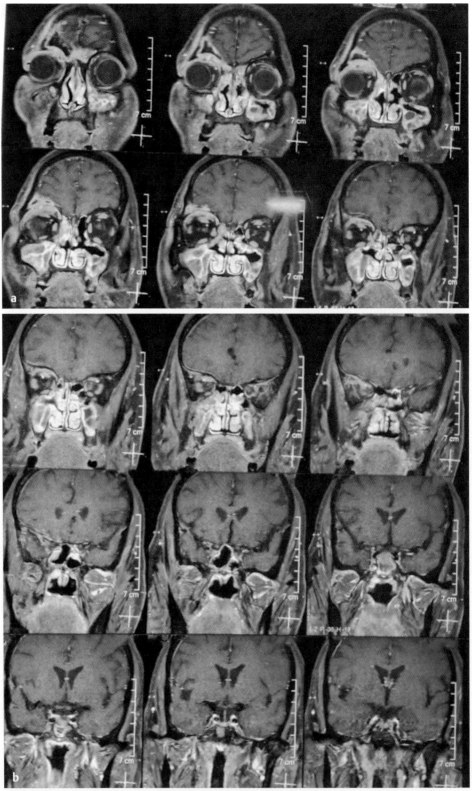

Fig. 11.231 (a, b) Magnetic resonance imaging (MRI) of the paranasal sinus (PNS) T1-weighted (T1W) contrast coronal images showing nonenhancing soft tissue in bilateral maxillary and ethmoid sinuses, osteomyelitis of the superolateral wall of the right orbit with extradural abscess. The right palate shows features of osteomyelitis.

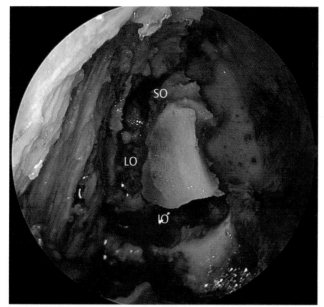

Fig. 11.232 Osteotomies for endoscopic Denker's procedure. (IO, inferior osteotomy; LO, lateral osteotomy; SO, superior osteotomy.)

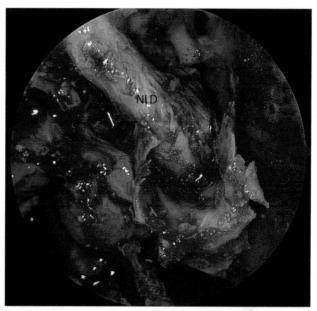

Fig. 11.233 Uncapping of the nasolacrimal duct (NLD).

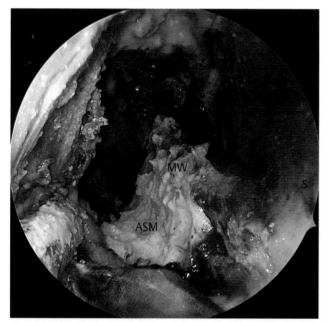

Fig. 11.234 Necrotic alveolar surface of the maxilla (ASM), medial wall of the maxilla (MW), and septum (S).

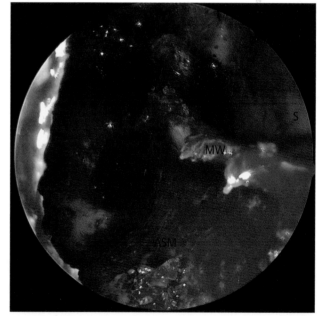

Fig. 11.235 Complete disease clearance from the alveolar surface of the maxilla (ASM), medial wall of the maxilla (MW), and septum (S) are marked.

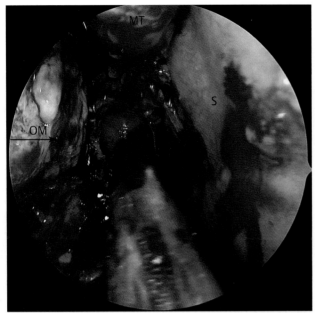

Fig. 11.236 Involved right medial wall of the orbit (OM; *black arrow*). (MT, middle turbinate; S, septum.)

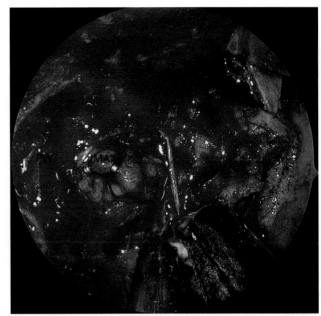

Fig. 11.237 Double clipping of the right internal maxillary artery (IMAX) and the posterior wall (PW) are marked.

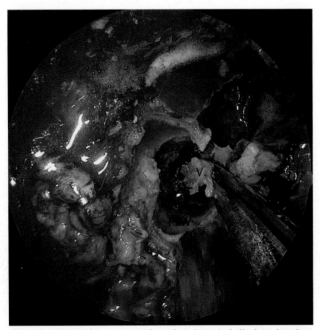

Fig. 11.238 Right pterygoid wedge (PTW) drilled and Vidian nerve (V) resected.

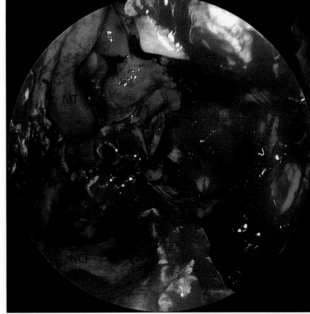

Fig. 11.239 Left post-Denker's cavity. (MT, middle turbinate; NCF, floor of nasal cavity; PW, posterior wall.)

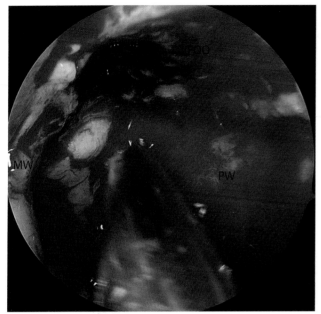

Fig. 11.240 Left floor of the orbit (FOO) found to be diseased. Medial wall (MW) and posterior wall (PW) of the maxilla.

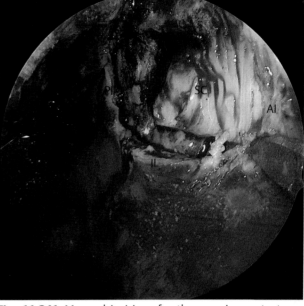

Fig. 11.241 Mucosal incisions for the superior septectomy for doing Draf III procedure. Anterior incision (AI), inferior incision (II), and posterior incision (PI) on the superior septal mucosa. (SC, septal cartilage.)

Step 4: Left EMD with Clearance of the Left Orbital Floor

An EMD procedure was performed to access the left maxilla (**Fig. 11.239**). The mucosa of the maxillary sinus was stripped off, and the left orbital floor was found to be diseased in its medial-most part (**Fig. 11.240**). The involved part of the orbital floor was removed; The periorbita was found to be free of disease. Following this, a complete sphenoethmoidectomy was done on the left side; the left ethmoid sinus was uninvolved.

Step 5: Endoscopic Modified Lothrop Procedure

Purulent secretion was seen coming from the right frontal sinus opening. To address the gross involvement of the frontal sinus, as planned before, an endoscopic modified Lothrop procedure was commenced. This involves removal of the superior part of the nasal septum, inferior portion of the interfrontal septum, and the floor of the frontal sinus till the lamina laterally. It creates a common median drainage pathway. The steps of the Draf III procedure are depicted in **Figs. 11.241** to **11.244**.

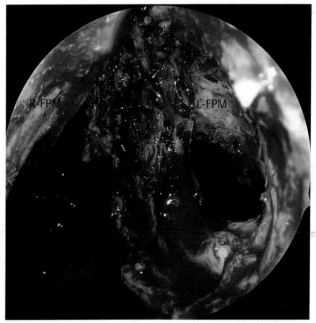

Fig. 11.242 Superior septectomy completed. (L-FPM, left frontal process of maxilla; R-FPM, right frontal process of maxilla.)

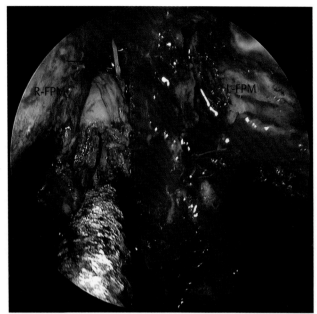

Fig. 11.243 Septal branch of the anterior ethmoid artery on the right side (*black arrow*). (L-FPM, left frontal process of the maxilla; R-FPM, right frontal process of the maxilla.)

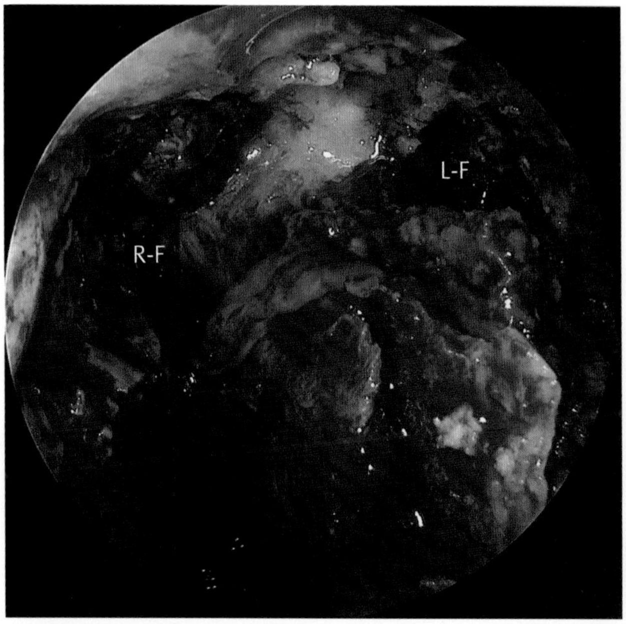

Fig. 11.244 Completed Draf III procedure. (L-F, left frontal recess; R-F, right frontal recess.)

Step 6: Right Orbital Transposition

The access to the medial half of the right superior orbital wall was achieved with coblation of the anterior ethmoidal artery entering from the orbit to the nasal cavity. The orbit was laterally transposed (**Figs. 11.245** and **11.246**). The periorbita of the right medial orbital wall was found to be necrosed (refer to **Fig. 11.235**). It was excised along with minimal orbital fat parallel to the medial rectus muscle (**Fig. 11.247**). The superior wall of the orbit was exposed by elevating the periosteum laterally. Extensive osteomyelitis of the superior wall of the orbit along the whole length was noted (**Fig. 11.248**). Thus, an external approach to excise the anterolateral part of the anterior cranial base was planned.

Step 7: Lynch–Howarth Procedure: Right Side

Incision was made at the inferior margin of the medial aspect of the eyebrow and was extended down toward the medial canthus. It was carried up to the level of the periosteum. The angular vessels were cauterized, and the supratrochlear and supraorbital bundles were preserved. The orbicularis oculi muscle was incised and the mucoperiosteum was elevated to visualize the anterior table of the frontal sinus. The anterior cranial base was found to be necrotic (posterior table of the frontal sinus and the superolateral wall of the orbit). Extradural abscess was let out from the undersurface of the superolateral wall of the orbit (**Figs. 11.249** and **11.250**). The same was sent for culture and sensitivity test.

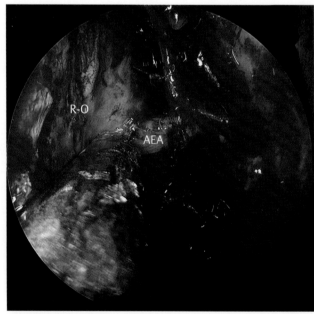

Fig. 11.245 Coblation of the anterior ethmoidal artery (AEA). (R-O, right orbit.)

The indocyanine green (ICG) dye was injected intravenously by the anesthetist at this point of time to see the viability of bone using Karl Storz IMAGE1 S Rubina camera. The Karl Storz IMAGE1 S Rubina endoscopic ICG fluorescence system uses near-infrared light and indocyanine

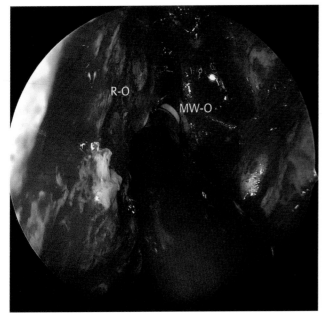

Fig. 11.246 Right orbital transposition. (MW-O, medial wall of orbit; R-O, right orbit.)

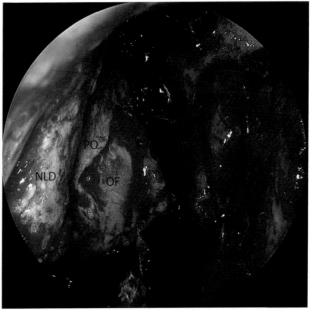

Fig. 11.247 Diseased periorbita of the right medial orbital wall removed. (NLD, nasolacrimal duct; OF, orbital fat; PO, periorbita.)

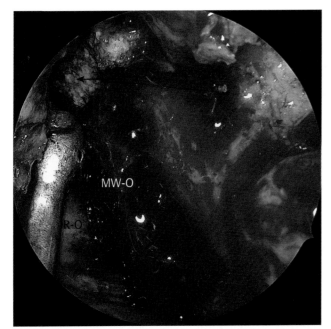

Fig. 11.248 Osteomyelitis of the superior wall of the orbit (*black arrow*). (MW-O, medial wall of orbit; R-O, right orbit.)

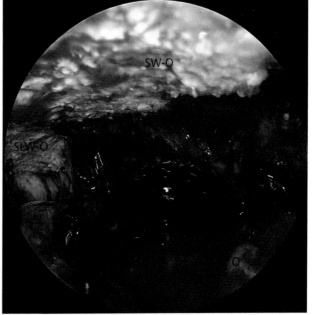

Fig. 11.249 Exposure after Lynch–Howarth procedure. Note the necrosed superior orbital wall (SW-O) and the superolateral wall (SLW-O).

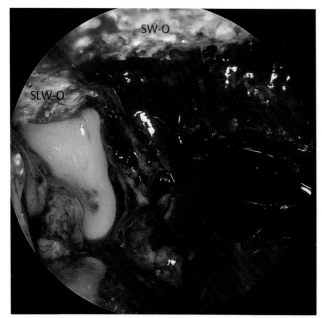

Fig. 11.250 Purulent abscess from the undersurface of the superolateral orbital wall (SLW-O). (SW-O, superior orbital wall.)

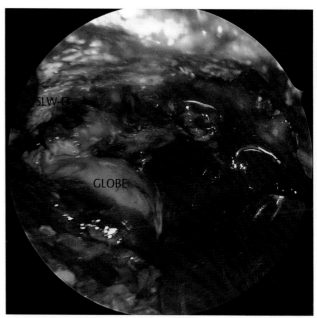

Fig. 11.251 Injection of indocyanine green (ICG). Note the *green dye* in the surgical field (SLW-O, superolateral orbital wall).

green dye (NIR/ICG) for fluorescence-guided imaging and is equipped with 4K resolution. It helps the surgeon to clearly distinguish between perfused and nonperfused areas, which is extremely helpful in terms of clearance of the osteomyelitic bone. The monochromatic mode is used for the same where the NIR/ICG signal is presented in white on a black background, thus providing clear demarcation (**Figs. 11.251** and **11.252**).

The necrotic bone was drilled completely under vision until healthy frontal dura was seen (**Figs. 11.253** and **11.254**).

The right upper alveolar teeth with necrotic hard palate were removed by the maxillofacial surgeon and the palatal mucosa was sutured primarily (**Video 11.14**).

Packing

Diluted amphotericin washes were given, and nasal cavity was packed with merocel 8 cm in both nostrils.

Postoperatively the patient's vision and proptosis improved.

Surveillance

The patient improved symptomatically on follow-up; no evidence of disease was seen on residual scan (**Fig. 11.255**). A

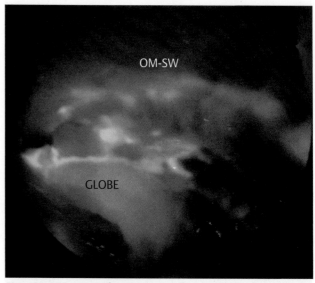

Fig. 11.252 Monochromatic mode showing clear demarcation of diseased areas in *black* on a white background. (OM-SW, superior orbital wall osteomyelitis.)

cumulative dose of 4.0 g of amphotericin with total 10 weeks of oral posaconazole was given for the patient.

Postoperative healing of bilateral nasal cavities is depicted in **Figs. 11.256** and **11.257**.

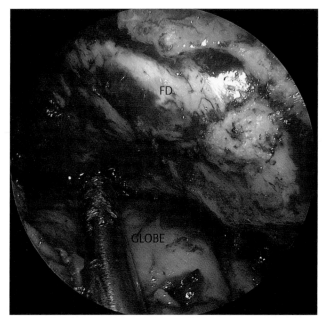

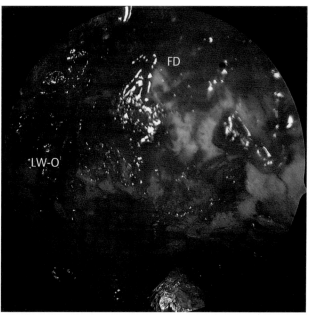

Fig. 11.253 Complete clearance of the posterior table of the frontal sinus. (FD, frontal dura.)

Fig. 11.254 Clearance of the lateral wall of the orbit (LW-O). (FD, frontal dura.)

Fig. 11.255 Postoperative scan showing resolution of the disease.

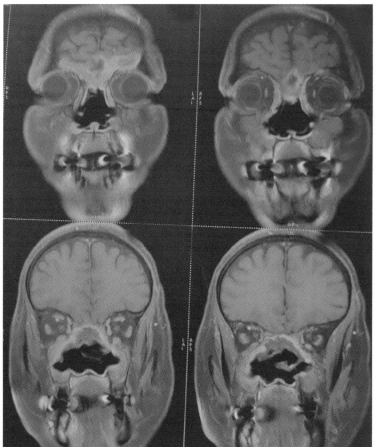

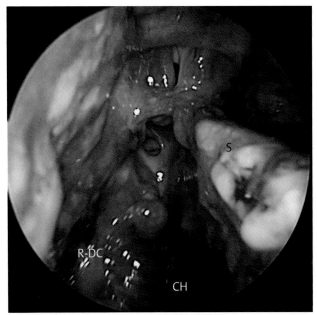 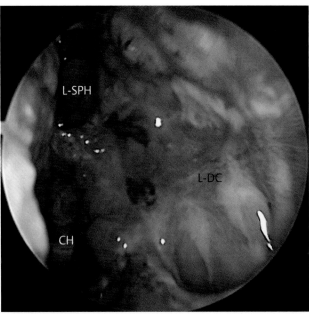

Fig. 11.256 Healing of the right nasal cavity. Right endoscopic Denker's cavity (R-DC) healed. (CH, choana; S, superior septectomy edge.)

Fig. 11.257 Healing of the left nasal cavity. Left endoscopic Denker's cavity (L-DC) healed. (CH, choana; L-SPH, left sphenoid sinus.)

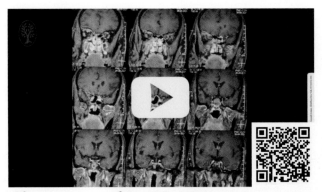

Video 11.14 A case of stage IVB—case 1.

Stage IVB (Case 2): Involvement of the Frontal Bone with Abscess

Case 15: A 59-year-old diabetic male patient was diagnosed with COVID-19 pneumonia and required treatment with systemic steroids and oxygen. One month after discharge, he developed headache and was diagnosed to have COVID-19-associated mucormycosis. The patient underwent left EMD procedure, posterior septectomy, and wide sphenoidotomy with bilateral full house FESS elsewhere. Two months later, the patient complained of intractable headache and frontal swelling for 2 weeks of duration (**Fig. 11.258**).

On examination, anterior rhinoscopy showed healing of the nasal cavity with bilateral post-FESS status and posterior septectomy, except mucosal crusting in the superior aspect of the septum extending into the bilateral frontal sinus and left lateral wall of the sphenoid (**Figs. 11.259** and **11.260**). The orbit and the palate were clinically uninvolved.

Evaluation at presentation included a detailed otorhinolaryngologic, ophthalmologic, neurologic, and maxillofacial examinations to assess the extent of disease. The proinflammatory marker values were recorded every alternate day. The hematological values are mentioned in **Table 11.15**.

MRI of the PNS, orbit, and brain including T1W, T2W, T2WFS, T1WFS postcontrast, and DWI was taken to study the extent of disease and to plan the surgical approaches and excision.

The coronal postcontrast T1 fat suppressed images showed nonenhancing soft tissue in bilateral frontal sinuses with gross osteomyelitis of the frontal bone and crista galli with extradural abscess. The hypodense lesions were seen in the sphenoid and the bilateral pterygoid wedge (**Figs. 11.261** and **11.262**).

Multidetector CT (MDCT) of the facial bones were taken to plan resection. It revealed gross erosion and destruction of the anterior and posterior tables of the frontal bone with the bilateral pterygoid wedge erosion (**Fig. 11.263**).

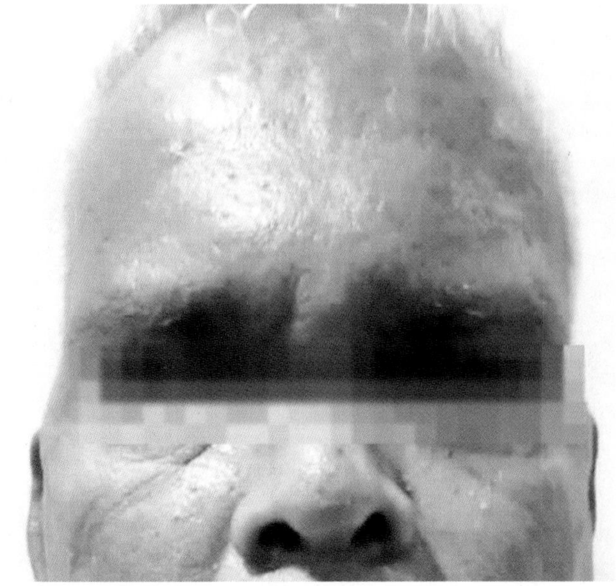

Fig. 11.258 Preoperative picture of a patient showing frontal swelling.

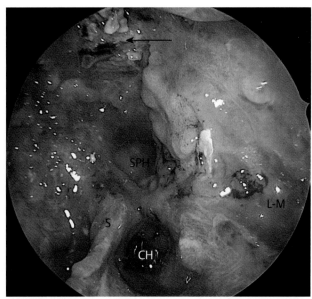

Fig. 11.259 Anterior rhinoscopy. Post functional endoscopic sinus surgery (FESS) status with posterior septectomy. (L-M, left maxilla; S, cut end of the septum SPH, sphenoid sinus.) Black arrow denotes the diseased superior cut end of septum.

Table 11.15 Hematological findings of the patient

	Total count (per µL)	CRP (mg/L)	D-dimer (ng/mL)	LDH (IU/L)	Ferritin (ng/mL)
Preoperative	7,000	250	2,500	290	305
Immediate postoperative	10,000	300	2,500	320	330
At discharge	6,000	50	250	190	95

Abbreviations: CRP, C-reactive protein; LDH, lactate dehydrogenase.

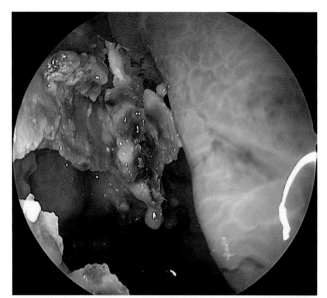

Fig. 11.260 Necrotic upper end of the septum. The region of the left frontal recess (L-F) is marked.

3D reconstruction pictures also confirmed similar findings (**Fig. 11.264**).

Considering the high chance for impending dural breach, the patient was immediately taken up for surgical debridement and abscess drainage. A bilateral EMD procedure, bilateral transpterygoid drilling, endoscopic modified Lothrop procedure, and an external bicoronal approach were planned for complete disease removal.

After orotracheal intubation, the CVP line was secured. The patient was placed in the reverse Trendelenburg position and hypotensive anesthesia was administered. The nasal cavities were examined, and swabs were taken for gram stain and KOH mount. Povidone-iodine nasal antiseptic washes (0.5%) were given before the onset of surgery. The bilateral nasal cavities were decongested with adrenaline-soaked gauze pieces (1:1,000).

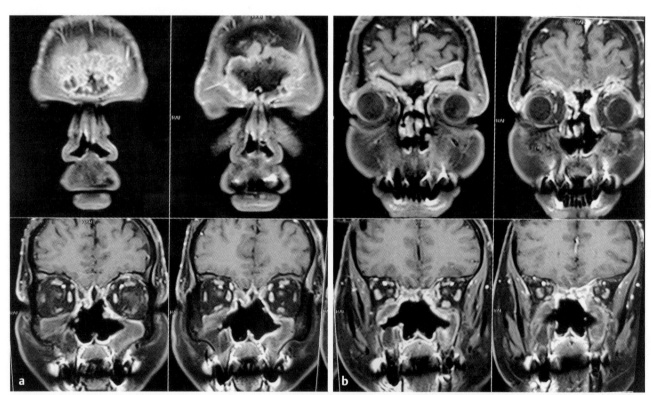

Fig. 11.261 (a, b) Coronal postcontrast T1 fat-suppressed (FS) image showing nonenhancing soft tissue in the bilateral frontal sinuses with gross osteomyelitis of the frontal bone and crista galli with an extra dural abscess.

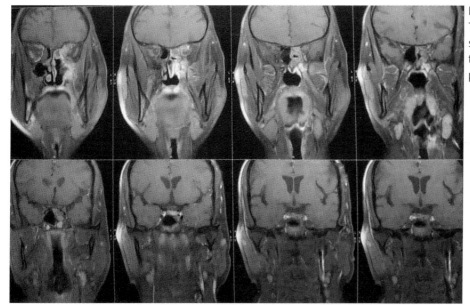

Fig. 11.262 Coronal postcontrast T1 fat-suppressed (FS) image showing hypodense lesion in the sphenoid sinus and bilateral pterygoid wedge.

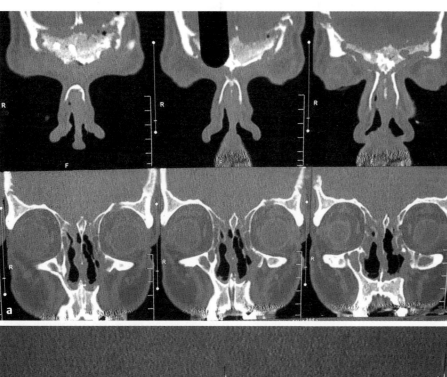

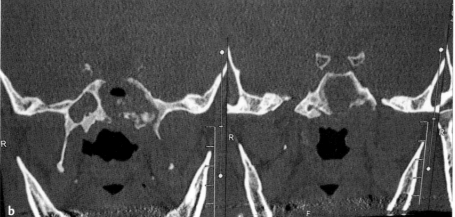

Fig. 11.263 (a, b) Multidetector computed tomography (MDCT) coronal images showing gross erosion and destruction of the anterior and posterior tables of the frontal bone with bilateral pterygoid wedge erosion.

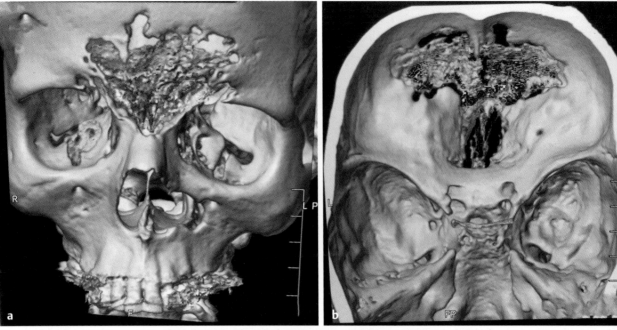

Fig. 11.264 (a, b) 3D reconstruction images of multidetector computed tomography (MDCT) showing gross erosion of the frontal bone.

Surgical Steps

Step 1: Bilateral Endoscopic Modified Denker's Procedure

The previously done Denker's procedure on the left side was revised and the maxilla was inspected. Granulation tissue over the posterior wall was removed. A right modified Denker's procedure was done to facilitate right transpterygoid drilling. The posterior wall of the left maxilla appeared normal.

The previously done posterior septectomy was also revised to facilitate the binostril approach (**Figs. 11.265–11.267**).

Step 2: Dissection of the Left ITF

At this stage, the surgeon shifts to the "four-handed technique," where the assistant holds the endoscope and the surgeon uses both hands to operate. The posterior wall of the left maxilla was drilled, and gross fat stranding was noted. The internal maxillary artery was identified and double clipped (**Fig. 11.268**). Using a coblator, the contents of PPF and ITF were dissected, pushed laterally, and removed.

Step 3: Left Transpterygoid Drilling

The vidian nerve and V2 branch of the trigeminal nerve were identified. Both were necrosed and hence resected. Transpterygoid drilling was commenced, and the pterygoid wedge appeared brittle and avascular. Using a curved

sharp elevator, it was detached from the GWS (**Fig. 11.269**). Transpterygoid drilling was completed, and the diseased left GWS was also drilled to give clearance (**Fig. 11.270**).

Step 4: Right ITF Dissection

The right posterior wall of the maxilla was also removed and identical to the left retroantral area. The right side was also grossly diseased. The internal maxillary artery was cauterized, and the contents of the fossa were debrided. It was noted that the roof of the maxilla on its posterior aspect was covered with granulation tissue and the same was removed and the bony margins were drilled till healthy bone was noted.

Step 5: Right Transpterygoid Drilling

On the right side, the vidian nerve and V2 branch of the trigeminal nerve were involved. Transpterygoid drilling was commenced after resecting both nerve bundles. The right pterygoid wedge was also lytic and diseased. It was drilled completely to achieve disease clearance (**Fig. 11.271**).

Step 6: Mid-Clival and Sellar Drilling

The posterior wall of the sphenoid was covered with unhealthy granulations from the level of the planum to the clivus. It was carefully removed using a curved elevator (**Fig. 11.272**).

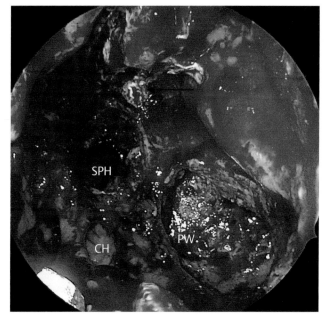

Fig. 11.265 Left endoscopic modified Denker's cavity. The *black arrow* points to the necrotic superior septum. (CH, choana; PW, posterior window; SPH, sphenoid sinus.)

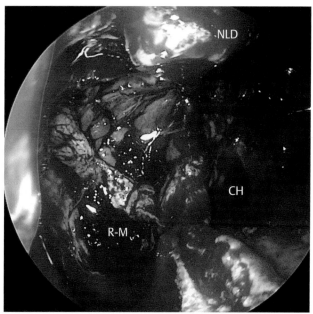

Fig. 11.266 Right endoscopic modified Denker's cavity. (CH, choana; NLD, nasolacrimal duct; R-M, right maxilla.)

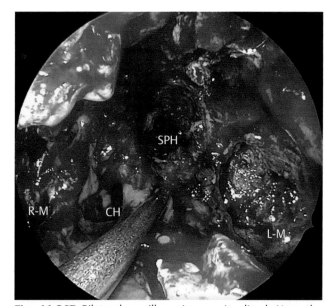

Fig. 11.267 Bilateral maxillary sinuses visualized. Note the posterior septectomy. (CH, choana; L-M, left maxilla; R-M, right maxilla; SPH, sphenoid sinus.)

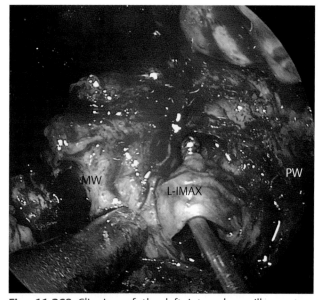

Fig. 11.268 Clipping of the left internal maxillary artery (L-IMAX), medial wall of the maxilla (MW), and the posterior wall (PW).

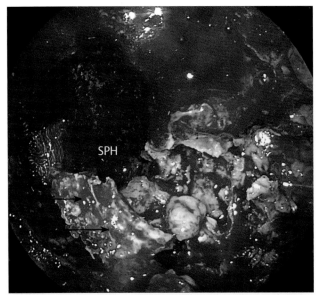

Fig. 11.269 Necrosed pterygoid wedge (*black arrows*) detached from the left greater wing of the sphenoid. (SPH, sphenoid sinus.)

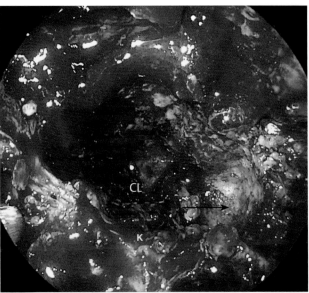

Fig. 11.270 Completed left transpterygoid drilling, clearance of the greater wing of the sphenoid (GWS; *black arrow*). (CL, mid-clivus.)

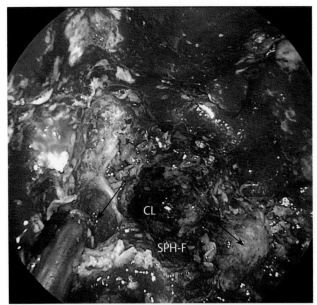

Fig. 11.271 Bilateral transpterygoid drilling (*black arrows* indicating the right and left sides). (CL, clivus; SPH-F, floor of the sphenoid sinus.)

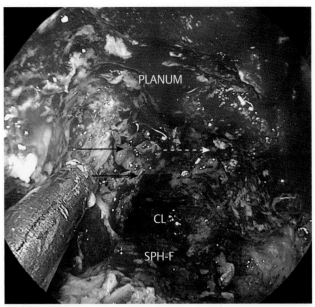

Fig. 11.272 Posterior wall of the sphenoid sinus covered with unhealthy granulations (*black arrows, broken white arrow*). (CL, clivus; SPH-F, floor of the sphenoid sinus.)

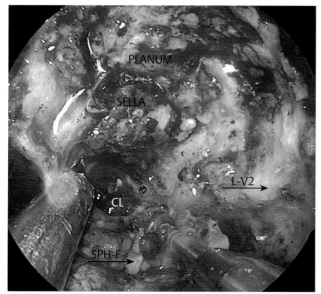

Fig. 11.273 Necrosed floor of the sphenoid (SPH-F), left V2 branch of the trigeminal nerve (L-V2), sella, and planum are marked.

The mucosa over the sphenoid sinus floor was also covered with granulation tissue. The same was removed, and the floor was found to be necrosed. It was drilled off completely (**Fig. 11.273**).

The bone over the sella appeared fragile and diseased. To achieve complete disease clearance, the anterior face of the sella was removed, and the sellar dura was preserved.

The mid-clival bone was also covered with diseased mucosa. The same was removed using Blakesley forceps and sent for HPE. Transclival drilling was done and the clival bone was noted to be avascular like the previously discussed cases (**Fig. 11.274**). Complete disease clearance of the posterior wall of the sphenoid and pterygoid wedge is depicted in **Fig. 11.275**.

Step 7: External Bicoronal Approach

The pericranial flap was harvested on the left side. Once the subgaleal flap was elevated, gross disease was seen covering the bilateral anterior table of the frontal sinus and bilateral supraorbital rim. The unhealthy granulation and purulent

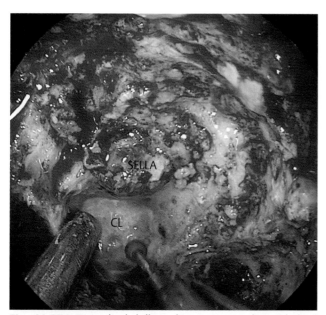

Fig. 11.274 Transclival drilling showing avascular mid-clival bone. (CL, clivus.)

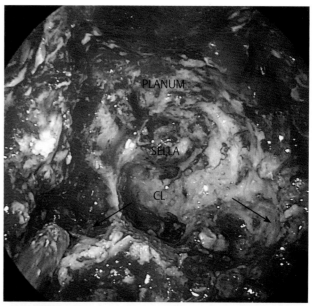

Fig. 11.275 Complete clearance of the posterior wall of the sphenoid with bilateral pterygoid wedge clearance (*black arrows*). (CL, clivus.)

discharge were cleared off to expose the bone underneath. It was entirely avascular, fragile, and necrotic. A depiction of a comparison of on-table findings with imaging findings is depicted in **Fig. 11.276**. Using a periosteal elevator, the frontal bone was carefully elevated off the frontal dura (**Figs. 11.277** and **11.278**). The extradural collection underneath the bone was fully evacuated and the diseased bony edges were drilled eggshell thin or until healthy bone was noted. The underlying dura appeared healthy and intact (**Fig. 11.279**).

After removal of the diseased bone and abscess clearance, the nasal endoscopic picture showed the basifrontal dura covered with disease. The granulations and slough were removed and the diseased dura was coblated (**Figs. 11.280** and **11.281**). The necrosed crista galli was drilled eggshell thin and removed by sharp dissection. The anterior skull base was repaired in a multilayer technique using fat, surgicel, fascia lata, and pericranial flap after antibiotic and amphotericin washes (**Fig. 11.282** and **Video 11.15**).

Packing

Complete hemostasis was achieved, diluted amphotericin washes were given, and nasal cavity was packed with merocel 8 cm in both nostrils.

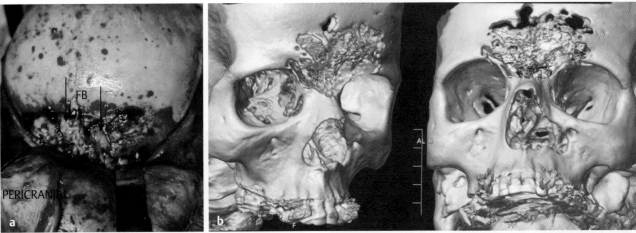

Fig. 11.276 (a, b) Comparative depiction of multidetector computed tomography (MDCT) picture with on-table finding of the frontal disease (*black arrows*). (FB, frontal bone.)

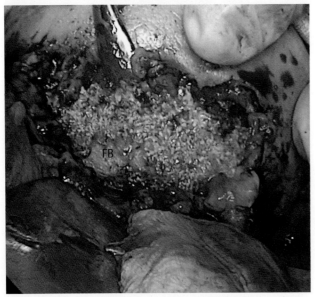

Fig. 11.277 After removal of the superficial granulation frontal bone (FB), necrosis is seen.

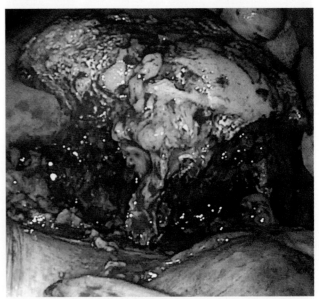

Fig. 11.278 The whole of the diseased frontal bone removed in toto.

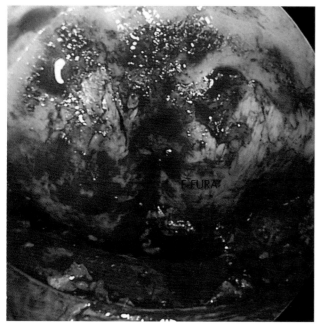

Fig. 11.279 Healthy frontal dura (F-DURA) after disease removal.

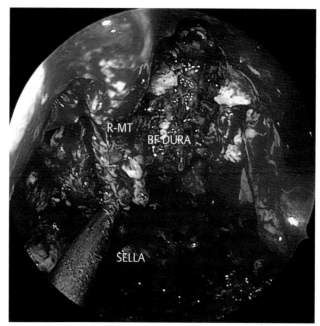

Fig. 11.280 Endoscopic view of the basifrontal dura (BF-DURA) covered with granulations. The right middle turbinate (R-MT) and sella are marked.

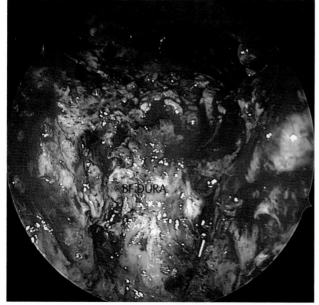

Fig. 11.281 After removal of the crista galli, and granulations, the basifrontal dura (BF-DURA) was bared. Superiorly the frontal sinus is seen connecting to the external incision.

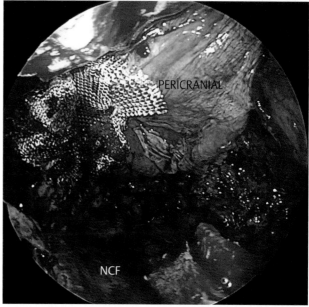

Fig. 11.282 Skull base repair using multilayered closure. The pericranial flap is marked.

Postoperative Management

Postoperatively the patient's frontal swelling disappeared (**Fig. 11.283**). He was treated with a cumulative dose of 4.5 g of liposomal amphotericin-B and 12 weeks of oral posaconazole medications. The patient was kept under strict glycemic control, and repeated endoscopic nasal cleaning was done at fortnightly intervals. Postoperative scan done 2 months later showed complete resolution of the disease (**Fig. 11.284**).

The endoscopic picture of the healed pericranial flap 2 months post-op is depicted in **Fig. 11.285**.

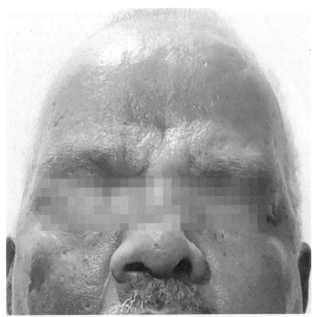

Fig. 11.283 Postoperative picture of a patient. Note that the frontal swelling has disappeared.

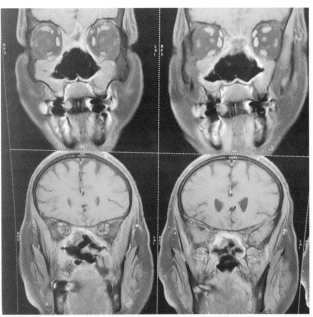

Fig. 11.284 Postoperative coronal T1-weighted (T1W) fat-suppressed (FS) magnetic resonance imaging (MRI) showing complete disease clearance.

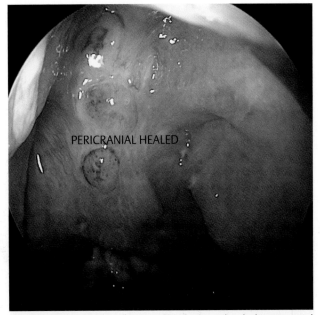

Fig. 11.285 Postoperative cavity showing healed pericranial flap.

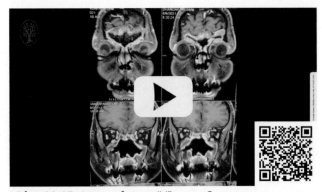

Video 11.15 A case of stage IVB—case 2.

Stage VA: Intracranial Intradural Abscess

Case 16: A 36-year-old male diabetic patient with the history of COVID-19 pneumonia in June 2021 presented 25 days after discharge with complaints of severe headache not relieved with medications. He was treated with intravenous steroids and oxygen during COVID-19 infection. At presentation, he had high-grade fever and the patient was in delirium. His GCS score was noted to be 12.

Nasal endoscopy revealed no positive findings. Orbital examination showed no abnormality. The palate was clinically not involved.

Evaluation at presentation included a detailed otorhinolaryngologic, ophthalmologic, and neurological examinations to assess the extent of disease. The neurosurgeon advised immediate surgery, considering the patient's condition.

The proinflammatory marker values were recorded every alternate day. The hematological values are mentioned in **Table 11.16**.

MRI of the PNS, orbit, and brain including T1W, T2W, T2WFS, T1WFS postcontrast, and DWI was taken to study the extent of disease and to plan the surgical approaches and excision.

The coronal T1 FS images showed features suggestive of osteomyelitis of the left pterygoid wedge and GWS with left temporal lobe abscess. The bilateral maxillary sinuses, orbit, and palate were uninvolved (**Fig. 11.286**).

The patient was immediately taken up for total excision considering the deteriorating neurological status. The surgical plan was based on the MRI findings of the left pterygoid wedge, GWS, and intracranial abscess. A left EMD procedure followed by transpterygoid drilling, drilling of the infratemporal surface of the greater wing, and drainage of abscess was planned. A contralateral nasoseptal flap was planned for dural reconstruction.

After orotracheal intubation, the central venous line was secured. The patient was placed in the reverse Trendelenburg position and hypotensive anesthesia was administered. The nasal cavities were examined, and swabs were taken for gram stain and KOH mount. The vibrissae were trimmed, and povidone-iodine nasal antiseptic washes (0.5%) were given before the onset of surgery. The bilateral nasal cavities were decongested with adrenaline-soaked gauze pieces (1:1,000).

Surgical Steps

Step 1: Left Endoscopic Modified Denker's Procedure

An EMD procedure was done on the left side. The left maxilla was found disease free, the mucosa over the posterior wall was elevated, and no gross bony involvement was seen. A complete sphenoethmoidectomy was also done on the left side (**Figs. 11.287** and **11.288**). The ethmoid sinus was disease free, and the polypoidal changes were noted in the left side sphenoid sinus.

Step 2: Harvesting the Right-Side Haddad Flap (Nasoseptal Flap)

This flap is considered the "workhorse" for anterior skull base reconstruction.

The right side septal mucosa was infiltrated with saline, vertical incision was made at the mucocutaneous junction, and the septal flap was carefully elevated posteriorly till the pterygosphenoid synchondrosis. Superior and inferior cuts were made over the mucosal flap and the nasoseptal flap was pushed down the right nasopharynx for safekeeping (**Fig. 11.289**). A complete ethmoidectomy and sphenoidotomy were also done on the right side.

Step 3: Wide Sphenoidotomy and Removal of the Keel

A posterior septectomy, bilateral wide sphenoidotomy, and posterior ethmoidectomies complete the nasal corridor. The pedicle of the hadad flap is carefully preserved during the posterior septectomy. The classical "owl's-eye appearance" was seen and triple osteotomy was done (**Fig. 11.290**). The rostrum and the anterior face of the sphenoid were completely removed. The mucosa inside the sinus was found to be polypoidal, but no frank disease was noted (**Fig. 11.291**), the sinus wall was stripped off the mucosa, and the posterior wall of the sphenoid was exposed. No bony changes were noted on the posterior wall (**Fig. 11.292**).

On elevation of the mucosa over the floor of the sphenoid sinus, gross osteomyelitis of the keel and part of the floor was noted and the same was resected (**Fig. 11.293**).

Table 11.16 Hematological findings of the patient

	Total count (per µL)	CRP (mg/L)	D-dimer (ng/mL)	LDH (IU/L)	Ferritin (ng/mL)
Preoperative	10,000	540	2,780	340	300
Immediate postoperative	8,000	235	2,500	350	285
At discharge	6,500	110	750	240	85

Abbreviations: CRP, C-reactive protein; LDH, lactate dehydrogenase.

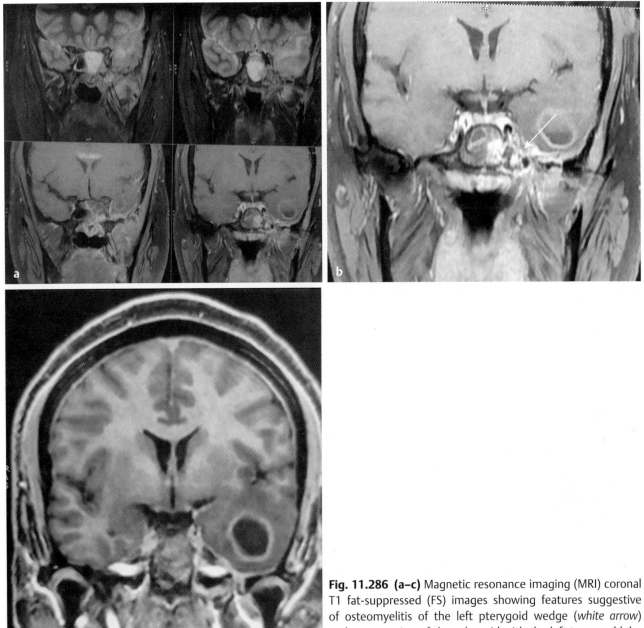

Fig. 11.286 (a–c) Magnetic resonance imaging (MRI) coronal T1 fat-suppressed (FS) images showing features suggestive of osteomyelitis of the left pterygoid wedge (*white arrow*) and greater wing of the sphenoid with the left temporal lobe abscess.

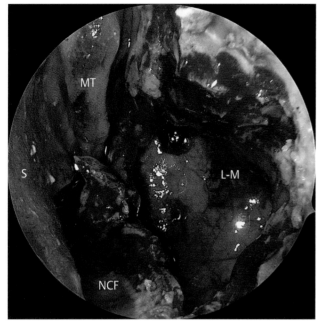

Fig. 11.287 Left maxilla (L-M), post-Denker's procedure. (MT, middle turbinate; NCF, nasal cavity floor; S, septum.)

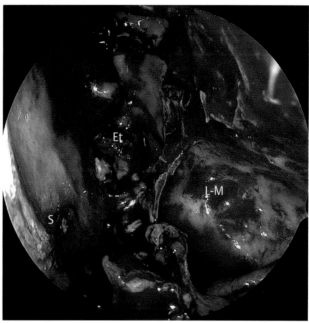

Fig. 11.288 Left maxilla (L-M) after the mucosa over the posterior wall is elevated. Left side functional endoscopic sinus surgery (FESS) is done. (Et, ethmoid; S, septum.)

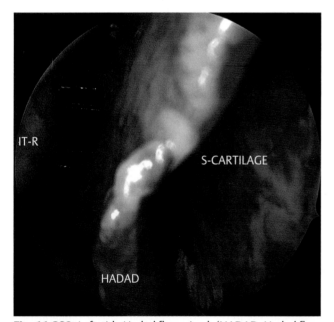

Fig. 11.289 Left-side Hadad flap raised. (HADAD, Hadad flap; IT-R, right inferior turbinate; S-CARTILAGE, septal cartilage.)

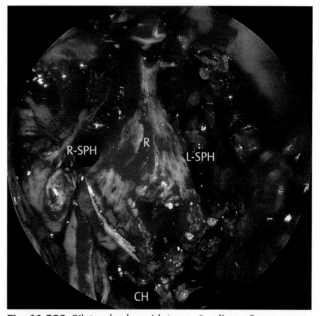

Fig. 11.290 Bilateral sphenoidotomy; "owl's eye" appearance. (CH, choana; L-SPH, left sphenoid; R, rostrum; R-SPH, right sphenoid.)

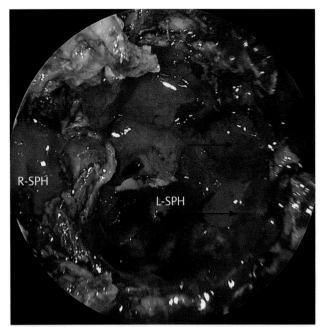

Fig. 11.291 Wide sphenoidotomy. *Black arrows* point to the polypoidal changes within the sinus. (R-SPH, right sphenoid; L-SPH, left sphenoid.)

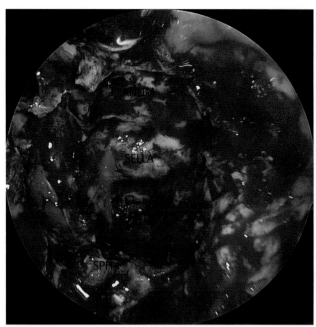

Fig. 11.292 Posterior wall of the sphenoid showing various landmarks. (CL, clivus; SPH-F, floor of the sphenoid.)

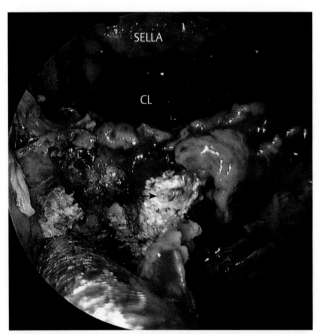

Fig. 11.293 Gross osteomyelitis of the keel (*black arrows*) and part of the floor of the sphenoid. The sella and clivus (CL) are marked.

Step 4: Dissection of the Left Infratemporal Fossa

The posterior wall of the maxilla was removed. The underlying periosteum appeared healthy (**Fig. 11.294**). The periosteum was opened, and the contents of PPF and ITF were examined and found to be grossly normal. The sphenopalatine and descending palatine arteries were coblated and the left internal maxillary artery was double clipped. The contents of the fossae were mobilized laterally and then dissected out (**Fig. 11.295**).

On further dissection posterior to the internal maxillary artery and lateral to the lateral pterygoid plate, a deep abscess was seen under the infratemporal surface of the GWS (**Fig. 11.296**). It was drained, and for further disease clearance, a transpterygoid drilling was commenced.

Step 5: Left Transpterygoid Approach

The lateral extension of the nasal corridor is achieved via a transpterygoid approach. The dissection of the ITF and PPF ensures access to the entire pterygoid base. A subperiosteal dissection is done to reduce bleeding from the pterygoid plexus of the veins, and the foramen Rotundum and the canal for the vidian nerve were identified. Both the nerve bundles

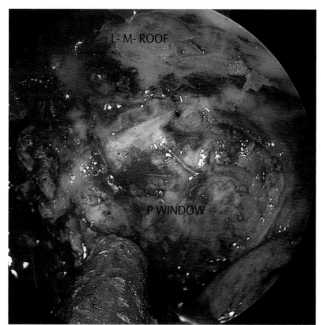

Fig. 11.294 A healthy-looking periosteum of the left pterygopalatine and infratemporal fossa (ITF). (L-M-ROOF, roof of left maxilla; P-WINDOW, posterior window.)

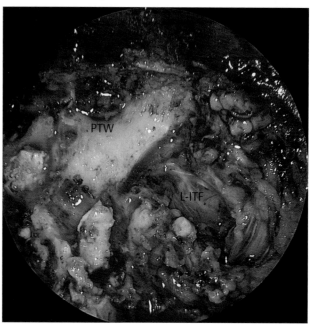

Fig. 11.295 Dissection of contents of the left infratemporal fossa (L-ITF); internal maxillary artery clipped. (PTW, pterygoid wedge.)

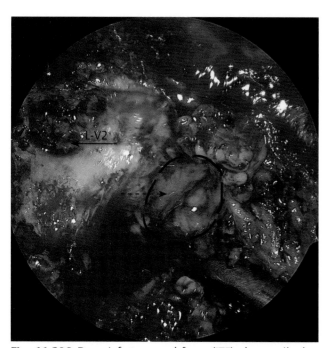

Fig. 11.296 Deep infratemporal fossa (ITF) abscess (*broken circle*) and the left V2 branch of the trigeminal nerve (L-V2).

were necrosed and the same were divided (**Fig. 11.297**). The vidian canal serves as the most important landmark to identify the petrous part of the ICA and thus the quadrangular space. The drilling commences in the inferior and medial aspects of the vidian canal, taking care to keep the drill in the inferior hemicircumference of it, because the ICA is superolateral to it. Bone around the foramen Rotundum is drilled till the point the V2 pierces the middle cranial fossa dura. In this case also, the pterygoid wedge appeared avascular and brittle unlike the normal bone (**Fig. 11.298**).

The mucosa over the medial pterygoid plate was elevated and it was found to be completely necrosed. It was followed up to the attachment to the pterygoid wedge and the whole bone was found to be diseased. Using a curved instrument, it was separated from its attachment to the GWS and removed in one piece and sent for HPE (**Figs. 11.299** and **11.300**).

The necrosed GWS was drilled and elevated off the base of the temporal lobe (**Fig. 11.301**). The presence of extradural abscess was noted. The same was drained and the greater wing was drilled lateral to the V3 branch of the trigeminal nerve (**Fig. 11.302**). During drilling, the dead and

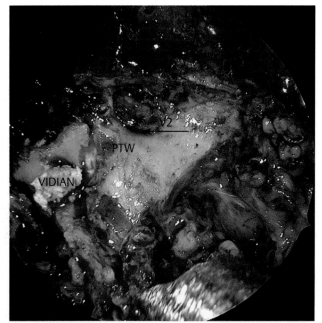

Fig. 11.297 Necrosis of the V2 and vidian nerves. (PTW, pterygoid wedge.)

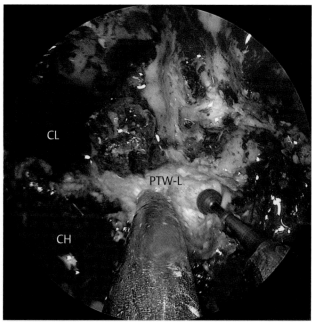

Fig. 11.298 Transpterygoid approach; drilling of the avascular left pterygoid wedge (PTW-L). (CH, choana; CL, clivus.)

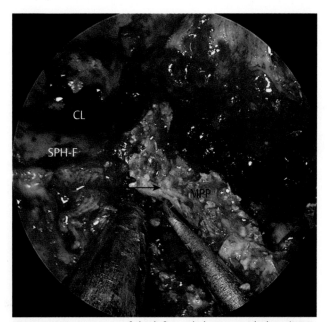

Fig. 11.299 Necrosis of the left medial pterygoid plate (MPP; *black arrow*). (CL, clivus; SPH-F, floor of the sphenoid.)

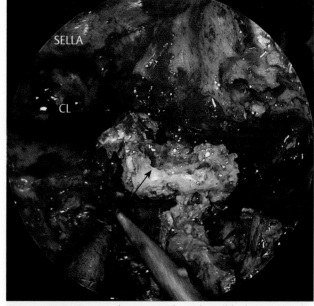

Fig. 11.300 Necrosed pterygoid wedge (*black arrow*). The sella is marked. (CL, clivus.)

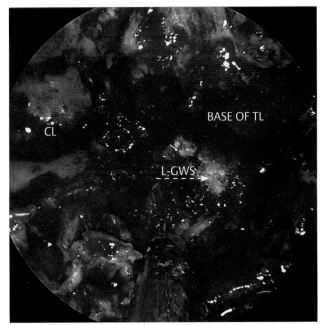

Fig. 11.301 Necrosed left greater wing of the sphenoid (L-GWS) and the base of the temporal lobe (BASE OF TL). (CL, clivus.)

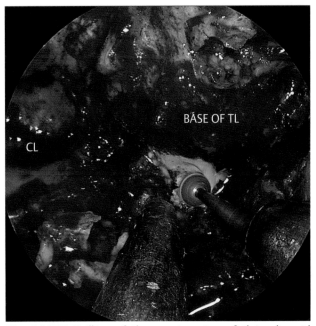

Fig. 11.302 Drilling of the greater wing of the sphenoid (GWS; *black arrow*). (BASE OF TL, base of the temporal lobe; CL, clivus.)

avascular bone dust was seen to be floating in the irrigation fluid resembling a "chalk powder" appearance (**Fig. 11.303**). Complete bony clearance was obtained at the level of the GWS (**Fig. 11.304**).

Using a carotid doppler, the petrous part of the carotid was mapped. A pseudoaneurysm was noted at the junction of the horizontal and vertical parts of the carotid (**Fig. 11.305**).

The quadrangular space was involved by the disease. This space is bounded inferomedially by the petrous and paraclival carotid arteries, laterally by V2, and superiorly by the abducens nerve. Bone over the quadrangular space was drilled and complete disease removal was obtained.

Step 6: Drainage of the Left Temporal Lobe Abscess

The area of the abscess was correlated with the MRI scan, a wide bore needle was inserted through the dura, and the presence of abscess was confirmed. Using a sharp knife, a dural incision was made and the abscess was let out (**Fig. 11.306**). The pus was sent for culture and sensitivity test. The abscess cavity was examined, and complete drainage was ensured (**Fig. 11.307**). Amphotericin-B washes were given, and dural leak was repaired in a multilayer fashion using surgicel (sterile cellulose-based thrombogenic material), fat, and the previously harvested nasoseptal (Hadad) flap (**Fig. 11.308**).

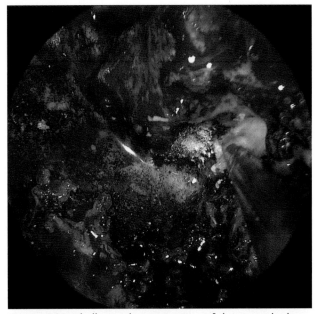

Fig. 11.303 Chalk powder appearance of the avascular bone of the greater wing of the sphenoid.

The uninvolved mucosa over the posterior maxillary wall was also draped over the watertight closure (**Fig. 11.309** and **Video 11.16**).

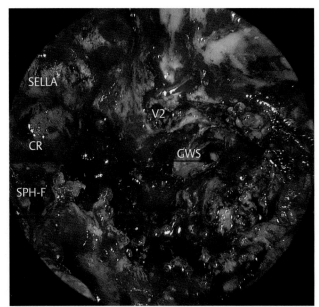

Fig. 11.304 Complete bony disease clearance on the left side. (CR, clival recess; GWS, greater wing of the sphenoid; SPH-F, sphenoid floor.)

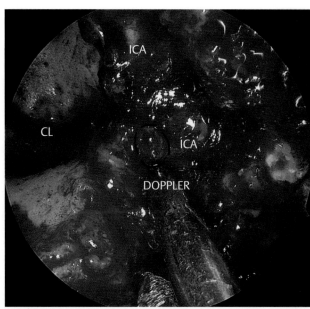

Fig. 11.305 Pseudoaneurysm (*broken circle*) at the junction of the petrous and paraclival carotid artery (ICA). (CL, clivus.)

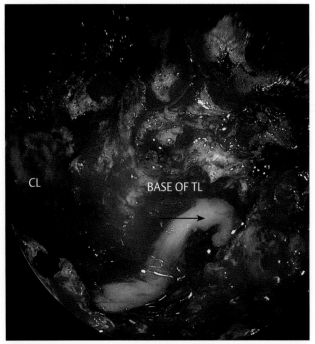

Fig. 11.306 Drainage of the left temporal lobe abscess. (BASE OF TL, base of the temporal lobe; CL, clivus.)

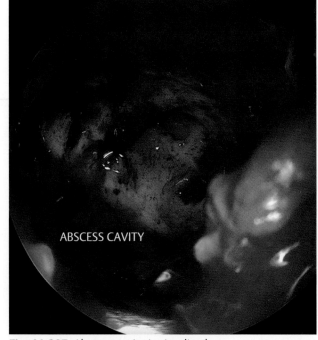

Fig. 11.307 Abscess cavity is visualized.

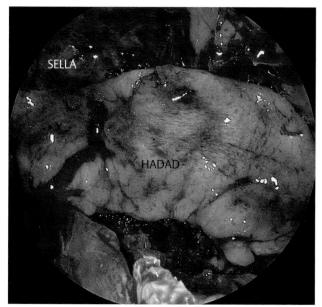

Fig. 11.308 Left anterior skull base repair with the Hadad flap. The sella is marked.

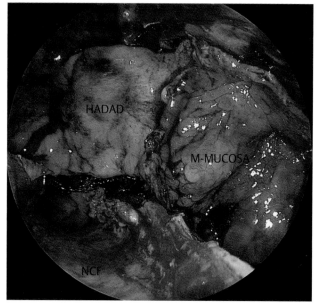

Fig. 11.309 Left posterior maxillary wall mucosa (M-MUCOSA) draped over the Hadad flap. (NCF, floor of the nasal cavity.)

Packing

After obtaining hemostasis, the nasal cavity was packed with merocel 8 cm in both nostrils.

Postoperative Management

The immediate postoperative CT of the brain showed complete resolution of abscess (**Fig. 11.310**). The patient was treated with systemic antibiotics and was kept in strict bed rest for 7 days. Supportive therapy with lower limb stockings and chest and limb physiotherapy was given. He clinically improved in the immediate postoperative period; his GCS score returned to 15.

Postoperatively the patient received a cumulative dose of 5.0 g of amphotericin-B with total 12 weeks' duration of 400 mg of posaconazole.

The follow-up scan done after 3 months showed complete resolution of disease (**Fig. 11.311**), and the postoperative healing of the nasal cavity is depicted in **Fig. 11.312**.

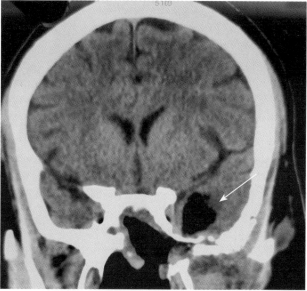

Fig. 11.310 Immediate postoperative computed tomography (CT) of the brain showing resolved abscess (*white arrow*) with no evidence of pneumocephalus.

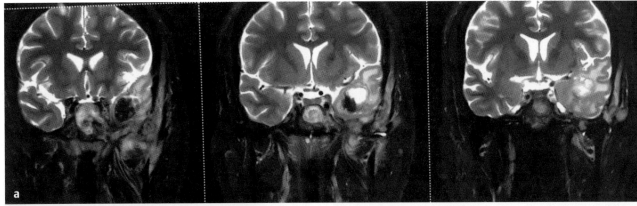

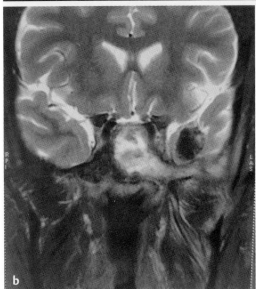

Fig. 11.311 (a, b) Postoperative T2-weighted (T2W) short tau inversion recovery (STIR) magnetic resonance imaging (MRI) of the brain showing complete resolution of abscess.

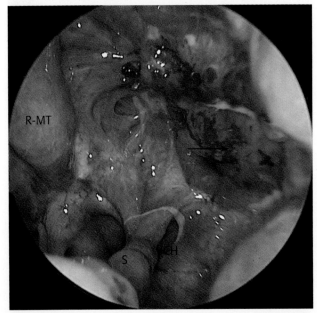

Fig. 11.312 Postoperative healing of the nasal cavity. Right middle turbinate (R-MT), Septum (S), Choana (CH). The *black arrow* shows healed Hadad flap.

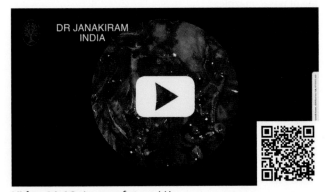

Video 11.16 A case of stage VA.

Stage VB: Intracranial Intradural Abscess

Case 17: A 57-year-old diabetic, hypertensive, and post-COVID-19 patient, who was treated with intravenous steroids, monoclonal antibodies, remdesivir, and oxygen by mask, was diagnosed with post-COVID-19 mucormycosis. He underwent FESS thrice and a frontal trephination surgery at a different hospital. A cumulative dose of 9.0 g of amphotericin-B was administered to the patient previously.

Currently, he was referred to the authors' center with frontal swelling, painful extraocular movements, and severe headache.

On examination, anterior rhinoscopy showed bilateral post-FESS status with multiple synechiae (**Fig. 11.313**).

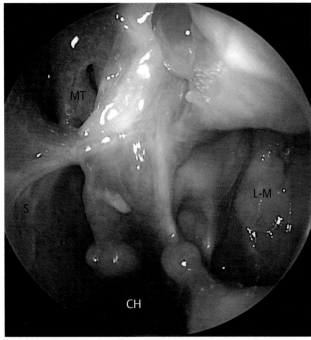

Fig. 11.313 Preoperative anterior rhinoscopy showing post functional endoscopic sinus surgery (FESS) status. (S, septum; MT, middle turbinate; L-M, left maxilla.)

Orbital examination showed bilateral compound myopic astigmatism. Palatal examination was within normal limits.

Evaluation at presentation included a detailed otorhinolaryngologic, maxillofacial, and neurological examinations to assess the extent of disease. The proinflammatory marker values were recorded every alternate day. The hematological values are mentioned in **Table 11.17**.

MRI of the PNS, orbit, and brain including T1W, T2W, T2WFS, T1WFS postcontrast, and DWI was taken to study the extent of disease and to plan the surgical approaches and excision.

The coronal postcontrast T1W and T2W STIR images showed nonenhancing soft tissue in the right maxillary sinus with bilateral ethmoiditis. T2 nonenhancing hypointense mucosal thickening in bilateral frontal sinuses was suggestive of fungal sinusitis. Erosion of the bilateral tables of the frontal bone and the right temporal bone with enhancing soft tissue and intracranial extra-axial soft tissue with a depth of 9 mm in the right frontotemporal lobes indicated underlying fulminant fungal disease. Erosion of the superolateral wall of the right orbit with intracranial extraconal abscess measuring 8 × 6 mm was also noted (**Fig. 11.314**).

MDCT with 3D facial reconstruction scan was taken. It revealed extensive bony destruction involving the bilateral frontal sinuses, superior part of the bony septum, right pterygoid wedge, GWS, floor of the anterior cranial fossa, right squamous temporal bone, and right lateral wall of the orbit (**Fig. 11.315**).

Considering the patient had extensive disease, he was immediately taken up for surgical debridement and abscess drainage. Right EMD, endoscopic modified Lothrop procedure, and external transcranial approach were planned.

After orotracheal intubation, the CVP line was secured. The patient was placed in the reverse Trendelenburg position and hypotensive anesthesia was administered. The nasal cavities were examined, and swabs were taken for gram stain and KOH mount. Povidone-iodine nasal antiseptic washes (0.5%) were given before the onset of surgery. Bilateral nasal cavities were decongested with adrenaline-soaked gauze pieces (1:1,000).

Table 11.17 Hematological findings of the patient

	Total count (per µL)	CRP (mg/L)	D-dimer (ng/mL)	LDH (IU/L)	Ferritin (ng/mL)
Preoperative	10,000	300	2,000	250	295
Immediate postoperative	11,000	310	2,500	300	300
At discharge	5,000	30	300	170	95

Abbreviations: CRP, C-reactive protein; LDH, lactate dehydrogenase.

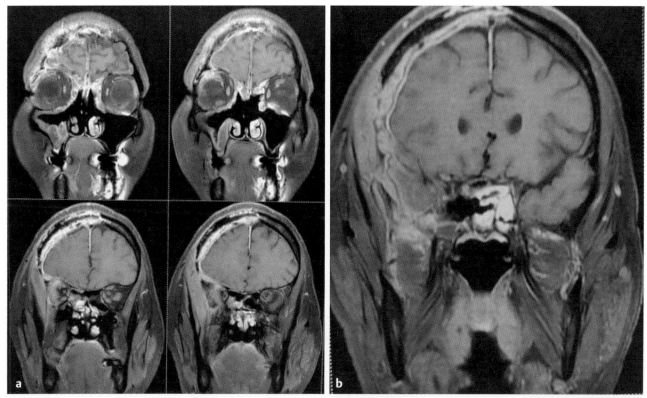

Fig. 11.314 (a, b) Preoperative T1-weighted (T1W) fat-suppressed (FS) images showing extensive fungal disease involving the right maxilla, bilateral ethmoid sinuses, and frontal sinuses with lytic destruction of the frontal tables and temporal bones with intracranial abscess.

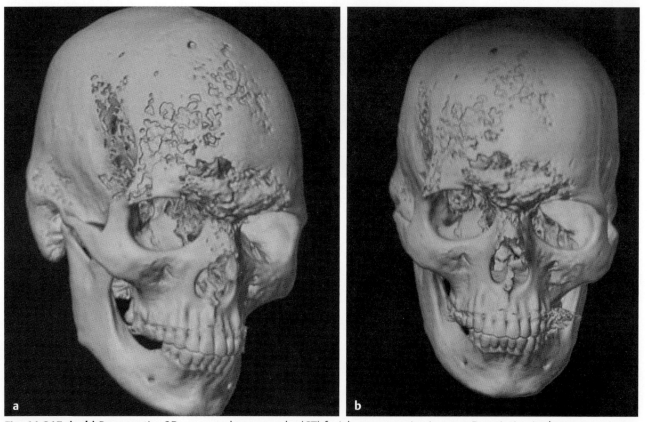

Fig. 11.315 (a, b) Preoperative 3D computed tomography (CT) facial reconstruction images. Description in the text.

Surgical Steps

Step 1: Right Endoscopic Modified Denker's Procedure with Bilateral Fess

A complete FESS was done on the left side (**Fig. 11.316**). During frontal sinusotomy, purulent discharge was noted coming out of the left frontal sinus. Similarly, a full house FESS was done on the right side. In addition, modified Denker's procedure was done on the right side. The right maxilla was filled with fungal debris (**Fig. 11.317**). It was debrided and complete clearance was achieved.

Step 2: Right Infratemporal Fossa Dissection

The right posterior wall of the maxilla was removed, and gross fat stranding was noted (**Fig. 11.318**). The internal maxillary artery was double clipped and coblated. The contents of the fossa were debrided off. Wide sphenoidotomy was done and polypoidal mucosa was removed completely. The part of the pterygoid wedge and the infratemporal surface of the right GWS were drilled off till healthy bone was encountered.

The surgeon has noted that unlike in other diseases, fungi infected bone when drilled, and the bone dust tends to float in the irrigation fluid. He has termed this as "Chalk Powder" appearance (**Fig. 11.319**).

Step 3: Endoscopic Modified Lothrop Procedure

Considering the extensive disease in bilateral frontal sinuses, an endoscopic modified Lothrop procedure was commenced. This involved removal of the superior part of the nasal septum, inferior portion of the interfrontal septum, and the floor of the frontal sinus till the lamina laterally. This creates a common median drainage pathway (**Fig. 11.320**). The nasal spine was found to be yellowish and necrotic and the same was drilled (**Fig. 11.321**). The crista galli was grossly lytic and the same was drilled eggshell thin and removed using sharp dissection. Once it was completed and frontal sinus was found to have gross disease.

Step 4: Transcranial Approach and Fronto-Parieto-Temporal Craniectomy

A bicoronal incision was made from the left helix to the right helix. On the right side, it was extended inferiorly in front of the tragus. The pericranial flap was harvested on the left side (**Fig. 11.322**). After raising the flap, the frontal bone on the right side and midline was found to be brittle, necrosed, and studded with what looked like fungal colonies (**Fig. 11.323**).

The right temporalis muscle was separated from its attachment to the temporal line and reflected laterally to access the zygoma, temporal fossa, and left lateral wall of the orbit.

A right fronto-parieto-temporal craniectomy was done by the neurosurgeon and the bone flap was elevated off the dura (**Fig. 11.324**). The undersurface of the bone flap was grossly infected with fungus (**Fig. 11.325**).

The frontoparietal dura was found to be covered in its entirety with thick unhealthy granulations (**Fig. 11.326**). The granulations were scraped off with a blunt elevator carefully and saline wash was given. Multiple rents were noted in the dura after removing the granulations.

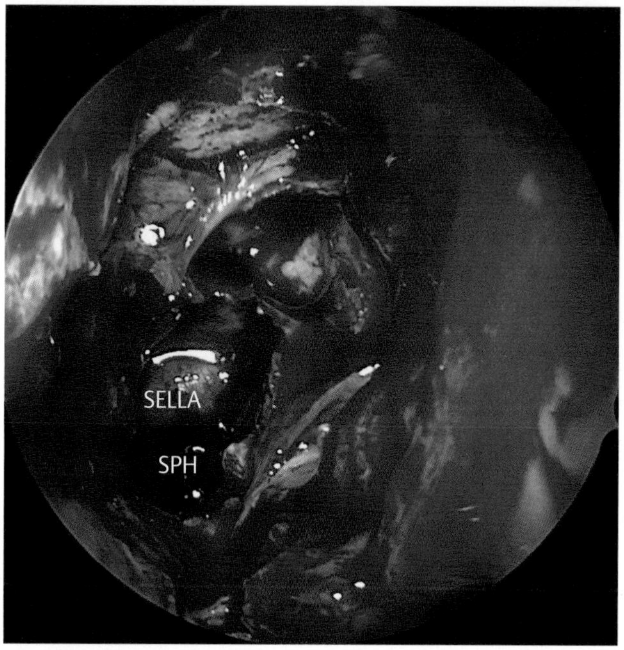

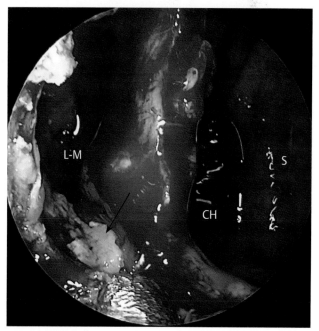

Fig. 11.316 Complete functional endoscopic sinus surgery (FESS) done on the left side with delineation of the skull base. The sphenoid sinus (SPH) and the sella are marked.

Fig. 11.317 Following right endoscopic Denker's procedure, the left maxilla (L-M) shows fungal debris (*black arrow*). (CH, choana.)

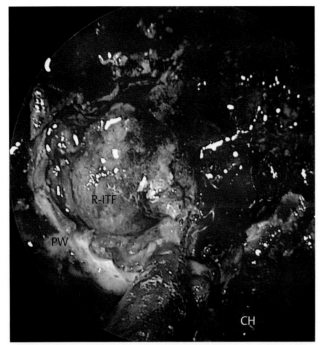

Fig. 11.318 Gross fat stranding noted in the right infratemporal fossa (R-ITF). (PW, posterior wall of the maxilla.)

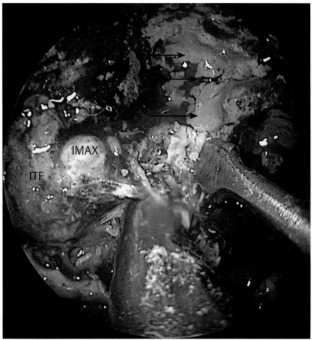

Fig. 11.319 *Chalk-powder sign* indicated by *black arrows.* (IMAX, internal maxillary artery; ITF, infratemporal fossa.)

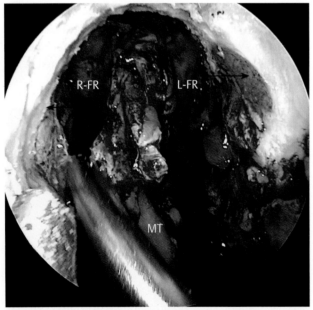

Fig. 11.320 Completion of endoscopic modified Lothrop procedure. Right frontal recess (R-FR), left frontal recess (L-FR), and skin over the lacrimal bone marking the lateral boundary of the Draf III procedure are marked with *black arrows.*

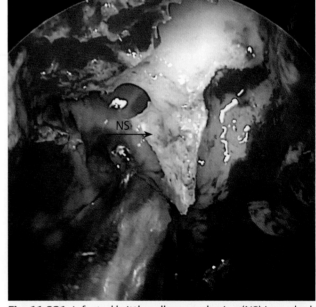

Fig. 11.321 Infected brittle yellow nasal spine (NS) is marked.

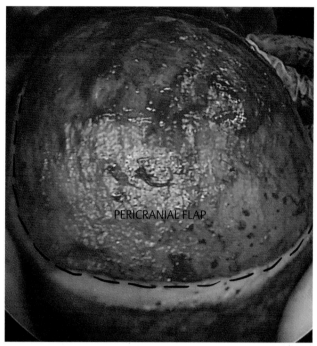

Fig. 11.322 Boundary of the pericranial flap is marked with a *broken black line*.

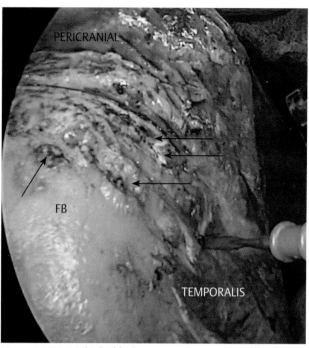

Fig. 11.323 *Multiple black arrows* showing fungal colonies over the right frontal bone (FB). The pericranial flap and temporalis muscle are marked.

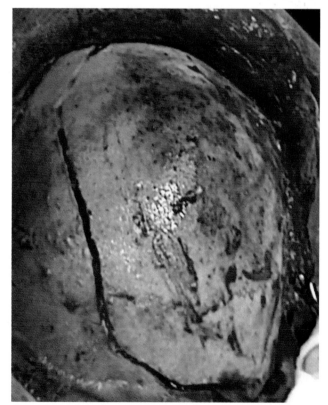

Fig. 11.324 Midline and right fronto-parieto-temporo-craniectomy osteotomies are marked.

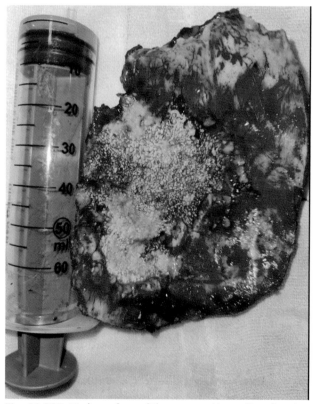

Fig. 11.325 Undersurface of the removed bone flap showing gross fungus and necrosis.

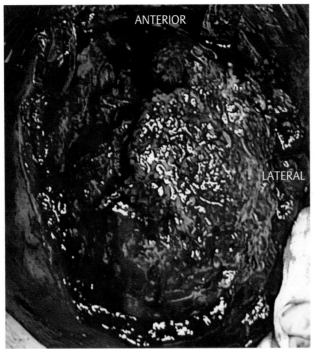

Fig. 11.326 Unhealthy frontoparietal dura covered with granulations. For orientation, anterior and right lateral sites are marked in *bold*.

Using a bone nibbler, the necrosed bilateral supraorbital rim was removed. The part of the superomedial orbital wall was also removed (**Fig. 11.327**). An abscess was noted under the right supraorbital rim. It was drained and pus was sent for culture and sensitivity.

The anterior-most part of the frontal bone attached to the nasal bone was completely necrosed and was removed in one triangular piece (**Fig. 11.328**). The frontoparietal dura following removal of granulations is depicted in **Fig. 11.329**.

The temporalis muscle was reflected laterally and retracted to expose the temporal fossa on the right side. It was found to be filled with necrosed temporal bone and temporalis muscle (**Fig. 11.330**). The necrosed bone was removed with a bone nibbler and drilled till healthy counterpart was seen, and the necrosed muscle was debrided off completely. The bilateral supraorbital rims were removed, and bone was drilled till healthy bleeding was seen. Complete clearance above the globe is shown in **Fig. 11.331**.

Once complete disease clearance was achieved, multiple amphotericin washes were given over the dura and intranasally. The temporoparietal flap on the right side was used for orbital reconstruction. The pericranial flap was tunneled through the frontal opening into the nasal cavity and draped over the gyrus recti for the anterior skull base repair (**Fig. 11.332** and **Video 11.17**).

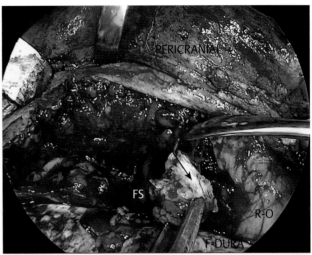

Fig. 11.327 Necrosed right superomedial orbital wall (*black arrow*) being removed. The frontal dura (F-DURA), right orbit (R-O), and pericranial flap are marked. (FS, frontal sinus.)

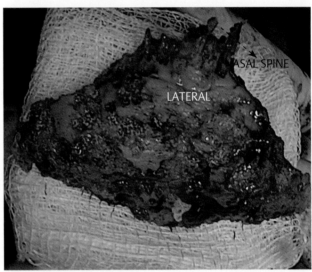

Fig. 11.328 Anterior-most part of the frontal bone attached to the nasal bone removed in one triangular piece. The glabella and nasal spine are marked.

Packing

Diluted amphotericin washes were given, and nasal cavity was packed with merocel at multiple levels.

Postoperative Management

Postoperatively the patient improved clinically in 2 weeks. The bone flap that was removed during the surgery was washed, sterilized, and returned to the patient for using as a template for reconstruction at a later date.

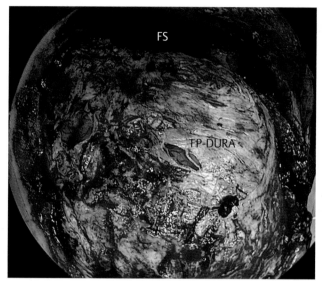

Fig. 11.329 Frontoparietal dura (FP-DURA) after removal of granulations. (FS, frontal sinus.)

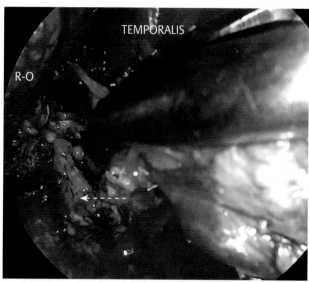

Fig. 11.330 Temporalis muscle (TEMPORALIS) on the right side reflected laterally to expose the necrosed temporal bone (*white arrow*). (R-O, right orbit.)

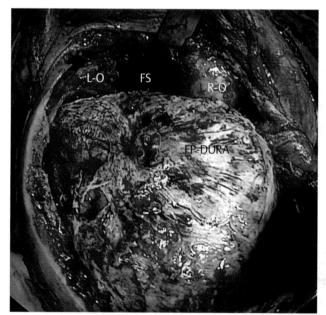

Fig. 11.331 Clearance after complete removal of all necrosed bone including bilateral supraorbital rims. (FP-DURA, frontoparietal dura; FS, frontal sinus; L-O, left orbit; R-O, right orbit.)

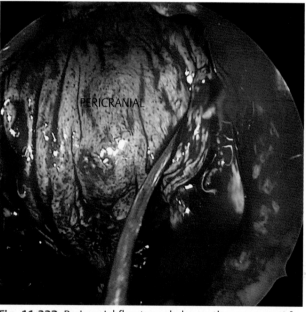

Fig. 11.332 Pericranial flap tunneled over the gyrus recti for anterior skull base repair.

He was treated with a total dose of 3.5 g of liposomal amphotericin-B and 12 weeks of oral posaconazole. He had intermittent episodes of hypokalemia and hypomagnesemia, which were treated with intravenous replacements after temporarily stopping amphotericin. The patient tolerated the treatment well.

Surveillance

The patient improved symptomatically on follow-up. No evidence of disease was seen on residual scan (**Fig. 11.333**). Postoperative endoscopic picture of the nasal cavity and the patient is depicted in **Figs. 11.334** and **11.335**. Note the craniectomy defect.

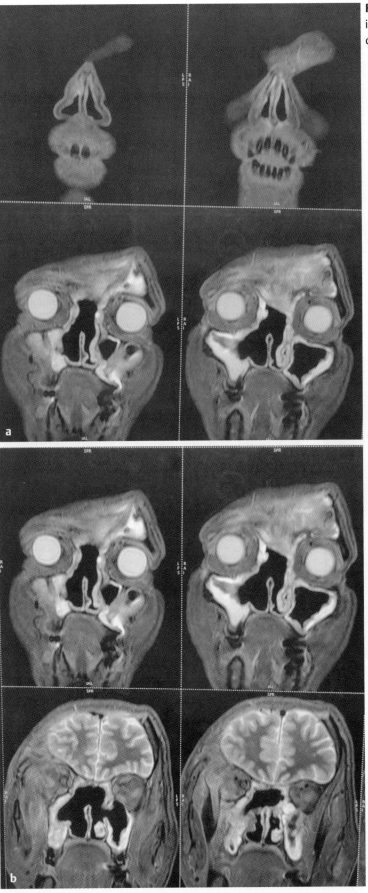

Fig. 11.333 (a, b) Postoperative magnetic resonance imaging (MRI) showing complete resolution of disease.

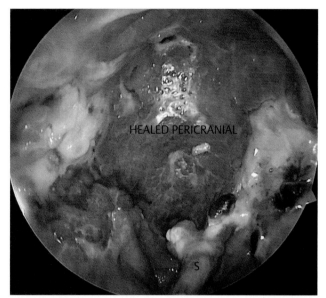

Fig. 11.334 Postoperative healing of nasal cavity depicted. The healed pericranial flap is marked in *bold*.

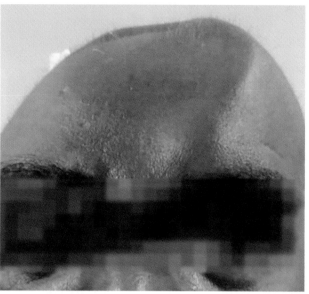

Fig. 11.335 Postoperative patient picture. Right craniectomy defect is evident.

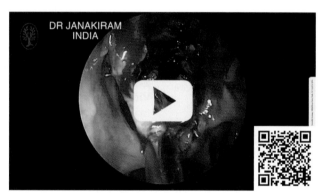

Video 11.17 A case of stage VB.

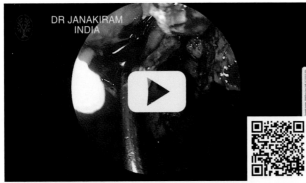

Video 11.18 A known case of coronary artery disease with post covid mucormycosis.

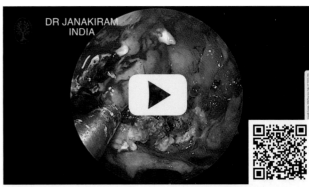

Video 11.19 A case of right orbital apex syndrome.

Interesting Cases

This chapter is a compilation of three other interesting cases treated at the authors' center. Due to space limitations, the authors did not expand it to a complete case discussion. Only the surgical videos are included here. The videos are self-explanatory.

The first case is a frontal lobe abscess drained endoscopically (**Video 11.18**). The second case is a case of OA syndrome with gross involvement of the GWS and the lesser wing of the sphenoid (**Video 11.19**). The last one is a case of crista galli involvement with gross necrosis of the pterygoid process and the GWS (**Video 11.20**).

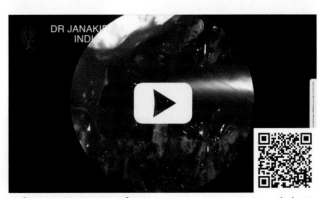

Video 11.20 A case of revision mucormycosis in a diabetic male.

References

1. Pandilwar PK, Khan K, Shah K, Sanap M, K S AU, Nerurkar S. Mucormycosis: a rare entity with rising clinical presentation in immunocompromised hosts. Int J Surg Case Rep 2020; 77:57–61

2. Singh AK, Singh R, Joshi SR, Misra A. Mucormycosis in COVID-19: a systematic review of cases reported worldwide and in India. Diabetes Metab Syndr 2021;15(4):102146

3. Khan MA, Quadri SAQ, Kazmi AS, et al. A comprehensive review of skull base osteomyelitis: diagnostic and therapeutic challenges among various presentations. Asian J Neurosurg 2018;13(4):959–970

4. Skiada A, Lass-Floerl C, Klimko N, Ibrahim A, Roilides E, Petrikkos G. Challenges in the diagnosis and treatment of mucormycosis. Med Mycol 2018;56(suppl_1):93–101

5. Dallan I, Castelnuovo P, de Notaris M, et al. Endoscopic endonasal anatomy of superior orbital fissure and orbital apex regions: critical considerations for clinical applications. Eur Arch Otorhinolaryngol 2013;270(5):1643–1649

6. Regoli M, Bertelli E. The revised anatomy of the canals connecting the orbit with the cranial cavity. Orbit 2017; 36(2):110–117

7. Ruiz-Valdepeñas EC, Julián JAS, Prat GP, et al. The quadrangular space, endonasal access to the Meckel cave: technical considerations and clinical series. World Neurosurg 2022; 163(2):e124–e136

8. Zanation AM, Snyderman CH, Carrau RL, Gardner PA, Prevedello DM, Kassam AB. Endoscopic endonasal surgery for petrous apex lesions. Laryngoscope 2009;119(1):19–25

9. Patel CR, Wang EW, Fernandez-Miranda JC, Gardner PA, Snyderman CH. Contralateral transmaxillary corridor: an augmented endoscopic approach to the petrous apex. J Neurosurg 2018;129(1):211–219

12

Postoperative Follow-Up and Management of Complications

Chapter 12

Postoperative Follow-Up and Management of Complications

Narayanan Janakiram, Shilpee Bhatia Sharma, Harshita Singh, and Lekshmy R. Kurup

Introduction

Post-COVID-19 mucormycosis at the author's center was effectively managed by a multidisciplinary team comprising otorhinolaryngologists, neurosurgeons, radiologists, ophthalmologists, orofacial maxillary surgeons, critical care physicians, nephrologists, anesthesiologists, neurophysicians, and rehabilitation specialists. This was critical to achieving the best surgical outcomes, thereby reducing overall complications, morbidity, and mortality.

The severity of the disease, the individual's immune status, and their response to systemic antifungals influence the likelihood of complications.

Complications are classified as anesthetic, medical, surgical, and psychological (**Flowchart 12.1**). Based upon duration of occurrence as intraoperative, perioperative, or postoperative, perioperative (within 1 week of surgery), early (between 1 week and 6 months), and delayed (beyond 6 months) are mentioned in **Table 12.1**.[1]

Early complications are more likely to resolve, whereas later complications are seen to persist. Even though longer follow-up is required, these findings highlight the importance of a patient's recovery and response to disease after surgery in the long term. All the complications are mentioned in **Flowchart 12.1**.

Preoperative Workup

All routine tests, including radiological imaging, complete blood profile, sugar levels with hemoglobin A1c (HbA1C), serum electrolytes, renal function tests, liver function tests, COVID-19 testing using reverse transcriptase polymerase chain reaction (RT-PCR) or rapid antigen test, and an electrocardiogram (ECG), were done in all patients. A complete 2D echocardiography was performed on the elderly and patients with underlying cardiovascular morbidity to ensure that all cardiac parameters were within normal limits.

For pulmonary assessment, computed tomography (CT) scan was performed to rule out active COVID-19 infection, in RT-PCR-negative individuals and evaluate post-COVID-19 sequelae. Airway assessment for anatomical distortion and evidence of fungal infection was done by the anesthetist. The majority of cases were categorized under difficult intubation.

Coagulation disorders were ruled out, and anticipating blood loss, cross-matching, and Rh typing were done for all cases. Informed consent was obtained after thorough discussion of all treatment options, including open, endoscopic, and combined surgical approaches and their associated risks and benefits.

Precautions to Minimize Postoperative Complications

- Strict blood sugar monitoring and administration of insulin before the surgery for optimization of sugar levels.
- Other comorbidities, like high blood pressure and asthma, were treated with supportive therapy.
- Preoperative sepsis was managed with antibiotics and antifungals.
- All anticoagulant drugs should be stopped.
- Patients were premedicated with anxiolytics, H2 blockers, and beta-blockers the night before as well on the day of surgery. Beta-blockers like metoprolol and atenolol are preferred. They improve the control over cardiovascular hemodynamic response and lowers the levels of stress-related catecholamine.[2] If beta-blockers are contraindicated, clonidine is preferred.
- After ensuring the use of adequate personal protective equipment and adequate aerosol control measures, in the operating theater, large-bore central venous lines are secured for administration of intraoperative drugs and postoperative systemic antifungal drugs.
- After preoxygenation, induction was done using remifentanil and propofol. Oral intubation was done. Tracheostomy tray or set was kept on standby whenever difficult intubation was anticipated.
- Maintenance of intraoperative anesthesia was done using sevoflurane, nitrous oxide, and vecuronium. Urinary catheterization was done in all patients for maintenance of input and output charts. Ventilation is maintained with normocapnia or mild hypocapnia (27 ± 2 mm Hg) to reduce bleeding and optimize the surgical field. Intermittent positive pressure ventilation (IPPV) was used as the mode of ventilation for all cases. Nasal packing was done using cotton pledgets

Table 12.1 Summary of postoperative complications

Duration	Anesthetic	Medical	Surgical						
			Sinonasal	Orbital	Oral	Otological	Neurological	Skin
Intraoperative	Difficult intubation TCR Bleeding Cardiopulmonary arrest		Bleeding					
Perioperative (0–7 d)		Cardiac failure (MI) Respiratory failure Acute renal failure Sepsis and shock UTI Amphotericin-related toxicity Multiorgan dysfunction Death	Pain Crusting Infection	Pain Reactionary chemosis Vision loss Ptosis	Pain Trismus Dysphagia Difficulty in phonation Wound dehiscence	Otalgia Heaviness of ear Facial palsy	Headache CSF leak Nerve palsy	Edema Hematoma Cellulitis
Postoperative								
Early								
Days 8–30		Thrombophlebitis Amphotericin-related toxicity	Crusting Anosmia PND Cough	Wound dehiscence	Trismus Dysphagia Residual		Nerve palsy	Cellulitis Abscess Sinus formation
1–3 mo		Pulmonary mucormycosis Malnutrition Weight loss	Crusting Anosmia SBO	Paresthesia	Oroantral fistula Cosmetic deformity	SOM	CSF leak Abscess	
3–6 mo		Liver failure Stoke Death	Anosmia SBO Postoperative empty nose syndrome	Epiphora Enophthalmos Cosmetic deformity		Hearing loss	Thrombosis	Cosmetic deformity
Delayed								
Beyond 6 mo till 15 mo			Residual Recurrence	Recurrence	Osteonecrosis Recurrence			

Note: Residual disease showed in our study anytime in early and delayed postoperative period. Recurrence of disease can occur anytime during the course of the postoperative period. Amphotericin-related toxicity develops bleeding at any duration throughout the course of the disease.

Abbreviations: MI, myocardial infarction; PND, post nasal discharge; SBO, surgical bed osteonecrosis; SOM; serous otitis media; TCR, trigemino cardiac reflex; UTI, urinary tract infection.

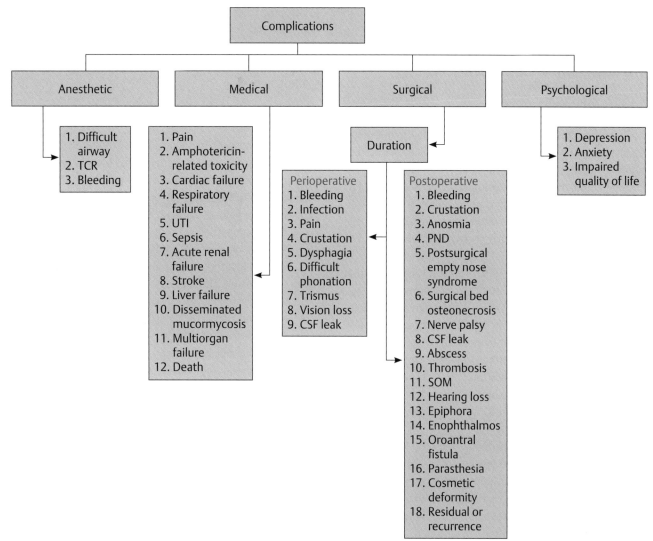

Flowchart 12.1 Flowchart depicting various complications associated with post-COVID-19 mucor. (CSF, cerebrospinal fluid; PND, post nasal drip; SOM, serous otitis media; TCR, trigeminocardiac reflex; UTI, urinary tract infection.)

soaked in a solution of xylocaine and adrenaline for nasal decongestion.

- The patient was placed in the reverse Trendelenburg position with the neck held in a neutral position, and the head slightly turned to the right. Drapes were used to cover the head and face, leaving the nose, eyes, and mouth open.

Protocol for Postoperative Management and Follow-Up

Following surgery, the patients are transferred to the intensive care unit (ICU) for optimal care.

They are kept under ICU observation for 2 to 5 days depending on the extent of the surgery and the condition of the patient. Systemic antifungal and antibiotics are administered and are actively monitored for its toxicity, urine output, and hydration. Proper nursing care is provided in its entirety.

After an endoscopic-guided pack removal and observation in the ICU, the patients are transferred to the postoperative ward. Once the general condition stabilizes, they are discharged with the advice to continue intravenous (IV) antifungals on outpatient department basis. They are also advised to continue other supportive therapies and saline nasal douching.

The follow-up care plan recommended is as follows: Weekly for 1 month, fortnightly for next 2 months, and monthly till 15 months.

Endoscopic assessment and suction clearance of nasal cavity is done at every visit. Serum inflammatory markers, electrolytes, and renal parameters are monitored during each visit. Radiological imaging with serial magnetic resonance imaging (MRI) is performed at the 1st, 3rd, 6th, and 12th month postsurgery. Cone beam CT (CBCT) was performed in the cases with any new palatal symptoms.

Intraoperative Complications

Trigeminocardiac Reflex

It is a well-studied, brainstem vagal reflex that manifests as bradycardia, asystole, hypotension, apnea, and gastric hypermotility.[3] This neurogenic response is due to stimulation and/or manipulation of the trigeminal nerve root or any of its peripheral branches. Trigeminocardiac reflex (TCR) is a well-known complication of craniomaxillary surgery, midfacial impaction, temporomandibular joint arthroscopies, and le Fort osteotomy.[4–6] Variants of TCR are the following:

- **Rhino-cardiac reflex (RCR):** This is a type of TCR that is most sensitive in the posterior nasal mucosa.[7]
- **Oculocardiac reflex (OCR):** Vagal bradycardia mediated via trigeminal nerve stimulation around the orbit, specifically tension on an extraocular muscle tendon through stretch or proprioceptors[8,9] during orbital injections or instrumentation.

Its clinical manifestations are bradycardia, nausea, faintness, and other cardiac arrhythmias. OCR has low latency and fatigability.[10–12]

Fig. 12.1 depicts the TCR pathway.[13–16]

The authors have observed TCR and its variants during disease removal from the infratemporal fossa, pterygopalatine fossa, quadrangular space, greater wing of the sphenoid, dissection around Meckel's cave, limited endoscopic orbital debridement, and transposition. In addition, it was also observed while raising the pericranial flap due to pressure effect on the supratrochlear ciliary branches of V1.[17]

To prevent TCR and OCR, surgeons are instructed to stop all surgical manipulations with immediate effect and pack the surgical field with 4% lignocaine solution and wait until sinus rhythm was achieved. The patients are administered an IV dose of an anticholinergic, that is, glycopyrrolate and/or atropine, to counter the bradycardia. If the TCR is refractory to atropine, then the treatment of choice is epinephrine.[14] A retrobulbar injection using 2 mL of 2% lidocaine could block the OCR reflex in all instances.[18] Of 193 patients operated on at author's center, 4 patients developed the above complication.

Bleeding

It is encountered both in the intraoperative and postoperative periods. Excessive bleeding is defined as bleeding more than 400 mL of blood or bleeding during a procedure that makes surgery difficult.[19] Bleeding can be classified as:

- Early/immediate bleeding: Epistaxis in the initial operating room or before discharge.[20]
- Delayed bleeding: Nose bleeds that occurred within the first 6 weeks after discharge.[20]

Factors responsible for bleeding are the following:

- Hypertension.
- Advanced age.
- Prolonged and unguarded steroid use.
- Extensive and prolonged use of anticoagulant agents for thromboprophylaxis in pateints with COVID-19 infection.[21]
- Reduced integrity of the blood vessel wall due to prior comorbidities.[22]
- Among patients at the author's center, those who received nonhumidified oxygen, a known risk factor for nasal dryness, crusting, and increased tendency of epistaxis, were also at high risk of bleeding.[23–25]

Current recommendations are to withhold both antiplatelets and anticoagulants. If the patient is at moderate to high risk of thromboembolic phenomena, the recommendation is to use LMWH to "bridge" the effect of the two anticoagulant therapies.[26]

Of the 193 patients who underwent surgery at the author's center, 25 patients presented with preoperative bleeding and about 50% patients developed excessive intraoperative bleeding. The majority of the patients with perioperative bleeding belonged to post-COVID-19 mucormycosis stage III and a patient with stage IVb disease presented with intractable bleeding for which external carotid artery ligation was performed. Early postoperative bleeding was encountered in a patient with stage IId disease, who died due to carotid blowout. All the cases were managed based upon protocol depicted in **Flowchart 12.2** and **Fig. 12.2**.

Postoperative Pain

Pain is the most common and debilitating symptom of COVID-19-associated mucormycosis. Both pre- and postoperatively, it significantly increases morbidity and mean hospital stay for patients. Various presentations included

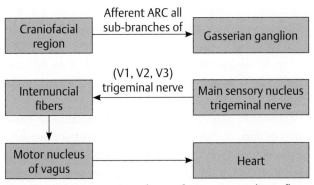

Fig. 12.1 Diagrammatic pathway of trigeminocardiac reflex.

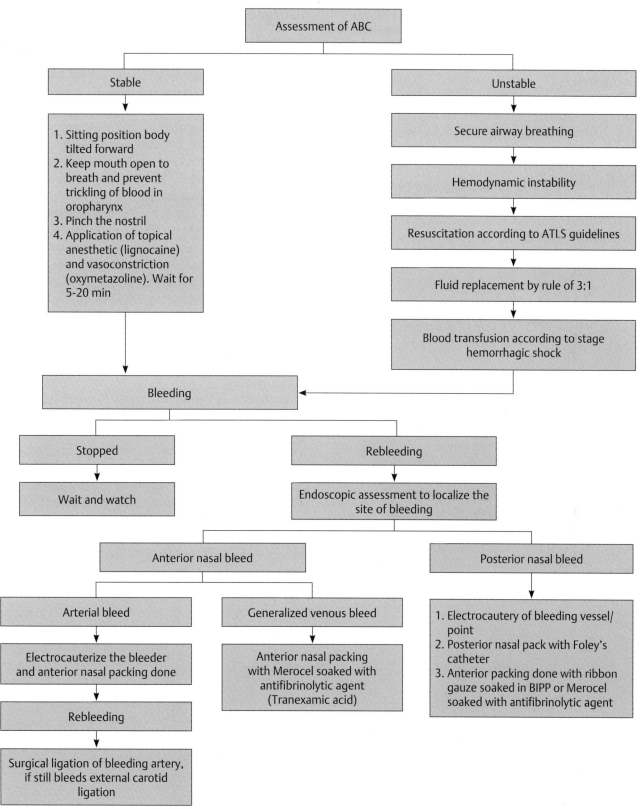

Flowchart 12.2 Algorithm depicting the protocol for management of bleeding. (ABC, airway, breathing, circulation; ATLS, advance trauma life support.)

facial pain (76%), toothache (35.2%), periorbital pain (28.5%), and headache (80.8%). Postoperatively its causes are the following:

- High level of cytokines circulating in post-COVID-19 patients.[27]
- Inflammatory response to soft-tissue and excessive bone debridement.
- Involvement and inflammation of multiple cranial nerves (CNs): optic (CN II), oculomotor (CN III), trigeminal nerve (CN IV), and all its branches, abducens, facial (CN VII), and cutaneous nerves supplying the face and higher structures.[28]
- Advanced stage of disease: Intracranial extension of disease involving the cavernous sinus and dural and meningeal layers of brain parenchyma.

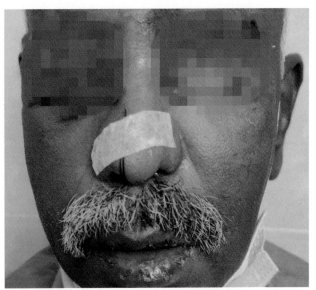

Fig. 12.2 Nasal pack in situ after postoperative nasal bleeding.

Management of Pain

Management of pain begins with optimal correction of systemic derangements such as hyperglycemia, ketoacidosis, aggressive surgical debridement, and prompt initiation of systemic antifungals. Treatment of pain is done according to World Health Organization (WHO) ladder of pain management and adjuvant therapy.

Pain was the most common immediate perioperative complication and lasted for a variable period ranging from 3 to 6 months depending on the extent of disease and patient's systemic response to antifungals and associated comorbidities. Every individual experienced a variable degree of pain throughout the course of the disease and its treatment.

Therapy is started with nonopioid analgesics (e.g., acetaminophen, nonsteroidal anti-inflammatory drugs [NSAIDs] and then work our way up to stronger analgesics until pain is relieved (**Table 12.1**). Some ladder versions include a fourth step for interventional procedures like nerve blocks or epidural infusions (**Fig. 12.3**).

Facial Edema

In an attempt to defend and repair damaged tissues, an inflammatory response to surgical procedure is initiated resulting in edema. Due to soft-tissue damage, the lymphatic system becomes inefficient at absorbing and transporting proteins.[37] The amount of blood lost during surgery is directly proportional to the degree of postoperative edema. In the author's study, almost all patients developed edema in the perioperative period, which settled by the first postoperative month. Massive facial edema was observed in patients with stage IV disease, followed by stage III, possibly because most of them underwent bicoronal/lynch–Howarth approaches (**Fig. 12.4**).

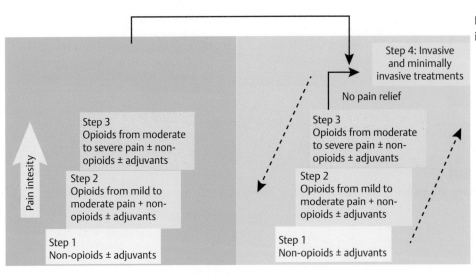

Fig. 12.3 World Health Organization pain relief ladder.

Pain intensity

Step 3
Opioids from moderate to severe pain ± non-opioids ± adjuvants

Step 2
Opioids from mild to moderate pain + non-opioids ± adjuvants

Step 1
Non-opioids ± adjuvants

Step 4: Invasive and minimally invasive treatments

No pain relief

Step 3
Opioids from moderate to severe pain ± non-opioids ± adjuvants

Step 2
Opioids from mild to moderate pain + non-opioids ± adjuvants

Step 1
Non-opioids ± adjuvants

Table 12.2 Drugs and their doses for management of pain

Drug	Class/Group	Grades of pain	Mode of delivery	Dosage	Side effects
Acetaminophen[29]	NSAIDs	Primary drug as well as combination with other drugs for mild to moderate pain (WHO step 1 analgesic) Action is limited in cases of severe pain	Oral or intravenous	4,000 mg/24 h in 4 divided doses Reduced dosage: 2,000 mg/24 h in 4 divided doses for patients with liver disease[30] FDA approved limited dose of acetaminophen about 325 mg per tablet in combination with opioids[31]	Hepatotoxicity Cautious use in patients with gastrointestinal, renal, and cardiovascular ailments
Tramadol	Opioids	Primary as well as combination therapy for moderate to severe pain (WHO step 2 analgesic)	Intravenous or intramuscular	300 mg/24 h (d)	Vomiting, gastritis, sedation, and respiratory depression
Morphine	Opioids	Primary as well as combination therapy for moderate to severe pain (WHO step 3 analgesic)	Oral, subcutaneous, intravenous, or intermittent intravenous through indwelling catheters, per rectal		Sedation, respiratory depression, and drug abuse
Fentanyl	Opioids	Moderate to severe pain (WHO step 3 analgesic)	Transdermal patch	25, 30, 50, 70 µg/h for 72 h	Irritation at local application site, sedation, and abuse
Fortwin-combination of Pentazocine and Phenergan (Promethazine)[32]	Opioid (pentazocine) and H1 blocker (promethazine)	Supportive therapy	Intramuscular	Ratio of 1:1 1 mL of pentazocine and 1 mL of promethazine	Nausea and drowsiness
Amitriptyline[33,34]	Tricyclic antidepressants inhibit norepinephrine and serotonin reuptake blocks various voltage-gated ion channels. Used as unconventional analgesic[35]	Neuropathic pain and in psychotherapy (adjuvant analgesic)	Oral	Administered as 10- or 25-mg tablet at night additionally would provide relief of depression	Orthostatic hypotension, weight gain, urinary retention, and drowsiness. May predispose to cardiac arrhythmias and heart block
Gabapentin	Analgesic inhibits Ca channel blockers, downregulates release of serotonin and inflammatory markers	Postoperative neuropathic pain (adjuvant analgesic)	Oral	Maximum of 3,600 mg/d in 3 divided doses[36] for 6–8 wk. 50–100 mg gradual reduction of dose over the next 4 wk	Dizziness, somnolence, gait disturbance, and substance abuse

(Continued)

Table 12.2 *(Continued)* Drugs and its doses for management of pain

Drug	Class/Group	Grades of pain	Mode of delivery	Dosage	Side effects
Carbamazepine	Analgesic: Acts via decreasing conductance in Na+ channels and inhibiting ectopic discharges	Postoperative neuropathic pain (adjuvant analgesic)	Oral	150- to 200-mg tablet twice daily. Dosages ranged from 300 to 2,400 mg/d in divided doses. Monitor serum electrolytes	Electrolyte imbalances, somnolence, dizziness, and gait disturbances
Alprazolam	Anxiolytic	Adjuvant therapy: Anxiety and insomnia	Oral	One 0.25- or 0.50-mg tablet at night as required	
Zolpidem	Anxiolytic	Adjuvant therapy: Anxiety and insomnia	Oral	One 10-mg tablet once at night	
Supportive adjuvant therapy					
Ondansetron	Antiemetic serotonin receptor antagonists	Adjuvant therapy	Oral or intravenous	8 mg twice a day	
Domperidone	Antiemetic	Adjuvant therapy	Intravenous/oral	30 mg/d with 10 mg stat, 20 mg sustained release	
Pantoprazole	Antacid—PPI		Intravenous or oral	40 mg once daily or 2 divided doses	
Multivitamins	Adjuvant therapy		Oral	One tablet at night	Altered taste and constipation
Combination of sodium picosulfate, milk of magnesia, and liquid paraffin	Laxative: Adjuvant therapy In severe cases, rectal suppository can be administered		Oral	10 mL at night	Nausea, altered taste, abdominal cramps, electrolyte imbalance, and rarely seizures Cautious use in patients with gastrointestinal ailments and electrolyte imbalances

Note: Patients taking NSAIDs for more than a week should also take a PPI. The peak effect of intravenous opioids occurs after about 10 minutes. The time required for opioids administered intramuscularly or subcutaneously varies, but it is usually between 20 and 30 minutes. Ibuprofen and aceclofenac are avoided due to less safety profile.
Abbreviations: FDA, Food and Drug Administration; NSAIDs, nonsteroidal anti-inflammatory drugs; PPI, proton pump inhibitor; WHO, World Health Organization.

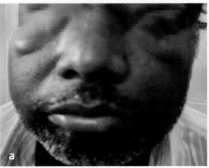 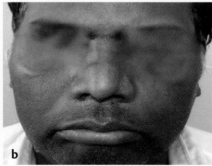

Fig. 12.4 (a) Facial edema at 10 days postoperatively. **(b)** Resolution of edema at 3 months postoperatively.

Management of Edema

- *Positioning*: A dorsal decubitus position with the head tilted by approximately 30 degrees aids in the control of edema.
- *Manual lymphatic drainage* (a mechanical method): Gentle pressure (30–40 mm Hg) helps in resolving edema by improving lymphatic drainage.[38,39]
- *Cryotherapy* is the therapeutic use of cold compressions for reducing skin and subcutaneous tissue temperature. It induces autonomic mediated vasoconstriction and controls inflammation, thus reducing pain and edema.[40,41,42]
- *Medical management*: It includes analgesics and NSAIDs. Corticosteroids are absolutely contraindicated in post-COVID-19 mucormycosis[43] (doses are given in **Table 12.1**).

Hematoma

Hematoma was noticed in patients who underwent bicoronal approach and temporalis muscle flap rotation. Thigh hematoma was noticed rarely in the cases where the fascia lata was harvested. This was managed with evacuation and tight compression dressing. At the author's center, 5 of 193 patients encountered this complication. The majority belonged to stage IV.

Infection

Surgery involving extensive soft-tissue debridement and removal of bone from the faciomaxillary region aggravates a very intense inflammatory reaction and makes the patient susceptible to infection, leading to cellulitis, abscess, and draining sinus. These complications arise during the early postoperative period.

It was noticed mostly 48 to 72 hours after surgery and was commonly seen in orbital exenterations and palatal primary closures. This was treated with culture-sensitive antibiotics, incision, and drainage following secondary suturing. Among the author's patients, three developed wound site infection in the early postoperative period and one patient operated on elsewhere presented with facial wound site abscess (**Figs. 12.5** and **12.6**).

Of 193 patients, 22 patients with stage Ib disease developed suture site infection.

Sinonasal Complications

Transnasal skull base debridement brings about inevitable damage to the nasal structures such as nasal septum and neighboring mucosa with decreased healing for weeks to even months after surgery.[23,24]

The four most common consistent signs and symptoms reported postoperatively, in order from most to least frequent, are briefly discussed here.

Nasal crusting: All patients experienced varying amount of nasal crusting initially; most of it healed by 12 to 14 weeks; delayed healing was seen in malnourished patients with poorly controlled diabetes and extensive skull base debridement (**Fig. 12.7**).

This was treated with a combination of hypertonic nasal saline and mupirocin ointment washes administered twice daily. Nasal saline irrigation (NSI) improves mucociliary clearance, decreases mucosal edema, and reduces the antigen load in the nasal cavity. Low-pressure, high-volume devices include NSI squeeze bottles and gravity-dependent irrigation pots. Hypertonic saline is the preferred option. The CDC recommends using cooled boiled water (boiled for at least 1 or 3 minutes). After each use, bottles must be sterilized or replaced every 3 months.[44] Saline nasal sprays are used to maintain nasal cavity humidification.

Consider osteonecrosis of the surgical bed or residual disease if nasal crusting persists for more than 6 months postsurgery.

Postnasal discharge (PND): It may be infectious or noninfectious in nature due to impaired mucociliary function.

To control PND-induced cough, an antihistamine is administered once at night along with an antitussive twice daily for 3 weeks. Depending on the severity of symptoms, mucolytic agents may or may not be prescribed.

Nasal airflow blockage: Nasal crusting and PND lead to a sense of obstruction.

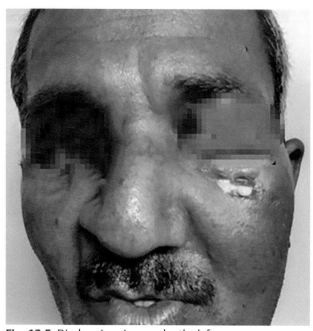

Fig. 12.5 Discharging sinus under the left eye.

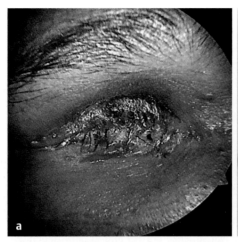
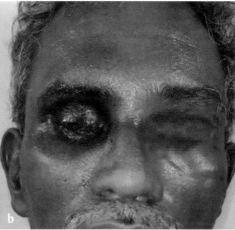

Fig. 12.6 Wound dehiscence after orbital exenteration at **(a)** Postoperative day 10 and **(b)** 4 months after surgery.

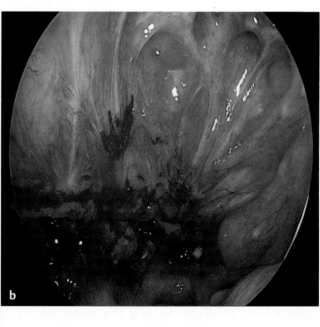

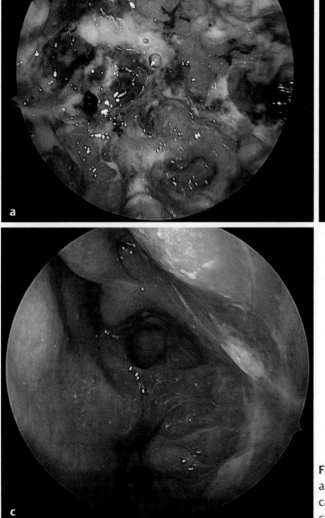

Fig. 12.7 (a) Endoscopic picture of nasal cavity showing crusting and discharge at 6 weeks postoperatively. **(b)** Endoscopic nasal cavity picture at 10 weeks postoperatively. **(c)** Endoscopic nasal cavity completely healed at 15 weeks postoperatively.

Anosmia or hyposmia: Varying degree of hyposmia/anosmia was seen in all patients who underwent extensive skull base dissections (stage III//IV/V). In the author's series, 42.3% patients experience hyposmia and 9.8% experienced anosmia.

Surgical Bed Osteonecrosis

Repeated endoscopic examination can pick up early osteonecrosis. Causes of osteonecrosis are compromised blood flow of underlying bone postsurgery, residual or recurrent disease whereby the primary site of infection is healed but the central infectious process in the bone marrow remains active (the fungal hyphae were identified in the necrotic areas and within the multinucleate giant cells[45,46] (**Fig. 12.8**). In all the patients in the author's series, this complication was encountered in stage IB (N = 12), stage III (N = 4), and stage V (N = 4).

After radiological evaluation, diseased bone was removed and histopathological corelation was done. If the results were in favor of mucormycosis, revision surgery was planned along with systemic antifungal therapy. If the results did not favor active infection, supportive therapy with tab posaconazole 200 mg twice a day was continued for an extended period of time until clinical and radiological examinations showed complete disease eradication.

Postsurgical Empty Nose Syndrome

It is an early complication that occurs 3 to 6 months after surgery. It manifests as paradoxical nasal obstruction despite a spacious nasal cavity as a result of extensive surgical debridement, resulting in impaired mucociliary function

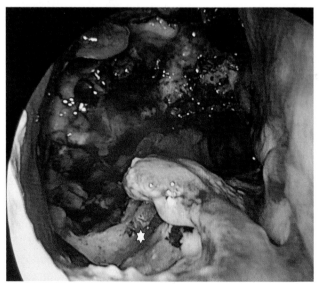

Fig. 12.8 Picture shows star mark osteonecrosis of the maxilla.

which leads to nasal dryness, rhinitis, sinusitis, decreased sense of nasal airflow, and foul smell.[47] In the author's series, 10% of patients experienced empty nose syndrome (maximum in stage III).

Treatment goals include adequate mucosal moisturization. It is achieved by means of hydration with saline or oil-based nasal preparations, adequate fluid intake, and periodic nostril closure. If the symptoms persist after a year of observation, surgery should be considered. Reconstruction of turbinatelike structure using bioimplants such as cartilage, collagen temporalis fibromuscular graft, silicone, hydroxyapatite cement, hyaluronic acid, and acellular dermal matrix has been tried.[48]

Otological Complications

Serous Otitis Media

It is a delayed complication of extensive skull base osteomyelitis of the frontal, sphenoid, and occipital bone, resulting in intense soft-tissue inflammation after surgery in and around the eustachian tube (ET), which is either physically obstructed or not functioning properly.[49,50] As a result, serous otitis media (SOM) develops resulting in otalgia, hearing loss, and generalized ear discomfort. It was encountered in five patients from the author's series.

It can be treated with local and systemic nasal decongestants. As it is recalcitrant to treatment, myringotomy with grommet insertion is done under local anesthesia.

Hearing Loss

In the patients in whom extensive skull base drilling was done, especially in the cases with medial petrous apex or clival involvement, the heat and sound of burr caused sensory neural hearing loss. In the author's series, one patient with stage IIIB typically presented with this complication, for which hearing loss was calibrated and hearing aid was advised.[51,52]

Neurological Complications

Cerebrospinal Fluid Leak

It can arise at any time in the intraoperative, perioperative, early, or delayed postoperative period. Intraoperative leaks are managed with the standard multilayer closure. Immediate postoperative leaks are managed conservatively in the initial period with supportive therapy. If the patient does not respond to treatment, they are taken under general anesthesia for localization and closure of leak. Following pack removal, they are advised to avoid any strenuous activities.

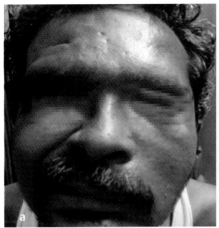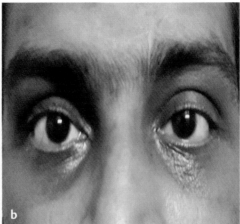

Fig. 12.9 (a) Left-sided facial palsy. **(b)** Left-sided sixth nerve palsy.

Cranial Nerve Palsy

CNs III, V, VI, and VII are commonly more affected compared to CN I, II, and IV less in rhino-orbito-cerebral mucormycosis (ROCM). The most common location is the cavernous sinus, where the third and sixth nerves are involved, but it can also occur at the orbital level. During COVID-19 Infection or the immediate post-COVID-19 period, the facial nerve (CN VII) was found to be involved at the level of the vidian canal in the nasal cavity or through perineural spread.[53] CNs I, II, and IV are affected due to direct involvement of disease as spread of mucormycosis is highly variable.

Nerve palsies may be transient, recover with time, or might be permanent with no signs of recovery (**Fig. 12.9**). There is no role for steroid therapy, an absolute contraindication in mucormycosis. If there are no signs and symptoms of disease progression after a year of follow-up, facial reanimation may be considered.

Eye care in facial palsy includes the following:
- Bandaging of eye at night.
- Antibiotic ointment application.
- Hydroxymethyl cellulose eye drops to prevent dryness of eyes.
- For lagophthalmos or lid lag, blepharoplasty or gold implants can be performed.

At the author's center, 5 of 193 patients presented with facial nerve palsy immediately after COVID-19 infection preoperatively, which did not show any signs of recovery.

Cerebral Abscess

Three of 193 patients at the author's center developed intracerebral abscesses following complete drainage of initial abscess. One patient developed occipital abscess and two other patients developed recurrent temporal lobe abscess. Serial MRI of the brain with diffusion-weighted imaging (DWI) sequence were taken in all patients to assess the development of abscess and the patients were monitored

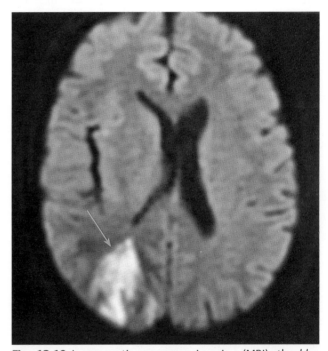

Fig. 12.10 In magnetic resonance imaging (MRI), the *blue arrow* shows the right-sided occipital lobe abscess.

for any new symptoms or signs. All three patients developed neurological symptoms and they underwent transcranial drainage of the abscess. There was no reported mortality in the author's series (**Fig. 12.10**).

Thrombosis

Mucormycosis is angiotropic, with preference for arterial elastic membranes. The spores multiply in the elastic lamina of the arteries; the hyphae erode the endothelium of the vessel walls, causing necrosis and extensive thrombosis of the main cerebral vessels such as the internal carotid artery (ICA), basilar artery, cavernous and dural venous sinuses.[54,55]

MRI with DWI, fluid-attenuated inversion recovery (FLAIR) sequencing, MR angiography, and venography

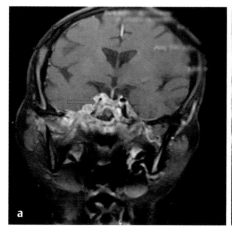
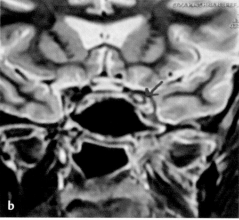

Fig. 12.11 Magnetic resonance imaging (MRI) plates. **(a)** Right carotid artery thrombosis (*bold blue arrow*). **(b)** Left cavernous sinus thrombosis (*red line arrow*).

were done to make a radiological diagnosis (**Fig. 12.11**). Anticoagulation therapy was initiated to prevent thrombus propagation, to aid in the recanalization of the lumen of occluded cerebral arteries and veins. Hence, preventing further complication such as deep venous thrombosis (DVT) and pulmonary embolism (PE).

Postoperative ICA thrombosis was seen in four of the author's patients. One patient developed pseudoaneurysm of the carotid artery and is asymptomatic. A total of eight patients had cavernous sinus thrombosis. Even though ICA thrombosis carries poor prognosis, all the author's patients survived, possibly due to chronicity of the condition and good collateral circulation.[49,55,56]

Oral Complications

Trismus

It is an early and most debilitating complication. At the author's center, about 18.6% patients witnessed trismus in the perioperative period and resolved within 3 months postsurgery (**Fig. 12.12**).

Swallowing Difficulty or Dysphagia

Initial gastrointestinal endoscopy was performed to rule out spread of disease followed by functional endoscopic evaluation of swallowing (FEES) to identify level of obstruction following extensive surgery involving skull base and oral cavity. For its further management, patients were referred to specialists for rehabilitation.

Protocol for Oral Cavity Care

- Patients are kept nil per oral for 2 days postoperatively Feeding is done through a Ryle tube.
- Initiation of clear liquid fluids with a straw from POD3 to POD5. Dairy items are strictly prohibited.

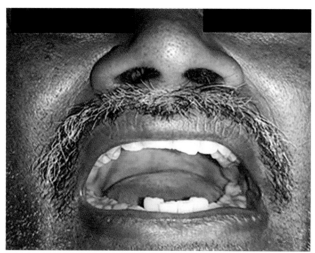

Fig. 12.12 Trismus in the first month postsurgery.

- Maintain adequate hydration and nutrition with protein-rich diet.
- Oral rinses in 1:1 dilution.
- Topical application of antibiotic ointment.
- Continue systemic antifungal, antibiotics, analgesic, and anti-inflammatory drugs.
- After POD10, start with mouth-opening exercises using therabite and massage of the face.
- New alternative therapy that can be tried is Botox injection. It is given intramuscularly and is believed to decrease pain, improve function, and mouth opening at doses ranging from 25 to 150 U into the temporalis and masseter muscles.[56]

Altered Taste

Altered taste is seen in few patients who underwent extensive sinonasal or faciomaxillary surgery. Nutritional supplementation and maintenance of oral hygiene help recover taste.

In addition, there is a high probability that the patient will not recover completely due to loss of sensation caused by disease-induced nerve (glossopharyngeal) damage and surgical debridement resulting in hyposmia. It was witnessed in all cases perioperatively and in the early postoperative period and improved by 6 months.

Difficulty in Phonation

A patient with difficulty in phonation is referred to a speech-language pathologist for rehabilitation.

Palatal Discoloration

It can occur at any time during the postoperative period and indicates disease progression, either residual or recurrence. A biopsy of the discolored segment is sent for potassium hydroxide (KOH) mounting and HPE (**Fig. 12.13**).

If the mucor fungi test is positive, a CBCT scan of the palate is performed to identify the areas involved in order to plan revision surgery in conjunction with medications. Supportive therapy with tab posaconazole is extended until mucosa heals.

Loose Tooth

It indicates compromised blood supply to the palate and disease progression. Osteonecrotic foci with removal of the teeth should be done and reconstruction with an obturator and prothesis is required. Active mucor infection warrants a revision surgery. In the author's study, seven patients presented with this complication, and they were managed accordingly.

Oroantral Fistula

A pathological epithelialized unnatural communication between the oral cavity and the maxillary sinus that is occupied by granulation and polyposis from a debrided sinonasal cavity is known as an oroantral fistula.

It usually happens 1 to 3 months after surgery. Surgery is planned based on the size of the fistula. CBCT is a precise investigation tool that can detect sinus floor discontinuity, sinus opacification, or communication between the oral cavity and the sinus (**Fig. 12.14**). Small fistulas spontaneously close. Buccal flaps are frequently used to close small to moderate-sized defects. A palatal mucoperiosteal rotation flap is best suited for a chronic oroantral fistula.[57]

Other options for oroantral fistula repair include free mucosal flaps, collagen, fibrin glue, auricular cartilage, tongue flap, temporalis fascia flap, dura, and bones such as zygoma, iliac crest, septal cartilage, as well as synthetic metals such as gold and titanium, depending on surgeon expertise.[58] At the author's center, six patients who encountered this issue belonged to stage III (N04) followed by stage Ib (N02).

Orbital Complications

Reactionary Chemosis

It is a perioperative complication caused by surgically induced inflammation of orbital structures. Complete visual examination, including movements in all directions, should be done. Topical antibiotic eye drops are given in tapering doses over a 7- to 10-day period. Cold compresses are given around the eyes as a form of supportive therapy. Almost all patients belonged to stage III (N26) followed by stage IV.

Infraorbital Nerve Paresthesia

This complication is common due to infraorbital nerve involvement after extensive surgical approaches such as the endoscopic modified Denker's procedure. Injury to the nerve can occur during drilling of the anterolateral wall of the maxilla or removal of infection from the infraorbital nerve in the superior part of the infratemporal fossa. It was witnessed in about 20% of all the patients in the author's study.

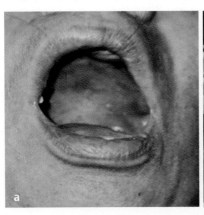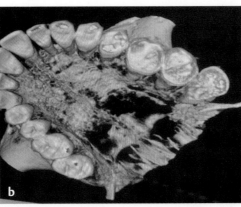

Fig. 12.13 (a) Palatal discoloration at 2 months postoperatively. **(b)** Cone beam computed tomography (CT) scan with 3D reconstruction shows palatal bone erosion.

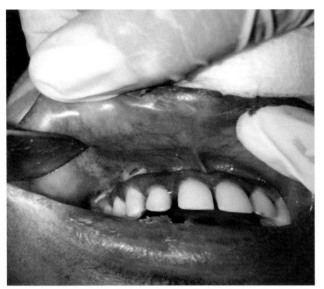

Fig. 12.14 Demonstrating oroantral fistula at 2 months postoperatively.

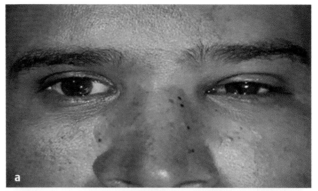

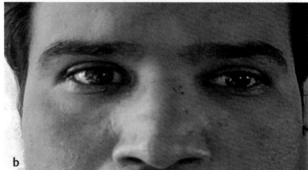

Fig. 12.15 (a) Perioperative ptosis and reactionary chemosis. **(b)** Demonstration of the recovery of ptosis and reactionary chemosis in the early postoperative period.

Loss of Vision

It is an irreversible complication caused by central retinal artery occlusion (CRAO). Depending on the involvement of the intraconal and extraconal compartments, and the patient's consent, orbital exenteration with or without a lid-sparing surgery is planned. At the author's center, eight patients went for orbital exenteration and two patients lost vision and did not give consent for the same.

Ptosis

It is an early complication caused by the involvement of CNIII or surgery-induced trauma. It is transient and will gradually recover within months. At the author's center, patients with stage II (N17), stage III (N12), and stage IV (N7) disease presented with ptosis and recovered within 3 months after surgery (**Fig. 12.15**). After a brief period of observation, if there are no signs of recovery, then surgical repair is best accomplished with frontal suspension using a silicone (silastic) rod.[59] Surgery was considered in two patients.

Enophthalmos

It develops within 3 to 6 months postoperation due to fibrosis and contracture of the orbital soft tissue. When the periorbita is intact and an isolated orbital wall such as lateral, medial, and roof is involved, no reconstruction is required.

Large defects of the periorbita should be repaired using the temporalis fascia or temporalis muscle sling. Removal of the orbital floor, more than two-thirds of bone, if excised, always requires a primary reconstruction. Sometimes 3D reconstruction of the orbit is considered.[60]

Of the 64 revision cases at the author's center, three patients belonged to stage IV. Reconstruction was done with the temporalis muscle sling along with titanium plates and screw to provide support to underlying structures (**Fig. 12.16**).

Ophthalmoplegia

At the author's center, only three of the patients developed ophthalmoplegia (**Fig. 12.17**).

Epiphora

It can be an early or delayed complication. Depending on the duration, epiphora can be early or delayed complication, either it is transient or permanent as a result of reflex to inflammation, mechanical blockage, or permanent anatomical damage to the nasolacrimal duct system.[61] If transient management is conservative, which resolves within weeks after the wait-and-watch protocol, repeated endoscopic nasal cleaning and proper nasal douching are advised. Endoscopic dacryocystorhinostomy was performed in one patient at 7 months postsurgery consistent with epiphora.

Cosmetic Deformity

This complication developed in the early postoperative period. At the author's center, about 50 patients suffered

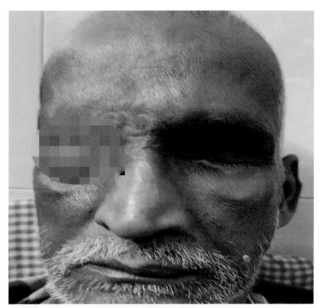

Fig. 12.16 Enophthalmos at 4 months postsurgery.

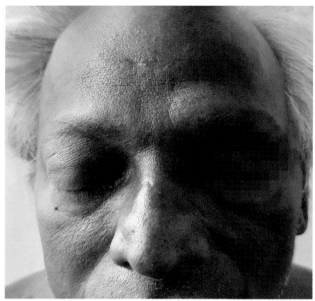

Fig. 12.17 The patient developed complete ophthalmoplegia immediately after surgery.

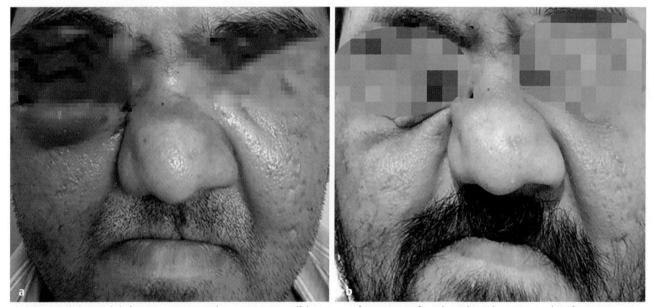

Fig. 12.18 (a) Facial deformity at 3 months postsurgery. **(b)** Picture of a patient after dental implant 6 months after surgery.

cosmetic deformity, with the majority in stage III, followed by stage IV and stage1B. The correction of cosmetic deformity after palatal resection is discussed in detail in Chapter 8 (**Fig. 12.18**). The rehabilitation of a patient with orbital exenteration done by fabricating a prosthesis that combines heat polymerized polymethyl methacrylate and room temperature vulcanizing silicone prosthetic material. Support the globe if it is preserved or fill the orbital cavity if the globe is exenterated. Depending upon the degree of defect, it is repaired using the radial forearm fasciocutaneous, osseocutaneous, or rectus abdominis myocutaneous flap. Structures such as the lips, eyelids, and nose should be reconstructed separately, usually with local flaps.[62,63] For bone defects as in stage IV, impression of bone should be obtained and constructed with mesh or bone cement. For reconstruction, no signs of residual or recurrent disease should be present and it should be done by specialists.

Residual Disease

It is defined as when a patient has symptoms and radiological evidence of mucormycosis without a disease-free interval due to incomplete disease clearance or improper healing and closure of the primary site of infection due to new bone formation.

Insufficient dose and inability of antifungals IV drugs to penetrate the site of infection due to the vaso-occlusive nature of the disease also result in a residual disease.[44]

At the author's center, 14 of 193 patients had residual disease, and 7 had revision surgery followed by antifungal therapy. The remaining seven patients who refused revision surgery were managed with extended medical therapy. All these patients are all doing well (**Fig. 12.19**).

Recurrence of Disease

Clinical symptoms or radiological evidence of mucormycosis may reappear after a brief disease-free interval following complete surgical resection until normal healthy tissue bleeding is observed or a disease-free healthy margin on HPE is observed and the recommended antifungal dose is administered. This is most likely because partial treatment resulted in healing and new bone formation at the primary site of infection while the central infective process in the bone marrow progressed.[46]

In the author's study of the 193 primary and secondary cases, 10 patients had disease recurrence. One patient each

witnessed progression of disease 2 months postsurgery in pulmonary mucormycosis and stroke in third month postoperatively. Management was done by both the physician and the otorhinolaryngologist simultaneously (**Fig. 12.20**).

Morbidity and Mortality

Postoperative discomfort is minimal for patients undergoing endoscopic skull base surgery when compared to transcranial and transfacial approaches, and several studies report good outcomes in quality-of-life measures as well as reduced hospital stay.[64]

The main advantages of an endoscopic and combined approach include reduced morbidity due to the avoidance of any brain retraction and osteotomies, resulting in a shorter mean hospital stay.[65,66,67]

At the author's center, 12 of 193 (0.06%) patients died. Of these, five (41.7%) were primary cases and seven (58.3%) were revision cases. The majority of patients belonged to stage III following stages V and IV of disease and died in period ranging from day 3 to 2 months post surgery.

All medical complications and amphotericin-B–related toxicity are discussed in **Tables 12.3** and **12.4**.

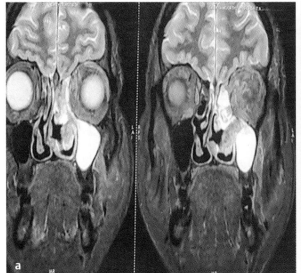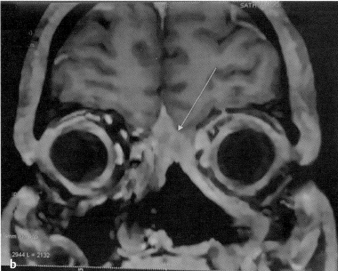

Fig. 12.19 (a) Magnetic resonance imaging (MRI) sequence showing mucormycosis in the left sinonasal orbital area. **(b)** MRI scan at 3 months of follow-up shows progression of disease in the left frontal area marked by the *white arrow*.

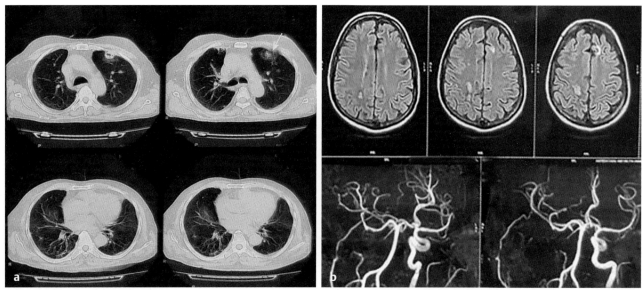

Fig. 12.20 (a) Infective foci in pulmonary mucormycosis (*yellow arrow*). **(b)** Magnetic resonance imaging (MRI) flair sequence shows hyperintense lesion in venous circulation in the parietal lobe leading to ischemia and stroke.

Table 12.3 Medical complications and its management

Sepsis and septic shock	ARF	Cardiac arrest (MI)	Respiratory failure	Stroke
Life-threatening organ dysfunction caused by a host response to infection. Sepsis-induced hypotension is regarded septic shock, and aggressively managed	ARF, defined as increase in serum creatinine level of 0.5 mg/dL or 50% in creatinine above the baseline, 50% decrease in the baseline GFR[3,4] or A sudden decline in GFR ranging from minutes to days resulting in acid–base disbalance, electrolyte imbalance, and accumulation of nitrogenous product[5]	It is a known complication in post-COVID-19 mucormycosis due angioinvasion of blood vessel by organisms resulting in septic thromboembolic phenomenon leading to MI. Stress cardiomyopathy can lead to sudden heart block	ARDS is defined as acute lung inflammation and increased permeability, leading to hypoxemic respiratory failure. On radiodiagnosis, bilateral pulmonary opacities may be noted	It arises due to thrombosis of cerebral artery leading to infarction leading to neurological deficits

(Continued)

Table 12.3 *(Continued)* Medical complications and its management

Sepsis and septic shock	ARF	Cardiac arrest (MI)	Respiratory failure	Stroke
Sepsis six protocol 1. Maintain high oxygen flow 2. Get blood culture report done 3. Send serum lactate and blood count 4. Start empirically IV antibiotics therapy 5. Start with fluid resuscitation 6. Monitor urine output	In authors' study, ARF is encountered as a result of amphotericin-B toxicity (leads to acute tubular necrosis). It leads to intrarenal type of ARF *Specific investigations to be done* 1. Urine osmolarity 2. BUN-to-creatinine ratio 3. Urine: Na concentration 4. Urine-specific gravity 5. FENa%	1. After securing airway, breathing, and circulation 2. ECG should be recorded 3. Based on it, MI should be differentiated between non-ST segment elevation and ST segment elevation MI and treatment based on AHA guidelines 4. In authors' study, MI caused by thromboembolic phenomenon, so discussed below 5. Thrombolytic therapy leads to dissolution of fibrin clot	1. Follows Berlin criteria 2. Treatment of precipitating factors 3. Get biomarkers tested, i.e., nitrous oxide	*Prethrombolysis treatment* 1. Intubation and supplement oxygen if SpO_2 < 75%, maintain breathing and circulation 2. Do not lower the blood pressure rapidly unless the patient is with known cardiac morbidity 3. Do not administer antithrombolytics unless hemorrhagic stroke is ruled out 4. Immediately neuroimaging, i.e., CT scan should be done
Consider intubation and ventilation CVP line → fluids <8 mm Hg / 8–12 mm Hg MAP → vasopressor <65 mm Hg / >65 mm Hg O_2 levels → transfuse blood if <70% / >70% ← less Hb treated ← Inotropic drug no Norepinephrine is drug of choice, followed by epinephrine and/or low-dose vasopressin as second line of drug	1. Maintain adequate hydration 2. Strictly maintain urine output 3. Serum metabolic acidosis is treated with sodium bicarbonate 4. Treatment of hyperkalemia by dietary restricts and resins 5. Consider hemodialysis 6. To increase renal perfusion vasopressor to be administered	*Drugs used in* 1. Alteplase tissue plasminogen activator given in a dose of 100 mg/h. 2. urokinase not specific for fibrin clot 3. streptokinase, many complications associated with it Along with antiplatelets drugs based on AHA guidelines	1. Management of ABC 2. Fluid restriction 3. Management of blood transfusion-related lung injury 4. Mechanical ventilation 5. Position of patient in prone position for 12 h 6. Nutritional support 7. Sedation 8. Neuromuscular blockade 9. Pulmonary artery vasoconstriction reversed by vasodilators drugs such as inhaled nitrous oxide and prostacyclin 10. Corticosteroids 11. Oxygen supplementation[6]	Femoral line to be established Consider intra-arterial urokinase or t-PA IV in dose of 0.9 mg/kg, monitor vitals and local for sites of bleeding If bleeding present, apply compression at local site. Consider transfusion of FFP, cryoprecipitate, and platelets Further management should be done by neurosurgeon, vascular surgeon, and neurophysician

Abbreviations: ABC, airway, breathing, circulation; AHA, American Heart Association; ARDS, acute respiratory distress syndrome; ARF, acute renal failure; CT, computed tomography; CVP, central venous pressure; ECG, electrocardiogram; FENa, fractional excretion of sodium; FFP, fresh frozen plasma; GFR, glomerular filtration rate; IV, intravenous; MI, myocardial infarction; t-PA, tissue plasminogen activator.

Table 12.4 Amphotericin-B–related toxicity and its management

Type of complications	Mechanism of action	Duration from therapy initiation	Clinical features	Treatment
Allergic reactions	Release of prostaglandin E2	Within 5 min	Bronchospasm, tachypnea, dyspnoea, flushing, urticaria, and severe laryngospasm	IV diphenhydramine 50 mg and hydrocortisone 100 mg IV IV epinephrine
Infusion-related toxicity	Release of proinflammatory cytokine from innate cells	Range: 45 min to 72 h	Fever, headache, chills, rigors, nausea, vomiting, myalgia, and arthralgia C-reactive proteins are elevated during rapid infusion, so daily monitoring of levels for the first 3 d, followed by alternate day monitoring	Slow infusion rate of Amp-B, hydration, NSAIDS, and ibuprofen (10 mg/kg) Meperidine (45 mg) IV for rigors given before 30 min In severe symptoms, injection IV hydrocortisone 100 mg given in selected patients
Thrombophlebitis	Irritation of veins by coagulation of colloid (5% dextrose)	2 wk and beyond	Pain and swelling at local site	1. Application of hot packs 2. Application of drug combination heparin and benzyl nicotinate 3 times 3. Slow infusion of drug over 4–6 h 4. Rotation of infusion site, preferred central line 5. Small size needle 6. Systemic heparin sodium (500–1,000 units) with infusion
Nephrotoxicity 1. Creatine increase 2. Hypokalemia 3. Hypomagnesemia 4. Hyponatremia 5. Hypophosphatemia 6. Hypernatremia 7. Hyperkalemia 8. Hypocalcemia	1. Vasoconstriction of smooth muscle in preglomerular complex results in reduced blood flow, hence reduced GFR and decreased renal clearance 2. Altered membrane permeability by oxidative stress, ionophoric action and forming pores in cells, more profound in renal tubules	Reversible damage starts within 2 wk of treatment	Oliguria, polyuria pedal edema, hypotension, cardiac abnormalities, drowsiness, altered mental status, seizures, generalized weakness, ascending paralysis, and paralytic ileus ECG conducted	1. Hydration pre- and postinfusion of 1 L (0.9%) normal saline before 60 min of amphotericin infusion Posthydration: 500 mL (0.9%) normal saline Or alternatively hydration with ORS can be done 2. Dose escalation over days and prolonged time of infusion of drug 3. Discontinue the concomitant nephrotoxic drugs such as diuretic, aminoglycosides All electrolyte deficits should not be corrected by rapid infusion over short duration

(Continued)

Table 12.4 *(Continued)* Amphotericin-B–related toxicity and its management

Type of complications	Mechanism of action	Duration from therapy initiation	Clinical features	Treatment
Hypokalemia Normal value: 3.5–5 mmol/mL	1. Intramembranous vacuolization of epithelial cells in renal tubules 2. Renal tubule acidosis 3. Reduced absorption from distal colon	Dose-dependent reversible damage beyond 2 wk of therapy	*Lab parameters* Mild: <3–3.5 mmol/mL Moderate: <2.5 mmol/mL Severe: <2 mmol/mL	*Mild to moderate loss* 1. Supplementation of potassium-rich food 2. Liquid preparation Syrup KCL (potassium chloride) 5 mL twice daily till the level is normal *Severe loss* 3. IV KCL 20 meq/L in 100 mL over 20–60 min or 1–2 mEq/KCL/d of potassium citrate or potassium bicarbonate over 2 divided doses 4. Potassium-sparing diuretic tab amiloride or spironolactone can be used
Hypomagnesemia Normal value: 1.46–2.68 mg/dL	1. Due to renal tubular acidosis and associated losses	Dose-dependent reversible loss beyond weeks of therapy	Mild: 1.2–1.4 mg/dL Severe: <1.2 mg/dL	*Mild to moderate loss:* Magnesium sulfate or chloride or citrate tablet in 15–20 mmol/d in 2 or more divided doses *Severe loss* 4 mEq/mL of IV magnesium sulfate diluted in 5% glucose: about 8–12 g in the first 24 h, followed by 4–6 g the next 3–4 d
Hyponatremia Normal value: 135 mmol/mL	1. Due to decreased absorption from renal tubules	Dose-dependent reversible loss beyond 6–10 wk of therapy	Mild: <132 mmol/mL Moderate: 121–130 mmol/mL Severe: <120 mmol/mL	1. Salt-rich diet 2. 3% nasal saline infusion 1 mL/kg/h over 6–8 h. Slowly 3. Tab demeclocycline 300 mg twice 4. Inj conivaptan 20 mg over 30 min on day 1 and 20–40 mg from day 2 onward
Amphotericin-induced SIADH	1. Inhibited action on ADH-dependent sodium reabsorption in renal tubules	Dose-dependent reversible beyond 2 wk of treatment or 10 g or more drug	Na >155 mmol/mL	1. Fluid restriction 2. Inj DDAVP (35 μg) IV
Hematological effects 1. Anemia 2. Thrombocytopenia 3. Leukopenia	1. Inhibition of erythropoiesis and erythropoietin production 2. Secondary renal toxicity	After 3 wk	Pallor, bleeding, increased WBC counts, infections	1. Add syrup hematinic 2. Blood transfusion, if required
Hepatoxicity (rare)	Secondary to renal toxicity; exact mechanism still unclear	Prolonged treatment beyond 4–6 wk	*Elevated levels of* 1. Alkaline phosphate 2. SGOT 3. SGPT 4. Bilirubin	1. Stop the drug at least 24–42 h 2. High-protein diet in the form of albumin

Abbreviations: Amp-B, amphotericin-B; DDAVP, desmopressin acetate; ECG, electrocardiography; GFR, glomerular filtration rate; inj, injection; IV, intravenous; KCL, potassium chloride; NSAIDs, nonsteroidal anti-inflammatory drugs; ORS, oral rehydration solutions; SGOT, serum glutamic-oxaloacetic transaminase; SGPT, serum glutamate pyruvate transaminase; SIADH, syndrome of inappropriate antidiuretic hormone secretion.

References

1. Naunheim MR, Sedaghat AR, Lin DT, et al. Immediate and delayed complications following endoscopic skull base surgery. J Neurol Surg B Skull Base 2015;76(5):390–396

2. Rahimzadeh P, Faiz SH-R, Alebouyeh MR. Effects of premedication with metoprolol on bleeding and induced hypotension in nasal surgery. Anesth Pain Med 2012;1(3):157–161

3. Chowdhury T, Sandu N, Sadr-Eshkevari P, Meuwly C, Schaller B. Trigeminocardiac reflex: current trends. Expert Rev Cardiovasc Ther 2014;12(1):9–11

4. Lübbers H-T, Zweifel D, Grätz KW, Kruse A. Classification of potential risk factors for trigeminocardiac reflex in craniomaxillofacial surgery. J Oral Maxillofac Surg 2010; 68(6):1317–1321

5. Kratschmer F. On reflexes from the nasal mucous membrane on respiration and circulation. Respir Physiol 2001; 127(2–3):93–104

6. Widdicombe J. Reflexes from the lungs and airways: historical perspective. J Appl Physiol 2006;101(2):628–634

7. Yang MB, Zhao HL, Lan JP, Qiu SQ. Nasal-cardiac reflex initiated by nasal packing (three cases report and literature review) [in Chinese]. Lin Chung Er Bi Yan Hou Tou Jing Wai Ke Za Zhi/J Clin Otorhinolaryngol 2012;26(3):120–122

8. Dunville LM, Sood G, Kramer J. Oculocardiac reflex. Treasure Island, FL: StatPearls Publishing; 2022

9. Bosomworth PP, Ziegler CH, Jacoby J. The oculo-cardiac reflex in eye muscle surgery. Anesthesiology 1958;19(1):7–10

10. Sires BS, Stanley RB Jr, Levine LM. Oculocardiac reflex caused by orbital floor trapdoor fracture: an indication for urgent repair. Arch Ophthalmol 1998;116(7):955–956

11. Smith RB. Death and the oculocardiac reflex. Can J Anaesth 1994;41(8):760

12. Arnold RW, Dyer JA, Gould AB Jr, Hohberger GG, Low PA. Sensitivity to vasovagal maneuvers in normal children and adults. Mayo Clinic Proc 1991;66(8):797–804

13. Schaller BJ, Filis A, Buchfelder M. Trigemino-cardiac reflex in humans initiated by peripheral stimulation during neurosurgical skull-base operations. Its first description. Acta Neurochir (Wien) 2008;150(7):715–717, discussion 717–718

14. Arasho B, Sandu N, Spiriev T, Prabhakar H, Schaller B. Management of the trigeminocardiac reflex: facts and own experience. Neurol India 2009;57(4):375–380

15. Kosaka M, Asamura S, Kamiishi H. Oculocardiac reflex induced by zygomatic fracture; a case report. J Craniomaxillofac Surg 2000;28(2):106–109

16. Lang S, Lanigan DT, van der Wal M. Trigeminocardiac reflexes: maxillary and mandibular variants of the oculocardiac reflex. Can J Anaesth 1991;38(6):757–760

17. Bainton R, Barnard N, Wiles JR, Brice J. Sinus arrest complicating a bitemporal approach to the treatment of pan-facial fractures. Br J Oral Maxillofac Surg 1990;28(2):109–110

18. Garrity JA, Yeatts RP. The oculocardiac reflex with an orbital tumor. Am J Ophthalmol 1984;98(6):818

19. Ramadan HH, Allen GC. Complications of endoscopic sinus surgery in a residency training program. Laryngoscope 1995;105(4, Pt 1):376–379

20. Zimmer LA, Andaluz N. Incidence of epistaxis after endoscopic pituitary surgery: proposed treatment algorithm. Ear Nose Throat J 2018;97(3):E44–E48

21. Lodigiani C, Iapichino G, Carenzo L, et al; Humanitas COVID-19 Task Force. Venous and arterial thromboembolic complications in COVID-19 patients admitted to an academic hospital in Milan, Italy. Thromb Res 2020;191:9–14

22. Thongrong C, Kasemsiri P, Carrau RL, Bergese SD. Control of bleeding in endoscopic skull base surgery: current concepts to improve hemostasis. ISRN Surg 2013;2013:191543

23. Poiroux L, Piquilloud L, Seegers V, et al; REVA Network. Effect on comfort of administering bubble-humidified or dry oxygen: the Oxyrea non-inferiority randomized study. Ann Intensive Care 2018;8(1):1–9

24. Miyamoto K, Nishimura M. Nasal dryness discomfort in individuals receiving dry oxygen via nasal cannula. Respir Care 2008;53(4):503–504

25. Strumpf DA, Harrop P, Dobbin J, Millman RP. Massive epistaxis from nasal CPAP therapy. Chest 1989;95(5):1141

26. Douketis JD, Woods K, Foster GA, Crowther MA. Bridging anticoagulation with low-molecular-weight heparin after interruption of warfarin therapy is associated with a residual anticoagulant effect prior to surgery. Thromb Haemost 2005;94(3):528–531

27. Pinto LG, Pinho-Ribeiro FA, Verri WA Jr. Cytokines and pain. Front Immunol 2021;12:788578

28. Mohindra S, Mohindra S, Gupta R, Bakshi J, Gupta SK. Rhinocerebral mucormycosis: the disease spectrum in 27 patients. Mycoses 2007;50(4):290–296

29. Groninger H, Vijayan J. Pharmacologic management of pain at the end of life. Am Fam Physician 2014;90(1):26–32

30. Bosilkovska M, Walder B, Besson M, Daali Y, Desmeules J. Analgesics in patients with hepatic impairment: pharmacology and clinical implications. Drugs 2012;72(12):1645–1669

31. Chun LJ, Tong MJ, Busuttil RW, Hiatt JR. Acetaminophen hepatotoxicity and acute liver failure. J Clin Gastroenterol 2009;43(4):342–349

32. Lalfamkima F, Debnath SC, Adhyapok AK. A study of promethazine hydrochloride and pentazocine intramuscular sedation along with 2% lidocaine hydrochloride and adrenaline and comparison to placebo along with 2%

lidocaine hydrochloride and adrenaline for surgical extraction of mandibular third molar. J Maxillofac Oral Surg 2015;14(1):90–100

33. Thompson DF, Brooks KG. Systematic review of topical amitriptyline for the treatment of neuropathic pain. J Clin Pharm Ther 2015;40(5):496–503

34. Moore RA, Derry S, Aldington D, Cole P, Wiffen PJ. Amitriptyline for neuropathic pain in adults. Cochrane Database Syst Rev 2015;7(7):CD008242

35. Lunn MP, Hughes RA, Wiffen PJ. Duloxetine for treating painful neuropathy, chronic pain or fibromyalgia. Cochrane Database Syst Rev 2014;1(1):CD007115

36. Mathieson S, Lin CW, Underwood M, Eldabe S. Pregabalin and gabapentin for pain. BMJ 2020;369:m1315

37. Ebert JR, Joss B, Jardine B, Wood DJ. Randomized trial investigating the efficacy of manual lymphatic drainage to improve early outcome after total knee arthroplasty. Arch Phys Med Rehabil 2013;94(11):2103–2111

38. Kasseroller RG. The Vodder school: the Vodder method. Cancer 1998;83(12, Suppl American):2840–2842

39. Rockson SG, Miller LT, Senie R, et al. American Cancer Society Lymphedema Workshop. Workgroup III: diagnosis and management of lymphedema. Cancer 1998;83(12, Suppl American):2882–2885

40. Greenstein G. Therapeutic efficacy of cold therapy after intraoral surgical procedures: a literature review. J Periodontol 2007;78(5):790–800

41. Osunde OD, Adebola RA, Omeje UK. Management of inflammatory complications in third molar surgery: a review of the literature. Afr Health Sci 2011;11(3):530–537

42. Beech AN, Haworth S, Knepil GJ. Effect of a domiciliary facial cooling system on generic quality of life after removal of mandibular third molars. Br J Oral Maxillofac Surg 2018;56(4):315–321

43. Yaedu RYF, Mello MdAB, da Silveira JSZ, Valente ACB. Edema management in oral and maxillofacial surgery. In: Kumar V, Salgado AA, Athari SS, eds. Inflammation in the 21st Century. London: IntechOpen; 2018

44. Succar EF, Turner JH, Chandra RK. Nasal saline irrigation: a clinical update. Int Forum Allergy Rhinol 2019;9(S1):S4–S8

45. Goel A, Kini U, Shetty S. Role of histopathology as an aid to prognosis in rhino-orbito-cerebral zygomycosis. Indian J Pathol Microbiol 2010;53(2):253–257

46. Kohut RI, Lindsay JR. Necrotizing ("malignant") external otitis histopathologic processes. Ann Otol Rhinol Laryngol 1979;88(5, Pt 1):714–720

47. Chand MS, MacArthur CJ. Primary atrophic rhinitis: a summary of four cases and review of the literature. Otolaryngol Head Neck Surg 1997;116(4):554–558

48. Kuan EC, Suh JD, Wang MB. Empty nose syndrome. Curr Allergy Asthma Rep 2015;15(1):493

49. Khan MA, Quadri SAQ, Kazmi AS, et al. A comprehensive review of skull base osteomyelitis: diagnostic and therapeutic challenges among various presentations. Asian J Neurosurg 2018;13(4):959–970

50. Johnson CM, Wise SR, Balough BJ, Johnson TE. Unilateral adult-onset otitis media with effusion—is flexible nasopharyngoscopy enough? AAO-HNS Poster; 2009

51. Samii M, Tatagiba M. Skull base trauma: diagnosis and management. Neurol Res 2002;24(2):147–156

52. van der Valk J, Treurniet F, Koopman JP, Koppen H. Severe daily headache as an uncommon manifestation of widespread skull base osteomyelitis. Case Rep Neurol 2019;11(2): 178–182

53. Swift AC, Denning DW. Skull base osteitis following fungal sinusitis. J Laryngol Otol 1998;112(1):92–97

54. Turunc T, Demiroglu YZ, Aliskan H, Colakoglu S, Arslan H. Eleven cases of mucormycosis with atypical clinical manifestations in diabetic patients. Diabetes Res Clin Pract 2008; 82(2):203–208

55. Takahashi S, Horiguchi T, Mikami S, Kitamura Y, Kawase T. Subcortical intracerebral hemorrhage caused by mucormycosis in a patient with a history of bone-marrow transplantation. J Stroke Cerebrovasc Dis 2009;18(5):405–406

56. Song PC, Schwartz J, Blitzer A. The emerging role of botulinum toxin in the treatment of temporomandibular disorders. Oral Dis 2007;13(3):253–260

57. Anavi Y, Gal G, Silfen R, Calderon S. Palatal rotation-advancement flap for delayed repair of oroantral fistula: a retrospective evaluation of 63 cases. Oral Surg Oral Med Oral Pathol Oral Radiol Endod 2003;96(5):527–534

58. Parvini P, Obreja K, Sader R, Becker J, Schwarz F, Salti L. Surgical options in oroantral fistula management: a narrative review. Int J Implant Dent 2018;4(1):40

59. Finsterer J. Ptosis: causes, presentation, and management. Aesthetic Plast Surg 2003;27(3):193–204

60. DeMonte F, Tabrizi P, Culpepper SA, Abi-Said D, Soparkar CN, Patrinely JR. Ophthalmological outcome following orbital resection in anterior and anterolateral skull base surgery. Neurosurg Focus 2001;10(5):1-6

61. Osguthorpe JD, Calcaterra TC. Nasolacrimal obstruction after maxillary sinus and rhinoplastic surgery. Arch Otolaryngol 1979;105(5):264–266

62. Miles BA, Sinn DP, Gion GG. Experience with cranial implant-based prosthetic reconstruction. J Craniofac Surg 2006;17(5):889–897

63. Santamaria E, Cordeiro PG. Reconstruction of maxillectomy and midfacial defects with free tissue transfer. J Surg Oncol 2006;94(6):522–531

64. McCoul ED, Anand VK, Bedrosian JC, Schwartz TH. Endoscopic skull base surgery and its impact on sinonasal-related quality of life. Int Forum Allergy Rhinol 2012;2(2):174–181

65. Su SY, Kupferman ME, DeMonte F, Levine NB, Raza SM, Hanna EY. Endoscopic resection of sinonasal cancers. Curr Oncol Rep 2014;16(2):369

66. Castelnuovo P, Battaglia P, Turri-Zanoni M, et al. Endoscopic endonasal surgery for malignancies of the anterior cranial base. World Neurosurg 2014;82(6, Suppl):S22–S31

66. Hagemann J, Roesner J, Helling S, et al. Long-term outcome for open and endoscopically resected sinonasal tumors. Otolaryngol Head Neck Surg 2019;160(5):862–869

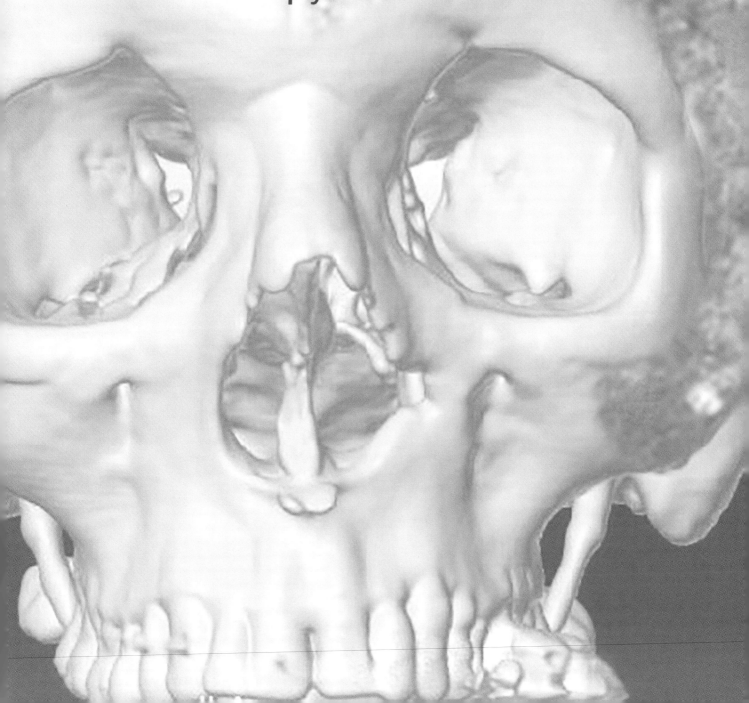

13

Postoperative Medical Therapy

Chapter 13

Postoperative Medical Therapy

Neha Mishra and Sampath Chandra Prasad Rao

The Organism and Pathogenesis

The Mucorales are ubiquitous in nature and grow rapidly in decaying soil and veg organic matter releasing large number of spores. The genera most commonly found causing human infections are *Rhizopus, Mucor,* and *Rhizomucor* (**Fig. 13.1**). Other species like *Cunninghamella, Absidia,* and *Saksenaea* may cause infection, but these are comparatively less frequent.[1]

Mode of transmission depends on the site of involvement:

- Rhino-orbito-cerebral (ROCM) and pulmonary mucormycosis is through inhalation of spores.
- Cutaneous mucormycosis is generally through inoculation of spores on a breached skin or mucosa.
- Renal mucormycosis is through unsterile scopes.
- It can show hematogenous spread to any remote site as well.

The infection through the agent of mucormycosis is an angioinvasive that leads to infarction of the vessels and causes necrotic eschar that is the hallmark of the disease.[2]

The intact innate immunity is important to prevent mold infection; therefore, only individuals with neutropenia and functional deficiency of polymorphonuclear leukocytes are at higher risk of developing this disease.[3] Intact phagocytic function is important to prevent the development of mucormycosis, although T cells are not necessarily responsible for this activity. Both polymorphonuclear and mononuclear phagocytes of healthy human being are responsible for the production of the cationic peptides and oxidative metabolites, which in turn are responsible for killing of the fungal spores.[4]

For cutaneous mucormycosis, intact skin and mucosa play the role of a barrier as agents of mucormycosis are typically incapable of penetrating the intact skin.[5]

Iron overload and usage of iron chelators like deferoxamine predispose to development of mucormycosis. The iron chelator acts as a siderophore that increases the iron uptake by the fungus stimulating fungal growth and leading to tissue invasion.[6]

Even patients with diabetic ketoacidosis have high serum iron levels, which may predispose them to infection in the presence of acidic pH.[7]

Normal human sera inhibits growth of Rhizopus, due to special ability to produce enzyme ketone reductase which allows them to thrive on high glucose levels, for example, conditions like diabetic ketoacidosis.[8]

Common risk factors predisposing an individual to develop mucormycosis are the following[9]:

- Diabetes and diabetic ketoacidosis.
- Steroid usage.
- Hematological malignancies and related transplants.
- Solid organ transplants.
- Iron overload and treatment with chelators like deferoxamine.
- Trauma and burn.

Management

Managing mucormycosis is a task that requires addressing multiple modalities. The aim of management is to reduce disease progression and further disease burden.

Management can be broadly divided into three categories, which are as follow (**Flowchart 13.1**):

- Addressing the predisposing factors.
- Medical management (antifungals).
- Surgical management.

One should address on each of them simultaneously in order to achieve optimal disease control and better patient outcome.

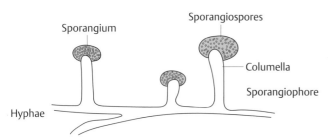

Fig. 13.1 The structure of *Rhizopus.*

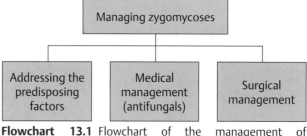

Flowchart 13.1 Flowchart of the management of mucormycosis.

Addressing the Predisposing Factors

Mucorales are ubiquitous in nature and not everyone who comes in contact with it develops the infection. There are certain risk factors that make an individual prone to this infection. Hematopoietic transplantation, malignancies, and uncontrolled diabetes are the most common risk factors predisposing to the development of this disease.[10]

Risk factors for developing mucormycosis should possibly be eliminated; if not, we must try and reduce it to bare minimum. For example, if the individual is diabetic, then we must try to achieve optimal glycemic index or if the patient is on immunosuppressive drugs, then the dose of medication should be reduced to as low as possible.

Antifungal Drugs

Amphotericin-B (AmB) is the first-line therapy drug for mucormycosis. Other azoles like posaconazole and isavuconazole may also be used as an alternative and/or continuation therapy.

Structure of a Fungal Cell and Sites of Action of Available Antifungals

The fungal cell wall is composed of chitin, glucans, glycoprotein, and mannans. This wall is important for fungal survival, and it also serves as a barrier. Most of the available antifungals works on the cell wall.

The cell membrane is made up of a phospholipid bilayer with ergosterol embedded in between the layers. It is a sterol responsible for cell membrane integrity and fluidity.

The antifungal drugs that are used for the treatment of mucormycosis belong to the polyenes and azoles group. Both these classes of antifungals primarily act on the cell wall and cell membranes of the fungal cell.

Mechanism of Action of Polyenes

AmB is the drug of choice for mucormycosis and the drug primarily acts by binding with ergosterol. It forms a complex that leads to breach in cell membrane by the formation of pores that causes leakage of monovalent ions, leading to cell death. AmB can also lead to oxidation reactions leading to production of free radicals, which further impairs the membrane's permeability and adds up to its fungicidal activity (**Fig. 13.2**).[11]

Mechanism of Action of Azoles

This group of drugs inhibits cytochrome P450 enzyme, 14α-demethylase, which catalyzes the conversion of lanosterol to ergosterol, thus preventing ergosterol biosynthesis. It primarily affects the integrity, morphology, and growth of fungal cell (**Flowchart 13.2**).[12]

Microbiology

The most common species responsible for invasive mucormycosis remains *Rhizopus*, *Mucor*, *Lichtheimia*, and *Rhizomucor*. AmB is a broad-spectrum antifungal with known activity against most fungi. Mucorales are sensitive to AmB if resistance leads to invasive spread of disease.[13]

Fungal organisms that are in vitro resistant to Mucormycosis are *Aspergillus terreus*, *Cladophialophoria carrionii*, *Candida lusitaniae*, *Scedosporium*, and *Fusarium*.[14,15,16,17]

C. auris has variable susceptibility with 10 to 15% reported resistance.

Among the azole posaconazole and isavuconazole are known to have lower minimum inhibitory concentrations (MIC) for Mucorales. Fluconazole is not known to have mold activity and voriconazole is known to have higher in vitro MIC against *mucor*. Although itraconazole has been found to

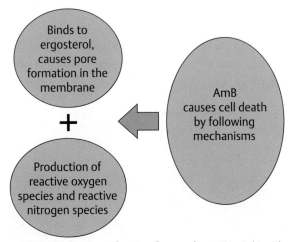

Fig. 13.2 Mechanism of action for amphotericin-B (AmB).

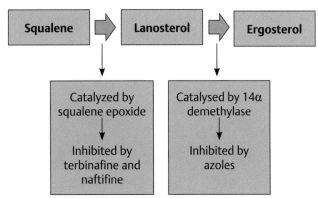

Flowchart 13.2 Mechanism of action of azoles: Inhibition of ergosterol production at various steps.

have good activity against *L. corymbifera* and *R. pusillus* in the available in vitro data, it is a drug with poor bioavailability and does not achieve desirable therapeutic levels. Hence, its utility is limited in this particular pathology.[13]

Medical Management

Medical management should start as soon as evidence of disease is confirmed. The best case scenario is a microbiologically and/or pathologically confirmed disease with evidence of tissue or angioinvasion. In some cases, with underlying hematological disease, for example, posttransplant patients with low platelets or increased risk of bleeding, it might be practically difficult to take a biopsy or confirm it on tissue basis. In such cases, the clinical picture including symptomatology along with the underlying risk factors and typical radiological signs should be looked upon and the decision should be taken after finding enough reasons to start antimold drugs.

The drugs used and the protocols generally followed are described in **Table 13.1** and **Flowchart 13.3**, respectively.

Drug of Choice

AmB has remained the first line of treatment until more data on the efficacy of other drugs used as first-line medication become available.

The reason for the enhanced antifungal activity of this molecule could be more than one antifungal effect on fungal cells. AmB is available in three types of formulations: liposomal (remains the drug of choice), lipid, and conventional formulations. Liposomal and lipid formulations are less nephrotoxic. The conventional formulation is the most nephrotoxic of the three formulations. The dosage of the drugs varies depending on the type of formulation being used.

The dosage ranges from 5 to 10 mg/kg. In available data, higher doses have been associated with better treatment response, but this can also lead to increased incidence of nephrotoxicity. Slow escalation of doses is generally discouraged and it is better to start at the adequately calculated weight-based doses from the beginning itself.[18] The dose of liposomal AmB (LAMB) may be increased depending upon the site of involvement. LAMB dose as high as 10 mg/kg can be used for central nervous system (CNS) disease. If the CNS is spared, then 5 mg/kg of body weight has proven to be beneficial.

The generally prescribed dose of conventional AmB is 0.5 to 1 mg/kg body weight. The major limitation of the deoxycholate formulation is its associated nephrotoxicity.[19]

Cost of lipid and liposomal formulations adds to the financial burden associated with the management of the disease.

Table 13.1 Protocol for drug administration and its toxicity

Drug	Dosage	Toxicity	Monitoring
Amphotericin-B*	• Liposomal (LAMB): 5-10 mg/kg once daily • Lipid complex: 5 mg/kg once daily • Conventional: 0.3-1 mg/kg once daily	• Nephrotoxicity (renal tubular damage and renal vasoconstriction) • Hypokalaemia • Hypomagnesemia • Severe rigors • Fever while infusion • Anemia • Cytopenia	• Monitor kidney function and serum electrolytes • Watch for enhanced renal toxicity when being used with other nephrotoxic drugs
Posaconazole	• Oral suspension – 200 mg four times a day • Delayed release tablets – 300 mg twice a day on first day, followed by once a day • Injection – 300 mg twice a day on first day followed by 300 mg once daily	• Nausea, vomiting, pain abdomen, diarrhea, headache, rash • Transaminitis • If treated for more than 6 months, then can lead to QTc prolongation, adrenal insufficiency, nephrotoxicity	• Check for interaction prior to initiation of the drug • Monitor liver functions
Isavuconazole	200 mg daily thrice on days 1 and 2 followed by 200 mg once daily	• Nausea, vomiting, pain abdomen, diarrhea, headache, backpain, hypokalemia, peripheral edema, cough, dyspnea • Deranged liver functions	• Monitor liver function tests • Check for interaction with other drugs

*Reconstitution of the drug should be done with 5% Dextrose, DO NOT reconstitute with saline.

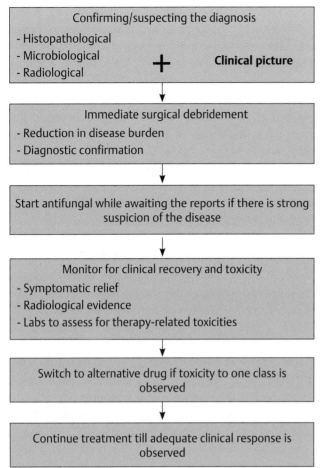

Confirming/suspecting the diagnosis
- Histopathological
- Microbiological
- Radiological

+ **Clinical picture**

Immediate surgical debridement
- Reduction in disease burden
- Diagnostic confirmation

Start antifungal while awaiting the reports if there is strong suspicion of the disease

Monitor for clinical recovery and toxicity
- Symptomatic relief
- Radiological evidence
- Labs to assess for therapy-related toxicities

Switch to alternative drug if toxicity to one class is observed

Continue treatment till adequate clinical response is observed

Flowchart 13.3 Flow diagram suggesting the protocol when mucormycosis is suspected and diagnosed

Lipid preparations do not contain deoxycholate, which is directly nephrotoxic. Liposomes allow delivery of the drug directly to the reticuloendothelial cells where the drug interacts with the trapped fungi, and delivery to the cholesterol-containing cells is limited. Hence, the toxicity is limited.[19]

Azoles like posaconazole and isavuconazole have been used for the treatment of mucormycosis either as a continuation therapy or as salvage therapy. These can be considered as first-line therapy drugs if there is underlying renal dysfunction or intolerance to AmB.

Combination Therapy

There are no data available to guide the usage of two antifungals concomitantly for mucormycosis. Dual antifungals have been tried in patients with isolation of more than one pathogenic mold. The available data are too limited to support for the combination of AmB with azole or echinocandins beyond a marginal recommendation. Moreover, the problem of enhanced toxicity, drug interaction, and additional cost remains while using the same combination of drugs.

We need to evaluate the outcomes and probably larger studies are necessary to prove the benefit of the combination of AmB with azole or echinocandins.[18]

Salvage Therapy

Only two drugs are available and the question of salvage comes only when the patient has intolerance to one class of drug, for example, when there is nephrotoxicity due to AmB or hepatotoxicity due to mold-active azole.

The other reason that may lead to switch of the therapy can be drug resistance to mucormycosis, which depends on the species and epidemiology.

Duration

The exact duration of treatment of this ailment is not known. Most of the guidelines suggest continuing the treatment till the immunosuppression is reversed, that is, till diabetes is controlled, neutropenia is resolved, and immunosuppressive therapy is complete. The drugs should be continued till the signs and symptoms are completely resolved. The imaging finding can be used as a guide to further look at the outcome.

As per the author's experience, it is better to treat it like an osteomyelitic disease and considering the duration of at least 4 to 6 weeks of intravenous therapy followed by oral medications, especially in ROCM. This is followed by complete clinical and radiological evaluation about the residual or reoccurrence of disease depending upon the diagnosis and duration of treatment of the disease.

Factors that may reduce AmB-related nephrotoxicity are the following:
- Salt loading helps in preventing AmB-related decline in glomerular filtration rate. Therefore, giving saline prior to administration of AmB prevents rise in creatinine.
- Avoid concomitant usage of nephrotoxic drugs like aminoglycosides.

It should be understood that it is a multimodality treatment and should simultaneously involve people from different specialties like an ENT (ear, nose, and throat) surgeon, skull base surgeon, plastic surgeon, infectious disease specialist, endocrinologist, nephrologist, radiologist, microbiologist, pathologist, physicians, etc.

The combined effort from all is required to tackle this particular ailment.

Other Modalities for Treatment of Mucormycosis

- *Hyperbaric oxygen therapy (HBOT)*: It is known to have benefits in nonhealing ulcers, osteomyelitis, and other diseases like decompression injuries, carbon monoxide poisoning, and radiation injuries. This technique involves inhaling 100% oxygen for a certain time at a certain pressure and it primarily works by reduction in edema by vasoconstriction and decrease in leucocyte chemotaxis and adhesion. It has been used as an adjunctive therapy in certain refractory cases of mucormycosis. The evidence available is in the form of case reports; therefore, more detailed and comprehensive studies are still required to prove the benefit of this therapy.[20,21,22]

- Recent analyses revealed that HBOT helps in reducing post-COVID-19 ROCM-associated mortality when used in patients who are generally nonresponsive to conventional therapy. Hence, it can be considered an adjunctive therapy in patients who are nonresponsive to surgical and medical management or do not tolerate the drugs due to their toxicity.[23]

- *Iron chelators*: Iron chelators that act as siderophore (e.g., deferoxamine) can increase the risk of mucormycosis by causing iron overload. Other iron chelators like deferasirox and deferiprone do not act as siderophore and hence have been tried in the management of mucormycosis. Most of the studies that have shown the benefits of iron chelators are animal-based studies. However, the DEFEAT Mucor trial done on humans has shown increased mortality when compared to the treatment of choice.[24]

- *Other antifungals*: Information available about the usage of other antifungals in such cases is very limited. Drugs like echinocandins have been tried earlier in experimental murine models and have demonstrated synergistic action when used in combination with AmB,[25,26] although larger human trials are necessary to prove the benefits of the same.

References

1. Roden MM, Zaoutis TE, Buchanan WL, et al. Epidemiology and outcome of zygomycosis: a review of 929 reported cases. Clin Infect Dis 2005;41(5):634–653

2. Greenberg RN, Scott LJ, Vaughn HH, Ribes JA. Zygomycosis (mucormycosis): emerging clinical importance and new treatments. Curr Opin Infect Dis 2004;17(6):517–525

3. Gil-Lamaignere C, Simitsopoulou M, Roilides E, Maloukou A, Winn RM, Walsh TJ. Interferon- γ and granulocyte-macrophage colony-stimulating factor augment the activity of polymorphonuclear leukocytes against medically important zygomycetes. J Infect Dis 2005;191(7):1180–1187

4. Ibrahim AS, Spellberg B, Walsh TJ, Kontoyiannis DP. Pathogenesis of mucormycosis. Clin Infect Dis 2012; 54(Suppl 1):S16–S22

5. Gartenberg G, Bottone EJ, Keusch GT, Weitzman I. Hospital-acquired mucormycosis (*Rhizopus rhizopodiformis*) of skin and subcutaneous tissue: epidemiology, mycology and treatment. N Engl J Med 1978;299(20):1115–1118

6. Maertens J, Demuynck H, Verbeken EK, et al. Mucormycosis in allogeneic bone marrow transplant recipients: report of five cases and review of the role of iron overload in the pathogenesis. Bone Marrow Transplant 1999;24(3):307–312

7. Singh AK, Singh R, Joshi SR, Misra A. Mucormycosis in COVID-19: a systematic review of cases reported worldwide and in India. Diabetes & Metabolic Syndrome: Clinical Research & Reviews. 2021;15(4):102146

8. Gale GR, Welch AM. Studies of opportunistic fungi. I. Inhibition of *Rhizopus oryzae* by human serum. Am J Med Sci 1961;241:604–612

9. McNulty JS. Rhinocerebral mucormycosis: predisposing factors. Laryngoscope 1982;92(10, Pt 1):1140–1143

10. Farmakiotis D, Kontoyiannis DP. Mucormycoses. Infect Dis Clin North Am 2016;30(1):143–163

11. Ahmad A, Wei Y, Syed F, et al. Amphotericin B-conjugated biogenic silver nanoparticles as an innovative strategy for fungal infections. Microb Pathog 2016;99:271–281

12. Scorzoni L, de Paula E Silva AC, Marcos CM, et al. Antifungal therapy: new advances in the understanding and treatment of mycosis. Front Microbiol 2017;8:36

13. Borman AM, Fraser M, Patterson Z, Palmer MD, Johnson EM. In vitro antifungal drug resistance profiles of clinically relevant members of the Mucorales (mucoromycota) especially with the newer triazoles. J Fungi (Basel) 2021;7(4):271

14. Steinbach WJ, Benjamin DK Jr, Kontoyiannis DP, et al. Infections due to *Aspergillus terreus*: a multicenter retrospective analysis of 83 cases. Clin Infect Dis 2004;39(2):192–198

15. Nucci M, Anaissie E. Fusarium infections in immunocompromised patients. Clin Microbiol Rev 2007;20(4):695–704

16. Meletiadis J, Meis JFGM, Mouton JW, Rodriquez-Tudela JL, Donnelly JP, Verweij PE; EUROFUNG Network. In vitro activities of new and conventional antifungal agents against clinical *Scedosporium* isolates. Antimicrob Agents Chemother 2002;46(1):62–68

17. Kontoyiannis DP, Lewis RE. Antifungal drug resistance of pathogenic fungi. Lancet 2002;359(9312):1135–1144

18. Cornely OA, Alastruey-Izquierdo A, Arenz D, et al; Mucormycosis ECMM MSG Global Guideline Writing Group. Global guideline for the diagnosis and management of mucormycosis: an initiative of the European Confederation of Medical Mycology in cooperation with the Mycoses Study Group Education and Research Consortium. Lancet Infect Dis 2019;19(12):e405–e421

19. Mistro S, Maciel I de M, de Menezes RG, Maia ZP, Schooley RT, Badaró R. Does lipid emulsion reduce amphotericin B

nephrotoxicity? A systematic review and meta-analysis. Clin Infect Dis 2012;54(12):1774–1777

20. Barratt DM, Van Meter K, Asmar P, et al. Hyperbaric oxygen as an adjunct in zygomycosis: randomized controlled trial in a murine model. Antimicrob Agents Chemother 2001;45(12):3601–3602

21. Ferguson BJ, Mitchell TG, Moon R, Camporesi EM, Farmer J. Adjunctive hyperbaric oxygen for treatment of rhinocerebral mucormycosis. Rev Infect Dis 1988;10(3):551–559

22. Memar MY, Yekani M, Alizadeh N, Baghi HB. Hyperbaric oxygen therapy: Antimicrobial mechanisms and clinical application for infections. Biomed Pharmacother 2019; 109:440–447

23. Sultan A. Mucormycosis (black fungus): newest threat post Covid-19 infection. Int J Oral Health Dent. 2021;7(2):75-76

24. Spellberg B, Ibrahim AS, Chin-Hong PV, et al. The Deferasirox-AmBisome Therapy for Mucormycosis (DEFEAT Mucor) study: a randomized, double-blinded, placebo-controlled trial. J Antimicrob Chemother 2012;67(3):715–722

25. Ibrahim AS, Gebremariam T, Fu Y, Edwards JE Jr, Spellberg B. Combination echinocandin-polyene treatment of murine mucormycosis. Antimicrob Agents Chemother 2008;52(4):1556–1558

26. Reed C, Bryant R, Ibrahim AS, et al. Combination polyene-caspofungin treatment of rhino-orbital-cerebral mucormycosis. Clin Infect Dis 2008;47(3):364–371

14

Exploring the Future

Chapter 14

Exploring the Future

Sampath Chandra Prasad Rao and Ananth Chintapalli

Introduction

With its prevalence increasing particularly in a developing country such as India to 0.14 cases per 1,000 population, which is 80 times higher than what it is in the developed countries, mucormycosis is indeed a disease of concern least to say. Newer risk factors such as postpulmonary tuberculosis and chronic renal disease are adding to the etiologies, and with the lifestyles of the populations at large changing rapidly and quite significantly, so is the incidence of lifestyle-related comorbidities such as diabetes mellitus which happens to be the main underlying disease globally particularly in India. Hematological malignancies and organ transplantation are the leading causes of mucormycosis in developed countries. The diagnostic tools are advancing and detecting newer species of fungi such as Apophysomyces or Saksenaea complex.

Due to newer fungal species (e.g., *Thamnostylum lucknowense*, *Mucor irregularis*, *Rhizopus homothallicus*, etc.) diagnosis of fungal diseases is becoming even more challenging. Time plays a vital factor in the outcome of mucormycosis as any delay in diagnosis of the condition has high rates of mortality. For long, the clinical evaluation even at best has a low sensitivity and specificity. Clinical examination, laboratory investigations such as radiological evaluation, histopathology, and microbiology still are essentially the mainstay of diagnosing the condition.

Diabetes Mellitus and Diabetic Ketoacidosis

As the leading cause of mucormycosis, diabetes mellitus has almost doubled in its prevalence from 4.7% in the 1980s to 8.5% in the adult population globally (age-standardized). The prevalence of diabetes mellitus is much more rapid in the low- and middle-income countries than in the high-income countries. A more recent review by Jeong et al suggests diabetes mellitus as the most common underlying condition in as much as 40% of the cases, 20% of which had ketoacidosis.[1] As the population of people with diabetes, especially uncontrolled type II, is expected to increase, so are the number of mucormycosis cases. In India, the apparent cases of mucormycosis is unveiling the underlying diabetes mellitus in as much as 12 to 31% of the cases.

With a complex disease process, diabetes mellitus has environmental and genetic factors playing significant roles in determining the deranged secretion of insulin from the beta cells of the pancreas and peripheral insulin resistance such as in the muscle, liver, and adipose tissue resulting in reduced response of these tissues to insulin. In those individuals who are at risk of developing type II diabetes mellitus, the body initially tries to compensate the reduced tissue sensitivity to insulin by secreting more of it by the beta cells of the pancreas, thus resulting in hyperinsulinemia in the initial stages, and it is later when these beta cells burn out and fail to compensate the levels of insulin required by the body that frank diabetes mellitus ensues. Despite significant involvement of molecular and genetic factors in the pathogenesis of diabetes mellitus, and significant progress being achieved in managing the condition, the genetic causes of insulin resistance still remain elusive.

Various genes involved in diabetes mellitus, especially which influence hepatic and peripheral insulin resistance, adipogenesis, and beta cell mass and their function, have been identified using candidate gene association, linkage, and genome-wide association studies focusing on the role of genetic factors in the development of type II diabetes mellitus. The loss of a gene, the high-mobility group A1 (HMGA1), which significantly increases the risk of developing type II diabetes mellitus in humans and mice has been newly identified and studied. The variants of these genes are identified to be associated with insulin resistance among certain human races such as the white Europeans, Chinese, and Americans with Hispanic pedigree, which indicates a vast scope for further research in genetics and molecular studies to learn and help better understand how to prevent type II diabetes mellitus and in turn infections associated with it such as mucormycosis.

Hematological Malignancies and Hematopoietic Stem Cell Transplantation

Unlike in India, hematological malignancies are mainly acute myeloid leukemia, and hematopoietic stem cell transplantation is the major underlying cause which leaves the patient highly susceptible to mucormycosis. Lymphoblastic leukemia, myeloblastic syndrome, non-Hodgkin's lymphoma, and other malignancies are the causes in a lesser number of cases. The risk of mucormycosis is significantly higher among those patients with prolonged neutropenia.

Solid Organ Malignancies and Solid Organ Transplantation

The prevalence of solid organ malignancies and their transplantation are less when compared to the hematological malignancies and hematopoietic stem cell transplantation. Nevertheless, these conditions leave the individuals vulnerable to develop mucormycosis. The incidence also varies among the organ transplanted, the highest incidence being among the individuals receiving lung transplantation, followed by heart, liver, and renal in that order. Tacrolimus, a calcineurin inhibitor class of drugs, given as an immunosuppressant to transplant recipients was associated with a lower risk of mucormycosis. Calcineurin plays an important role in virulence and pathogenicity of several opportunistic fungi.

Corticosteroids and Other Immunosuppressive Agents

The immune suppressing effect of corticosteroids used in the medical management of autoimmune disorders, malignancies, and transplant recipients plays an important role in the etiopathogenesis of mucormycosis. Usage of high-dose systemic corticosteroids for more than 3 weeks significantly increases the risk of contracting mucormycosis. There are several reports of mucormycosis even with usage of short course of high-dose systemic corticosteroids. Administration of high doses of systemic corticosteroids to the patients affected with COVID-19 infection has significantly increased the incidence of mucormycosis. Prolonged usage of corticosteroids will lead to drug-induced diabetes and derange the functional capacity of the macrophages by impairing their ability of migration, ingestion, and phagolysosome fusion in the macrophages.

Breakthrough Mucormycosis

Breakthrough mucormycosis is when an individual receiving antifungal therapy for instance as a prophylactic measure as in an immune suppressed patient of transplant recipient develops mucormycosis. Reports suggest that patients receiving prophylactic voriconazole and echinocandins while being highly efficient against *Aspergillus* might actually increase the virulence of certain Mucorales.[2] Prophylactic therapy with the newer azole group of antifungals like posaconazole and isavuconazole has also witnessed breakthrough

invasive mucormycosis, despite their proved activity against the Mucorales. Factors which influence breakthrough mucormycosis depend on the specific mold active antifungal used, patient characteristics, and local epidemiology.

Going Forward

From the times since its initial reports and medical documentation, the understanding of mucormycosis has indeed evolved to a great extent as evident in the advanced therapeutics, albeit with a constant progress and yet significant mortality and morbidity, in treating the dreaded condition. In the COVID-19 era, it is now more than ever deemed appropriate to identify the disease in advance. With significant developments in understanding the pathophysiology of the disease, and with all the evidence, it is now clear that mucormycosis, as the medical world understands, is essentially a "cause–effect" analogy. The research must focus more, as is already, on the lines of averting mucormycosis than treating it, enriching its early detection in the vulnerable population. Demographics indeed have a significant role to play and so does the genetic constitution, the role of food that is consumed, and the pharmacokinetics of the drugs, both targeting the fungal disease and those used in treating the etiological factors in different populations, need to be meticulously researched.

Surgical Aspects

Surgical dimension of managing rhino-orbito-cerebral mucormycosis (ROCM) will always remain the mainstay treatment. Extensive and prompt debridement of the necrotic and toxic tissue from the involved areas significantly reduces the toxic burden and improves the outcomes quite significantly. With the latest advances in the surgical equipment and the anterior skull base approaches becoming more and more less invasive, the shift of the focus needs to be more toward salvaging the organs and healthy tissue without compromising on disease clearance.

Management of the orbit in ROCM plays a crucial role, and whether the globe needs to be debrided is a decision-making facet of the disease. Although orbital exenteration improves the prognosis of the patient, total removal of the orbital contents is cosmetically challenging for the patient and the treating surgeon alike. The indications for it remaining unclear, without concrete protocols, it is often a surgical challenge to decide.

With newer minimally invasive and less radical surgical principles being developed, owing to the development of newer pharmacological molecules against the pathogen, better understanding of the pathogen, and newer precision surgical equipment and better radiological studies, it is now becoming more feasible to adopt procedures that are less debilitating. The main concern of addressing the orbit is the potential of intracranial spread of the fungus if any infected tissue is left unattended. Ommaya reservoir is a synthetic dome placed extracranially and its catheter intracranially for drug delivery. The reservoir can be placed around the orbit or the frontal sinuses and the antifungal drug Amphotericin-B Liposomal (LAMB) be delivered into the cerebrospinal fluid (CSF) space, thus reducing the intracranial dissemination of the fungus.

Increasing Role and Significance of Neuronavigation

The anterior skull base procedures have now become more conservative and less invasive, and the shift has been from more radical and more open procedures to less invasive and less functionally and cosmetically debilitating approaches. Rigid endoscopes have become the conventional mode of access for the modern sinus and anterior skull base surgery. The anatomical landscape of this area has always been intriguing because of its variations and compact architecture. Nevertheless, the complication rates of routine endoscopic sinus surgery have been low given the wide use and accessibility of these techniques in most of the training centers. However, more advanced and complicated procedures are required for extensive diseases especially where the anatomical landmarks are distorted due to the disease or as in a revision surgery that needs a guidance tool for reducing the intraoperative complications during the procedure.

When operating based on a two-dimensional magnified image, the localization of the instruments within the sinonasal cavity and in the skull base essentially depends on the tactile feedback and largely upon the depth of penetration of the instrument. This often gets more complicated and difficult when the anatomy is distorted by the disease especially in cases of extensive sinonasal polyposis, sinonasal and skull base tumors, and in revision surgery.

Navigation technology improves the three-dimensional localization of the surgical instruments introduced into the surgical field by projecting it on the radiology scan (computed tomography [CT] or magnetic resonance imaging [MRI] scan) of the patient being operated.

Tracking Technology

Tracking is a method of dynamically following the movement of an instrument used during the surgery in relation to the patient being operated and projecting the location of the instrument onto an imaging study. There are two tracking systems used in neuronavigation—optical and electromagnetic based systems.

Both systems are highly accurate to within a few millimeters and both systems account for intraoperative head position by fastening a headset to the patient. Electromagnetic systems track instruments using a radiofrequency transmitter within a special headset and a receiver positioned within the instrument whereas the optical systems use infrared light and a camera positioned 6 ft (approximately 1.8 m) above the patient's head to track instruments, thus providing a wireless mechanism of instrument localization. Neuronavigation has a significant positive impact on the outcome of the surgery. As the surgical field is completely mapped and monitored throughout the surgery, the disease clearance is always complete when neuronavigation is used and the complications reduced, especially in skull base surgery where most of the newer navigation technologies are compatible with fusion imaging of the preoperative CT and MRI images.

Orbital Reconstruction

ROCM patients post orbital exenteration present with cosmetic deformity, persistent nasoorbital fistulas, which might need orbital reconstructions. A successful rehabilitation of anophthalmic socket needs a socket reconstruction with exenteration prosthetic fitting that mimics the contralateral globe. Various free flaps have been used to reconstruct the anophthalmic eye. Temporalis fascia is the most commonly used flap. Other flaps used are radial artery free forearm flap, dorsalis pedis flap, gracilis free flap, and latissimus dorsi or rectus muscle free flap. However, flaps have limitations of their pedicle length, inability to provide bulk of tissue, and donor site morbidity. Prosthetic rehabilitation with custom-made ocular prosthesis yields better and more satisfactory results both esthetically and psychologically as compared to a stock eye prosthesis. Advantages of custom-made ocular prosthesis are it retains the shape of the socket, prevents accumulation of fluid in the cavity, and maintains palpebral opening similar to natural eye.

Transcutaneous Retrobulbar Injection of Amphotericin-B in Rhino-Orbital-Cerebral Mucormycosis

Several case reports have described transcutaneous retrobulbar injection of amphotericin-B (TRAMB) and conservative orbital debridement with or without irrigation with amphotericin-B as a viable option in halting orbital progression and providing an opportunity to avoid orbital exenteration.[3] Randomized clinical studies are required to prove the success rate of TRAMB; however, it can be used as an adjunctive treatment after adequate sinus debridement.

Pharmacotherapy

The pharmacotherapeutic aspect of mucormycosis has always been a subject of great interest and an epicenter of research of the disease. Recent advancement of the pharmacological research has focused on targeting the polyene binding to ergosterol in the fungal cell membrane, rendering the cell more porus; inhibition of the cytochrome p450 14-alpha-demethylase by posaconazole, blocking the membrane stabilizing ergosterol; inhibition of cross-linking of beta-glucan in the fungal cell wall by echinocandin; and deferasirox, an iron chelating agent, which efficiently blocks the iron uptake by the fungus. Recent advancements have begun to enhance the host immune by granulocyte transfusion and cytokine therapy. Recombinant cytokines such as granulocyte colony-stimulating factor (G-CSF), granulocyte macrophage colony-stimulating factor (GM-CSF), and interferon-gama can be used to activate the granulocytes, which have the potency to damage the fungal cell wall. The role of neutropenia as a factor of mucormycosis and the synergistic action of neutrophils and lipid formulations of amphotericin-B in damaging the hyphae of *Rhizopus* species, as is well established, created research interest in delivering polymorphonuclear leukocytes by granulocyte transfusion.

Drugs for COVID-19 Infection

Fusion inhibitor group of antivirals acts by inhibiting the fusion process during the viral entry into the host cells and is demonstrating antiviral activity against the SARS-CoV-2. Drugs belonging to this class include umifenovir and camostat mesylate among others.

The entry of the SAR-CoV-2 into the host cells, similar to the other viruses, is through receptor-mediated endocytosis, which is regulated by AP2-associated protein kinase 1 (AAK1). Hence, the disruption of AAK1 will not only block the entry of the virus into the host cell but also help in reducing the intracellular viral assembly. Hence, baricitinib, a Janus kinase inhibitor with high potential to bind to and inhibit AAK1, can be used both to inhibit the viral entry into the host cell and reduce the inflammatory response associated with the COVID-19 infection.

Some protease inhibitors such as lopinavir, darunavir, and atazanavir have the potential to be used against COVID-19.

The combination of lopinavir and ritonavir (both used as HIV protease inhibitors) inhibited the main protease (M^{Pro})

of SARS-CoV-2. Studies showed that specific combination of lopinavir–ritonavir (Kaletra) demonstrated antiviral effects against SARS-CoV-2 both in vitro and in clinical trials.[4]

Another strategy to combat SARS-CoV-2 infection involves targeting the reverse transcription step by blocking RdRp and therefore preventing viral replication. A few potential inhibitors are nucleotide reverse transcriptase inhibitors (NtRTIs), non-nucleoside reverse transcriptase inhibitors (NNRTIs), nucleoside reverse transcriptase translocation inhibitors (NRTTIs), and nucleoside reverse transcriptase inhibitors (NRTIs).

Remdesivir is a monophosphoramidate prodrug, an NtRTI drug, that is worthy of a "solidarity" clinical trial for COVID-19, according to the WHO. Viral genomic RNA replication and production decline as it alters functions of viral exonuclease which disturbs the proof reading. Previous studies found that remdesivir was effective against MERS-CoV; it reduced the viral loads in the affected part in mice; therefore, it supported to regain the normal pulmonary functions and was also proposed as a therapeutic agent against SARS-CoV-2.[5] A preliminary study found that the viral load in nasopharyngeal and oropharyngeal swabs reduced significantly after 12 days of remdesivir administration.[6] An *in vitro* study reported that a combination of remdesivir and chloroquine, an antimalarial drug, effectively inhibited SARS-CoV-2 growth in Vero E6 cells.[7] Clinical trials are ongoing to assess the efficacy of remdesivir for COVID-19 in the US, Norway, and France. Remdesivir has been used to treat COVID-19 cases in the USA and Singapore. The first case of COVID-19 in the USA was recovered using intravenously administered remdesivir.

Role and Development of Vaccination

Vaccinations play a huge role in shaping the outcome of the pandemic. The vaccines are essentially based upon inactivated or live attenuated viruses, protein subunit, or virus-like particles. Each of these vaccines, viral vector (replicating and nonreplicating), DNA, RNA, and nanoparticles, has its own advantages. The immuno-informatics approach is also used for the epitope identification for the SARS-CoV-2 vaccine candidates. It can be used to identify the significant cytotoxic T cell and B cell epitopes in the viral proteins.

Outline of the vaccine production platforms for SARS-CoV-2 and their advantages and limitations are highlighted in **Table 14.1**.[8]

Radiological Advances

Despite providing excellent structural resolution for visualizing advanced diseases, CT and MRI have limited value in detecting mucormycosis early in its course. Mucormycosis

Table 14.1   Advantages and limitations of vaccine production platforms for SARS-CoV-2

S.No.	Vaccine platform	Advantages	Limitations
1	LAV/the whole virus	• It has the intrinsic ability to stimulate the immune system by inducing the TLRs, namely, TLR 3, TLR 7/8, and TLR 9, of the innate immune system that involves B cells, CD4, and CD8 T cells • It can be derived from "cold adapted" virus strains, reassortants, and reverse genetics	• LAV requires an extensive accessory testing to establish safety and efficacy • There is a probability of nucleotide substitution during viral replication, resulting in the creation of recombinants post vaccination
2	Inactivated virus vaccine	• Stable and safer as compared to the LAVs • It has pre-existing technology and infrastructure required for its development • It has already been tested for SARS-CoV and various other diseases • It can be used along with adjuvants to increase its immunogenicity	• It requires booster shots to maintain the immunity • Furthermore, large amounts of viruses need to be handled and the integrity of the immunogenic particles must be maintained
3	Subunit vaccine	• It does not have any live component of the viral particle • Thus, it is safe with fewer side effects	• It induces an immune response • Memory for future responses is doubtful
4	Viral vector-based vaccine	• It shows a highly specific gene delivery into the host cell with a vigorous immune response • It avoids handling of any infectious particle, and it has been used widely for MERS-CoV with positive results from the trials	• The host may possess immunity against the vector due to prior exposure, reducing the efficacy • It may lead to cancer due to the integration of the viral genome into the host genome
5	DNA vaccines	• The synthetic DNA is temperature stable and cold-chain free • It can be developed at an accelerated pace • It does not require handling of the infectious viral particle	• Although it elicits both cytotoxic and humoral immunity, the titers remain low • Insertion of foreign DNA into the host genome may cause abnormalities in the cell • It may induce antibody production against itself
6	RNA vaccines	• The translation of mRNA occurs in the cytosol of the host cell averting the risk of any sort of integration into the host genome	• Safety issues with reactogenicity have been reported for various RNA-based vaccines • It also shows instability

Abbreviation: LAV, live attenuated vaccine; TLRs, toll-like receptors.

being a saprophytic pathology, the disease process progresses with a metabolic pathogenesis which has specific radiological footprint. Hence, for early diagnosis and treatment, metabolic and functional imaging techniques complement the role of anatomic imaging modalities for optimal management of these patients. Studies have shown that fludeoxyglucose (FDG) get accumulated at the sites of infection aiding in localization and finding the extent of the involvement.[9] The mechanism of increased uptake of FDG by the inflammatory cells is because of the upregulation of cellular glucose metabolism secondary to respiratory burst. Several studies have shown optimistic outcomes in monitoring the disease based on fluorodeoxyglucose–positron emission tomography (FDG-PET) scan.[10]

References

1. Jeong W, Keighley C, Wolfe R, et al. The epidemiology and clinical manifestations of mucormycosis: a systematic review and meta-analysis of case reports. Clin Microbiol Infect 2019;25(1):26–34

2. Lamoth F, Kontoyiannis DP. Therapeutic challenges of non-aspergillus invasive mold infections in immunosuppressed patients. Antimicrob Agents Chemother 2019;63(11): e01244-19

3. Nair AG, Dave TV. Transcutaneous retrobulbar injection of amphotericin B in rhino-orbital-cerebral mucormycosis: a review. Orbit. 2022;41(3):275-286

4. Cao B, Wang Y, Wen D, et al. A trial of lopinavir–ritonavir in adults hospitalized with severe Covid-19. The New England Journal of Medicine 2020;382(19):1787-1799

5. Sheahan TP, Sims AC, Leist SR, et al. Comparative therapeutic efficacy of remdesivir and combination lopinavir, ritonavir, and interferon beta against MERS-CoV. Nat Commun 2020; 11:222

6. Biancofiore A, Mirijello A, Puteo MA, Di Viesti MP, Labonia M, Copetti M, De Cosmo S, Lombardi R; CSS-COVID-19 Group. Remdesivir significantly reduces SARS-CoV-2 viral load on nasopharyngeal swabs in hospitalized patients with COVID-19: A retrospective case-control study. J Med Virol. 2022;94(5):2284-2289

7. Wang M, Cao R, Zhang L, et al. Remdesivir and chloroquine effectively inhibit the recently emerged novel coronavirus (2019-nCoV) in vitro. Cell Res 2020;30:269–271

8. Ning W, Jian S, Shibo J, Lanying D. Subunit vaccines against emerging pathogenic human coronaviruses. Frontiers in Microbiology. 2020

9. Longhitano A, Alipour R, Khot A, Bajel A, Antippa P, Slavin M, Thursky K. The role of 18F-Fluorodeoxyglucose positron emission tomography/computed tomography (FDG PET/CT) in assessment of complex invasive fungal disease and opportunistic co-infections in patients with acute leukemia prior to allogeneic hematopoietic cell transplant. Transpl Infect Dis. 2021;23(3):e13547

10. Altini C, Niccoli Asabella A, Ferrari C, Rubini D, Dicuonzo F, Rubini G. (18)F-FDG PET/CT contribution to diagnosis and treatment response of rhino-orbital-cerebral mucormycosis. Hellenic J Nuclear Medicine. 2015;18(1):68-70

Suggested Readings

1. Ho YH, Wu BG, Chen YZ, Wang LS. Gastric mucormycosis in an alcoholic with review of the literature. Tzu Chi Med J 2007;19:169–172

2. Petrikkos G, Skiada A, Lortholary O, Roilides E, Walsh TJ, Kontoyiannis DP. Epidemiology and clinical manifestations of mucormycosis. Clin Infect Dis 2012;54(Suppl 1):S23–S34

3. Roden MM, Zaoutis TE, Buchanan WL, et al. Epidemiology and outcome of zygomycosis: a review of 929 reported cases. Clin Infect Dis 2005;41(5):634–653

4. Walsh TJ, Skiada A, Cornely OA, et al. Development of new strategies for early diagnosis of mucormycosis from bench to bedside. Mycoses 2014;57(Suppl 3):2–7

5. Samet JD, Horton KM, Fishman EK. Invasive gastric mucormycosis: CT findings. Emerg Radiol 2008;15(5):349–351

6. Thomson SR, Bade PG, Taams M, Chrystal V. Gastrointestinal mucormycosis. Br J Surg 1991;78(8):952–954

7. El Hachem G, Chamseddine N, Saidy G, Choueiry C, Afif C. Successful nonsurgical eradication of invasive gastric mucormycosis. Clin Lymphoma Myeloma Leuk 2016; 16(Suppl):S145–S148

8. Feldman M, Friedman L, Brandt L. Sleisenger and Fordtran's Gastrointestinal and Liver Disease. 10th ed. Elsevier; 2016:875

9. Sharma P, Mukherjee A, Karunanithi S, Bal C, Kumar R. Potential role of 18F-FDG PET/CT in patients with fungal infections. AJR Am J Roentgenol 2014;203(1):180–189

10. Altini C, Niccoli Asabella A, Ferrari C, Rubini D, Dicuonzo F, Rubini G. (18)F-FDG PET/CT contribution to diagnosis and treatment response of rhino-orbital-cerebral mucormycosis. Hell J Nucl Med 2015;18(1):68–70

11. Liu Y, Wu H, Huang F, Fan Z, Xu B. Utility of 18F-FDG PET/CT in diagnosis and management of mucormycosis. Clin Nucl Med 2013;38(9):e370–e371

12. Wang N, Shang J, Jiang S, Du L. Subunit vaccines against emerging pathogenic human coronaviruses. Front Microbiol 2020;11:298

Index